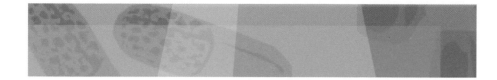

Drugs, Alcohol, and Tobacco

Learning About Addictive Behavior

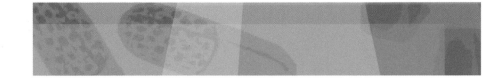

Drugs, Alcohol, and Tobacco

Learning About Addictive Behavior

Volume

1

A to Dri
Index

Rosalyn Carson-DeWitt, M.D.,
Editor in Chief

MACMILLAN
REFERENCE
USA ™

THOMSON
✦
™
GALE

New York • Detroit • San Diego • San Francisco • Cleveland • New Haven, Conn. • Waterville, Maine • London • Munich

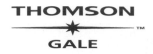

Drugs, Alcohol, and Tobacco: Learning About Addictive Behavior

Rosalyn Carson-DeWitt, M.D.

For permission to use material from this
product, submit your request via Web at
http://www.gale-edit.com/permissions, or you
may download our Permissions Request form
and submit your request by fax or mail to:

Permissions Department
The Gale Group, Inc.
27500 Drake Rd.
Farmington Hills, MI 48331-3535
Permissions Hotline:
248-699-8006 or 800-877-4253 ext. 8006
Fax: 248-699-8074 or 800-762-4058

LIBRARY OF CONGRESS CATALOGING-IN-PUBLICATION DATA

Drugs, alcohol, and tobacco: learning about addictive behavior /
Rosalyn Carson-DeWitt, editor in chief.
   p. cm.
     Includes bibliographical references and index.
     ISBN 0-02-865756-X (set: hardcover : alk. paper) — ISBN
     0-02-865757-8 (v. 1) — ISBN 0-02-865758-6 (v. 2) — ISBN 0-02-865759-4
     (v. 3)
     1. Drug abuse—Encyclopedias, Juvenile.   2. Alcoholism—
Encyclopedias, Juvenile.   3. Tobacco habit—Encyclopedias, Juvenile.
   4. Substance abuse—Encyclopedias, Juvenile.   5. Compulsive
behavior—Encyclopedias, Juvenile.   6. Teenagers—Substance use—
Encyclopedias, Juvenile. I.

Carson-DeWitt, Rosalyn.
HV5804 .D78 2003
613.8—dc21

2002009270

Printed in Canada
1 2 3 4 5 6 7 8 9 10

Preface

In 1995 Macmillan Reference USA published the outstanding *Encyclopedia of Drugs and Alcohol*, edited by Jerome Jaffe. An extensively revised second edition, entitled *Encyclopedia of Drugs, Alcohol, and Addictive Behavior*, was published in 2001. Now Macmillan Reference USA is drawing from the fine work done for these prior encyclopedias to publish *Drugs, Alcohol, and Tobacco: Learning About Addictive Behavior*, a three-volume set targeted towards general and younger readers.

Alcohol, drugs, and tobacco have myriad ill effects on the lives of children and teenagers. Babies are born addicted to crack or harmed by exposure to alcohol while in the womb. Children live in poverty and chaos, at high risk of neglect, abuse, and homelessness because of their parents' drug and/or alcohol problems. Increased school dropout rates, a high risk of psychiatric problems, and a greater chance of severe injury or death due to violence, motor vehicle accidents, and self-injury endanger the worlds of children and teens raised amid substance abuse. Furthermore, children from substance-abusing homes are more likely to turn to smoking, drugs, or alcohol. Then comes the convergence of the genetic propensity for substance abuse, the availability of alcohol and drugs, and peer pressure, all factors that increase a child's risk of engaging in substance abuse or addictive behaviors.

Drugs, Alcohol, and Tobacco: Learning About Addictive Behavior was the brainchild of Hélène Potter, director of new product development at Macmillan Reference USA. Aware that initiating substance use prior to the age of fifteen carries a greater risk of severe problems, and aware that prevention must begin with thorough education, Ms. Potter conceived of and pushed through this valuable project. Designed to engage, interest, and educate children and teens, this work provides information on specific drugs (such as nicotine, alcohol, marijuana, and ecstasy), risk and protective factors for addiction, diagnosis and treatment of addictions, medical and legal consequences of both casual use and addiction, costs to families and society, drug production and trafficking, policy issues, and other compulsive disorders (including gambling, cutting, and eating disorders).

Although the *Encyclopedia of Drugs, Alcohol, and Addictive Behavior* was used as a structural basis for this present work, the entire table of contents was revised to focus the new work on the needs and interests of young students. An impressive cadre of experts and academics was commissioned to review, revise, rewrite, and refocus every article from the original collection, or to produce new articles pertinent to the project's goals and relevant to children and teenagers. New ancillaries provide additional resources that will be particularly helpful to children and teenagers researching topics for school or for their own personal use.

The result is *Drugs, Alcohol, and Tobacco: Learning About Addictive Behavior*, a collection of over 190 alphabetically arranged articles intended to reach out to an audience of children and teenagers with information that can help them understand issues surrounding addictive behavior on both an academic and a personal level. The thoughtful, visually interesting design of the text includes call-out definitions in the margins of articles (so that young students do not have to flip to a separate glossary, although that is provided as well); lively marginalia that highlights interesting facts or makes reading suggestions for fiction that deals with topically similar issues; and more than 200 full-color illustrations that help young readers to organize and to compare and contrast information. Articles are followed by cross-references. Appendices include a wide-ranging list of organizations (including their addresses, phone numbers, and web sites) from which readers can seek more information or obtain contacts for personal help; a complete glossary of terms; and an annotated bibliography that will point students toward further research, assist teachers with class preparation, and guide individuals who are struggling with the effects of addiction in their personal lives.

Many fine people deserve considerable thanks for contributing to the birth of this new work, beginning with Hélène Potter, whose vision and guidance were essential throughout the production process. Editor Oona Schmid slaved over every aspect of the project and supported everyone else's work with competence and good humor. Jan Gottschalk consulted on the project, sharing her considerable experience with middle-school students, and providing excellent input regarding relevancy of material, fit with middle-school curriculum, and appropriateness for middle-school readers. Copyeditor Jessica Hornik Evans put in countless hours to make entries suitable in length, scope, and reading level for middle-school students. Amy Buttery worked to ensure that data presented were up-to-date and pertinent to young teenagers. And once again, my husband Toby, and our children Anna, Emma, Isabelle, and Sophie, graciously tolerated the presence of a fifth child in the guise of an encyclopedia in our home.

In closing, I would like to acknowledge the efforts of clinicians who are working on the front line to treat families grappling with addiction in their lives; academics who teach about substance abuse and its effects on individuals, society, and the international community; researchers who are studying issues that may lead to better ways to diagnose, treat, and prevent addiction; policymakers who struggle to find ways to protect society from the crime and violence associated with addictions; and the many individuals who awaken each day to face the effects of addiction wreaking havoc on their lives and to try once again to find their way free of addiction's stranglehold.

Rosalyn Carson-DeWitt, M.D.
Editor in Chief

July 2002

Contributors

The text of *Drugs, Alcohol, and Tobacco: Learning About Addictive Behavior* is based on the second edition of Macmillan's *Encyclopedia of Drugs, Alcohol, and Addictive Behavior*, which was published in 2001. We have updated material where necessary and added original entries that are of particular importance to the general public and younger students. Articles have been condensed and made more accessible for a student audience. Please refer to the List of Authors at the back of volume three in this set for the authors and affiliations of all those whose work appears in this reference. Here we wish to acknowledge the writers who revised entries and wrote new articles specifically for this set:

Peter Andreas

Linda Wasmer Andrews

Christopher B. Anthony

Samuel A. Ball

Robert Balster

Amy Buttery

Kate B. Carey

Jonathan Caulkins

Allan Cobb

Roberta Friedman

Jessica Gerson

Frederick K. Grittner

Angela Guarda

Becky Ham

Carl G. Leukefeld

Jill Max

Thomas S. May

Tom Mieczkowski

Cynthia Robbins

Heather Roberto

Ian Rockett

Joseph Spillane

Michele Staton Tindall

Marvin Steinberg

Michael Walsh

Michael Winkelman

Jill Anne Yeagley

Table of Contents

Accidents and Injuries from Alcohol

In the United States, injuries are the fourth-leading cause of death, exceeded only by heart disease, stroke, and cancer. Of all deaths from injury in the United States, about 65 percent are classified as unintentional or accidental. The other 35 percent are intentional injuries, occurring as a result of fights, assaults, suicide, **homicide**, and other crimes. Alcohol-related fatalities have been estimated to be about 43 percent of all unintentional injuries.

homicide murder

Studies show that an amazing number of those injured and killed every year have high levels of alcohol in their blood. This may be because the drinking accident victim engaged in risky behavior, such as not wearing a seat belt or motorcycle helmet. People who tend to take safety risks, act impulsively, and engage in thrill seeking are likely to both drink alcohol and to suffer from injuries. Alcohol is known

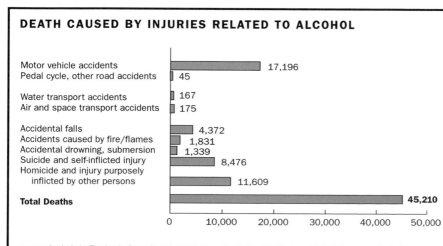

DEATH CAUSED BY INJURIES RELATED TO ALCOHOL

Motor vehicle accidents	17,196
Pedal cycle, other road accidents	45
Water transport accidents	167
Air and space transport accidents	175
Accidental falls	4,372
Accidents caused by fire/flames	1,831
Accidental drowning, submersion	1,339
Suicide and self-inflicted injury	8,476
Homicide and injury purposely inflicted by other persons	11,609
Total Deaths	**45,210**

SOURCE: Analysis by The Lewin Group based on data from the National Institute on Alcohol Abuse and Alcoholism. <http://www.nida.nih.gov/EconomicCosts/Table5_3.html>.

The majority of deaths caused by injuries related to alcohol are the result of motor vehicle accidents.

to decrease both motor coordination and balance, and to interfere with one's ability to pay attention and use good judgment.

Estimates of Alcohol's Involvement

Emergency room (ER) studies test patients admitted for injuries for blood alcohol level (BAL) or **blood alcohol concentration (BAC)**. In studies done on weekend evenings, when a large number of people would be expected to be consuming alcohol, close to 50 percent of people admitted to the ER had alcohol in their blood at the time of admission.

Motor Vehicle Accidents

Motor vehicle crashes are the leading cause of death from injury—and the greatest single cause of all deaths for those between the ages

blood alcohol concentration (BAC) amount of alcohol in the bloodstream, expressed as the grams of alcohol per deciliter of blood; as BAC goes up, the drinker experiences more psychological and physical effects

Roslyn Cappiello was paralyzed from the neck down because of an accident caused by a drunk driver.

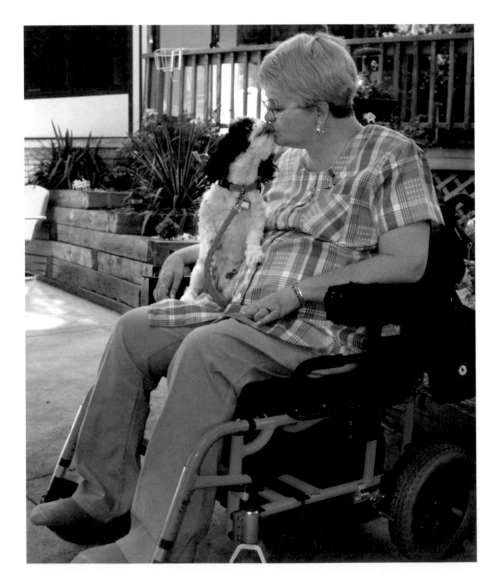

of 1 and 34 in the United States. About half of all unintentional injuries occur during the course of motor vehicle accidents. It has been estimated that 7 percent of all crashes and 44 percent of fatal crashes involve alcohol use. The risk of a fatal crash is estimated to be from three to fifteen times higher for a drunk driver (one with a BAC of at least 0.10 to 100 milligrams of alcohol for each 100 milliliters of blood—the legal limit in most U.S. states) than for a nondrinking driver. Alcohol is more frequently present in fatal than in nonfatal crashes. About 25 to 35 percent of those drivers requiring ER care for injuries resulting from such crashes have a BAC of 0.10 or greater.

Motorcyclists are at a greater risk of death than are automobile occupants, with up to 50 percent of fatally injured motorcyclists having a BAC of at least 0.10. Pedestrians killed or injured by motor vehicles are also more likely to have been drinking than those not involved in such accidents.

Home and Recreational Accidents

An estimated 22 to 30 percent of all nonfatal injuries that occur in the home involve alcohol.

Falls. Falls are the most common cause of nonfatal injuries in the United States, accounting for over 60 percent, and the second-leading cause of fatal accidents. Alcohol is involved in 21 to 48 percent of fatal falls and 17 to 53 percent of nonfatal falls. Alcohol may increase the likelihood of a fall as much as sixty times in those well over the legal limit for intoxication, compared with those having no alcohol exposure.

Fires and Burns. Fires and burns are the fourth-leading cause of accidental death in the United States. Studies show that alcohol is involved in as many as half of these deaths. Alcohol exposure is most frequent among victims of fires caused by cigarettes.

Drowning. Drowning ranks as the third-leading cause of accidental death in the United States. Alcohol is consumed in relatively large quantities by many of those involved in water-recreation activities, especially boating, and studies suggest that those involved in aquatic accidents are more likely to be intoxicated than those not involved in such accidents.

Violence-Related Injuries

Violence commonly causes both fatal and nonfatal injuries. These injuries are more likely to be alcohol-related than injuries from any other cause, for men and for women, regardless of age. Such injuries are considered intentional, such as those resulting from assaults, fights, homicides, and suicides.

Alcoholism versus Unwise Drinking

Problem drinkers and those diagnosed as alcoholics are at a greater risk of both fatal and nonfatal injuries than are those in the general population who may drink prior to an accident. Alcoholics and problem drinkers are significantly more likely than others to be drinking, and to be drinking heavily, prior to an accident. Alcoholics have also been found to experience higher rates of both fatal and nonfatal accidents even when sober. Daily drinking, binge drinking (consuming five or more drinks per occasion), and heavier drinking (fourteen or more drinks per week) increase the likelihood of injury as the underlying cause of death. The risk of accidental death has been estimated to be from three to sixteen times greater for alcoholics than for nonalcoholics. SEE ALSO ALCOHOL: COMPLICATIONS OF PROBLEM DRINKING; BLOOD ALCOHOL CONCENTRATION; DRIVING, ALCOHOL, AND DRUGS; WORKPLACE, DRUG USE IN.

Accidents and Injuries from Drugs

Injury is a major cause of death across the age spectrum, and the leading killer of Americans aged 1 through 44 years. Scientists frequently identify the causes of injury as a combination of risky behavior and hazardous environments. Risk-taking behavior and injury are especially common during adolescence and young adulthood. Drug use contributes to injuries among adolescents and young adults because it has negative effects on perception, judgment, and reaction time. A young person under the influence of drugs also has less respect for the welfare of self and others.

The field of research that explores the relationship between injury and drugs other than alcohol is relatively new. This research has been greatly aided by improved drug testing, which allows investigators to detect drugs in samples of blood, urine, saliva, sweat, or hair. Most of this research occurs in facilities such as hospital trauma centers and emergency departments, where more severely injured victims receive treatment. Other important research is conducted by medical examiners who test for the presence of drugs during an autopsy, which is the close investigation of a deceased person's body to determine the cause of her or his death. In the case of questionable deaths, autopsy results can lead medical examiners to conclude that injury was the

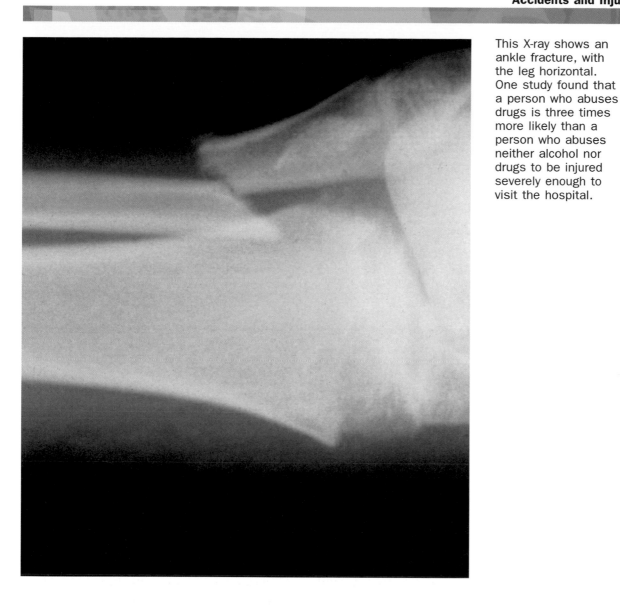

This X-ray shows an ankle fracture, with the leg horizontal. One study found that a person who abuses drugs is three times more likely than a person who abuses neither alcohol nor drugs to be injured severely enough to visit the hospital.

cause. They can then rule these injury deaths as **homicides** or suicides (intentional injury) or accidents (unintentional injury).

homicide murder

Driving Incidents

Just as drinking and driving create a dangerous mix, illegal drug use poses severe threat of injury to drivers and others on the road with them. A landmark Tennessee study found that over half of drivers stopped by police for reckless driving who tested negative for alcohol use were actually **intoxicated** with drugs. The drugs most frequently detected were cocaine and marijuana. The United States and many other countries are reporting rising numbers of injured motorists testing positive for marijuana, cocaine, **amphetamines**, or other illegal drugs. These trends probably reflect both real changes in driving under the influence of drugs and the improving capability of police to test drivers for drugs.

intoxicated a state during which physical or mental control has been diminished

amphetamine central nervous system stimulant, used in medicine to treat attention-deficit/ hyperactivity disorder (ADHD), narcolepsy (a sleep disorder), and as an appetite suppressant; may be abused

Injuries

An American study on nonfatal injury compared 15,000 substance abusers between the ages of 10 and 64 with a group of 75,000 non-abusers to see if their injury patterns varied. Abusers were more likely to be injured than non-abusers. Of subjects categorized as both drug and alcohol abusers, 58 percent sustained an injury over the three years of observation. This compared to 49 percent of those who had abused drugs only, 46 percent of those who had abused only alcohol, and 39 percent of those who had abused neither. With non-abusers as the base of comparison, the likelihood of hospitalization for an injury was four times higher among the combined drug and alcohol abuse group, three times higher among the drug abusers, and twice as high among the alcohol abusers.

Violent Deaths

barbiturate highly addictive sedative drugs that decrease the activity of the central nervous system

intravenously performed, entering, or occurring through a vein

methadone potent synthetic narcotic, used in heroin recovery programs as a non-intoxicating opiate that blunts symptoms of withdrawal

opioid substance that acts similarly to opiate narcotic drugs, but is not actually produced from the opium poppy

benzodiazepine drug developed in the 1960s as a safer alternative to barbiturates; most frequently used as a sleeping pill or an anti-anxiety medication

ecstasy designer drug and amphetamine derivative that is a commonly abused street drug

Another study conducted in three large metropolitan areas of the United States showed that illegal drug use strongly increased the likelihood that users would meet a violent death—in other words, die from intentional injury. This study looked at marijuana, cocaine, heroin, amphetamines, and **barbiturates**. The study found that drug users were seven times more likely than non-users to commit suicide, and five times more likely to be murdered. Subjects using both drugs and alcohol were seventeen times more likely to commit suicide, and twelve times more likely to die from homicide than non-users.

Overdoses

A drug overdose is the misuse of drugs in amounts so high that a person can fall asleep, become unconscious, lapse into a coma, or die. Overdoses are in fact a form of poisoning. Most drugs can be deadly when taken in large quantities, whether swallowed, inhaled, or injected **intravenously**. Drugs such as heroin, **methadone**, cocaine, **opioids**, **benzodiazepines**, amphetamines, and "designer" or "club" drugs such as **ecstasy** can all lead to an overdose. Combining drug and alcohol use is an extremely common cause of overdoses. Even caffeine, a drug that public health professionals consider relatively harmless in terms of causing injuries, has caused fatal overdoses when people have taken huge doses in the form of pills. Whether unintentional or intentional, drug poisonings are especially harmful to the young.

Injuries Are not Accidents

An unintentional injury is not an accident. Both unintentional and intentional injuries can be predicted and prevented. For example, routine use of trained lifeguards and secured locks at public swimming pools would help prevent drowning caused by drug intoxication. Drug screening, prevention, and treatment programs must be central parts of a comprehensive public health strategy aimed at reducing, and eventually eliminating, the burden of injury on society as a whole. SEE ALSO ACCIDENTS AND INJURIES FROM ALCOHOL; DRIVING, ALCOHOL, AND DRUGS; MEDICAL EMERGENCIES AND DEATH FROM DRUG ABUSE; SUICIDE AND SUBSTANCE ABUSE.

Addiction: Concepts and Definitions

Understanding the nature of addiction depends on understanding several related concepts. The following discussion explains and clarifies those concepts.

Abuse and Misuse

In everyday English, abuse is understood to mean practices that are in some way improper or cruel, as in the term "child abuse." As applied to drugs, however, the term is difficult to define and carries different meanings in different situations. Some drugs, such as morphine, have medical purposes. If they are used for other reasons, or in unnecessarily large quantities, then the term "drug abuse" is applied. Other substances, such as alcohol, are legal but do not serve

SCHEDULE OF DRUGS BY POTENTIAL FOR ABUSE

DEA Schedule	Abuse Potential	Examples of Drugs Covered	Some of the Effects	Medical Use
I	highest	heroin, LSD, hashish, marijuana, methaqualone	unpredictable effects, severe psychological or physical dependence, or death	no accepted use; some are legal for limited research use only
II	high	morphine, PCP, cocaine, methadone, methamphetamine	may lead to severe psychological or physical dependence	accepted use with restrictions
III	medium	codeine with aspirin or Tylenol®, some barbiturates, anabolic steroids	may lead to moderate or low physical dependence or high psychological dependence	accepted use
IV	low	Darvon®, Talwin®, Equanil®, Valium®, Xanax®	may lead to limited physical or psychological dependence	accepted use
V	lowest	over-the-counter or prescription cough medicines with codeine	may lead to limited physical or psychological dependence	accepted use

SOURCE: Adapted from the Drug Enforcement Administration *Drugs of Abuse* (1996) and *Schedules of Controlled Substances*, revised as of April 1, 1998.

Heroin, LSD, and marijuana are among the drugs that have the highest potential for abuse, while drugs such as over-the-counter cough medications with codeine have a very low risk of being abused.

therapeutic healing or curing

a **therapeutic** purpose. Using alcohol to a degree that is hazardous or damaging, either to the user or to others, is also understood as abuse. Any use of illegal substances that have no recognized medical purpose is generally regarded as abuse. Thus the best general definition of drug abuse is the use of any drug in a way that does not follow medical advice or that does not conform to a particular culture's accepted usage. The term "misuse" refers specifically to the use of a therapeutic drug in any way other than what is seen as good medical practice.

Recreational or Casual Drug Use

When a person's reason for using a drug is to obtain effects that give the user some kind of pleasure or rewarding sensation—even if that use has potential risks—this is known as recreational use. When an individual takes a drug occasionally rather than regularly, this is called casual use. The term implies that the user is not dependent or addicted (see following), but it does not indicate the motive for use or the amount used on any occasion. Thus, a casual user might become intoxicated (see next section) or suffer an **acute** adverse effect on occasion, even if these are infrequent.

acute having a sudden onset and lasting a short time

A person might occasionally use a drug to achieve a specific short-term benefit under special circumstances. This kind of drug use is known as circumstantial (drug use prompted by certain circumstances) or utilitarian (drug use that serves a particular purpose). The utilitarian use of amphetamines might include students who want to increase their endurance and postpone fatigue when studying for a test, truck drivers who need to stay awake on long hauls, athletes competing in endurance events, or military personnel on long missions. Most observers consider the first three examples to be abuse or misuse of a drug. The fourth example is not seen as abuse, because military authorities prescribe such drug use to achieve necessary combat goals under unusually dangerous circumstances.

impair to make worse or to damage, especially by lessening or reducing in some way

hallucination seeing, hearing, feeling, tasting, or smelling something that is not actually there, like a vision of devils, hearing voices, or feeling bugs crawl over the skin; may occur due to mental illness or as a side effect of some drugs

Intoxication

Intoxication occurs when the actions of a drug **impair** a person's normal functioning. Consumption of a high dose of drug on one occasion would cause acute intoxication. Chronic (long-term) intoxication is caused by repeated use of doses large enough to maintain a very high drug concentration in the body over a long period of time. Some drugs cause disturbances of speech, memory, and reflexes. Others raise blood pressure and heart rate and cause mental disturbances such as **hallucinations** and **convulsions**.

convulsion intense, repetitive muscle contraction

Habits

All people have habits, or behaviors that are repeated so often that they become almost automatic. In this sense habit is not necessarily good or bad. As applied to drug use, however, habit refers to regular, persistent use of a drug in amounts that may create some risk for the user, and over which the user does not have complete voluntary control. A drug habit implies that the drug use has become a concern on the part of the user or friends, family, or coworkers, but it may not yet be clear that the user needs treatment.

Problem Drinking

Problem drinking refers to drinking alcohol at an average daily level that causes problems in an individual's life, most often in terms of the person's health, relationships with others, finances, or compliance with the law. The actual level of consumption will vary with the individual. A drinker who might not meet the criteria of dependence (see following) or who might be reluctant to accept a medical diagnosis of alcoholism or addiction can often accept the description "problem drinker" and thus be encouraged to seek help for that problem.

Addiction and Dependence

The term "addiction" was used in everyday and legal English long before its application to drug problems. In the sixteenth century the bondage of a servant to a master was called an addiction. The term came also to describe a practice or habit that could not be broken. In both senses, it implied a loss of liberty of action. At the beginning of the twentieth century the term was used more specifically for habitual and excessive use of a drug. An addict was someone who could not voluntarily stop taking drugs or, in the case of alcohol addiction, stop drinking. It was understood that obtaining and using the drug dominated such a person's life.

In 1957 the Expert Committee of the World Health Organization defined addiction as a state of **periodic** or chronic intoxication produced by the repeated consumption of a drug (natural or **synthetic**). By this definition, the characteristics of addiction include:

periodic occuring at regular intervals or periods

synthetic something produced artificially

- an overpowering need (compulsion) to continue taking the drug and to obtain it by any means
- a tendency to increase the dose
- a psychic (psychological) and generally a physical dependence on the effects of the drug
- a harmful effect on the individual and on society.

Drugs vary in their effects on individuals, but overall a specific drug has the potential to make users dependent, experience withdrawal symptoms, become tolerant to the drug's effects, seek reinforcement, and intoxicate themselves.

COMPARING ADDICTIVE QUALITIES OF POPULAR DRUGS (HIGHER SCORE INDICATES MORE SERIOUS EFFECT)

Dependence: How difficult it is for the user to quit, the relapse rate, the percentage of people who eventually become dependent, the rating users give their own need for the substance, and the degree to which the substance will be used in the face of evidence that it causes harm.

Withdrawal: Presence and severity of characteristic withdrawal symptoms.

Tolerance: How much of the substance is needed to satisfy increasing cravings for it, and the level of stable need that is eventually reached.

Reinforcement: A measure of the substance's ability, in human and animal tests, to get users to take it again and again, and in preference to other substances.

Intoxication: Though not usually counted as a measure of addiction in itself, the level of intoxication is associated with addiction and increases the personal and social damage a substance may do.

SOURCE: Jack E. Henningfield. National Institute on Drug Abuse, "Is Nicotine Addictive?" 1994. <http://www.taima.org/en/risks.htm#fn01>.

euphoria state of intense, giddy happiness and well-being, sometimes occurring baselessly and out of sync with an individual's life situation

Regular, heavy use of a drug results in physical dependence, an altered physical state in which the body cannot function normally unless the drug is present. When drug use is abruptly discontinued or withdrawn, the user suffers from physical and mental disturbances known as a withdrawal syndrome. The body and mind experience changes usually the opposite of the effect of the drug. For example, if cocaine causes prolonged wakefulness and **euphoria**, the withdrawal syndrome will include profound sleepiness and depression. Resuming use of the drug or of a substitute drug with a very similar pattern of actions will end the withdrawal syndrome but may increase dependence.

Reinforcement and Its Relation to Dependence

A drug causes dependence if it produces some effect that makes the user want to use the drug again and thus try to get more of it. Such a drug sets off a chemical action in the brain that alters the user's thinking, feelings, and activities in a way that is usually (but not always) experienced as pleasurable or rewarding. The user wants to have that experience again, so the act of taking the drug is reinforced. Thus the drug is called a reinforcer.

A drug must have a reinforcing effect if it is to become addictive, but it is important to recognize that reinforcement is not the same as addiction. Reinforcement is an essential mechanism for survival, learning, and adaptation. Drinking water because we are thirsty, eating food because we are hungry, and escaping so as to avoid harm are all types of reinforcement by natural and necessary behaviors. Addictive drugs, although they produce a reinforcing effect, serve no necessary biological function.

Craving

Craving refers to an intense desire for a drug. A user craving a drug thinks constantly about it and its desired effects. The person feels an acute **deprivation** that can be relieved only by taking the drug and thus an urgent need to obtain it. Craving is also known as drug hunger. An urge is similar to a craving but is less intense.

deprivation situation of lacking the basic necessities of life (e.g., food or emotional security)

Craving directs all of the person's thoughts and activities towards obtaining and using a new supply of the drug. Drug-seeking behavior includes searching drawers and cupboards for possible remnants of the drug, getting money (whether by legal or illegal means), contacting the sources of supply, buying the drug, preparing it for use, and pretending to be ill or in pain in order to get a prescription for a drug of abuse. The more intense the craving, the more urgent, desperate, or irrational this behavior tends to become.

Tolerance and Sensitization

Tolerance refers to a state in which the drug user becomes less sensitive to the drug's effects over time. The user must take larger amounts of the drug to produce the desired effect. Tolerance comes about because of physiological changes in the nervous system, but it is also strongly influenced by learning. This means that the user has learned to perform certain tasks while under the influence of the drug. For example, a drug that when first used makes the user sleepy will no longer have that effect after the drug has been used for a while. The individual is said to tolerate the drug because certain normal activities, such as household chores or work-related activities, can be performed even while the individual is under the influence of the drug. Furthermore, tolerance to some effects of a drug does not mean tolerance to all effects of a drug. As a user increases the dose to continue to achieve what he or she perceives as the original pleasurable effects of the drug, the chance for other dangerous side effects may also be increased at the higher dose.

Taking drugs can also produce an effect that is the opposite of tolerance. Sensitization occurs when the same dose of a particular drug is taken repeatedly. With sensitization, the exact same dose of the drug begins to produce a larger, rather than smaller, effect. For example, a user might take a particular dose of amphetamine. At first, that dose might only cause a slight increase in the person's energy level or physical activity. After the same dose has been repeated several times, however, that dose might begin to cause intense **hyperactivity** or even a seizure. Because of its unpredictable nature, sensitization can be quite dangerous. Furthermore, research suggests that the effects of sensitization on the nervous system may be involved in the progression of drug users from soft gateway drugs (e.g., nicotine and alcohol) to hard drugs such as cocaine. SEE ALSO DIAGNOSIS OF DRUG AND ALCOHOL ABUSE: AN OVERVIEW; TOLERANCE AND PHYSICAL DEPENDENCE.

Addictive Personality

Many alcoholics and other substance abusers have similar personality features. They are often **impulsive** and immature—like children, they are dependent, with constant needs. They also tend to have a low tolerance for frustration and are frequently anxious and depressed. These features have been grouped under the term "addictive personality." However, when the alcoholic or substance abuser stops using drugs and/or alcohol for long periods of time (periods called **abstinence**), many of these personality characteristics disappear. Thus it may be that the drug abuse itself, or the life that goes along with it, produces these characteristics rather than the individual's actual personality.

Addictive personality has also been used to refer to similar characteristics in a person before he or she began using drugs. Some researchers have thought that certain personality traits might, then, predict when a person has a higher risk of becoming an addict.

Studies of addictive personality in alcoholics have shown that these individuals tend to display certain characteristics more strongly than others. Some alcoholics seem to drink to escape the pain of frustration, while other alcoholics seem to need to drink in order to satisfy childish needs. Some alcoholics appear to drink to reduce guilt and anxiety, and other alcoholics appear to use alcohol as a way to escape from life's disappointments. Socially isolated individuals find a kind of alternate life through drinking. Similar patterns of behavior have been observed in the personalities of other types of drug abusers.

Psychometric studies of addictive personality have helped researchers identify some of the common mental disturbances that ac-

hyperactivity overly active behavior

impulsive acting before thinking through the consequences of the action

abstinence complete avoidance of something, such as the use of drugs or alcoholic beverages

psychometric relating to the technique of measuring mental abilities

company alcohol or drug abuse, such as **antisocial personality disorder** and **depression**. SEE ALSO ANTISOCIAL PERSONALITY; CHILDHOOD BEHAVIOR AND LATER DRUG USE; PERSONALITY DISORDER; RISK FACTORS FOR SUBSTANCE ABUSE.

Adolescents, Drug and Alcohol Use

Adolescence is a time of many changes—physical, mental, social, and emotional. Most adolescents adapt to these changes in healthy ways. Others experience turmoil and conflict. They become deeply unsettled and confused as they attempt to cope with this time in their lives. This unhappiness and confusion may lead them toward dangerous or deviant behavior, such as drug use. A single episode of drug use does not necessarily lead to further use, but several episodes may lead to ever-increasing use, resulting in **abuse** and **dependence**. Continued drug use can have serious consequences, not only during adolescence but into adulthood as well.

Whether a young person continues to use a drug depends on three major factors: age of first use, type of drug used, and reasons for use. Younger adolescents who try one type of drug may go on to sample a number of other substances. An adolescent may start by trying cigarettes, for instance, which can lead to daily smoking of both cigarettes and marijuana. That habit may lead to regular use of multiple drugs, such as weekend drinking and smoking or daily **uppers** and **downers**. By late adolescence, this type of drug-taking could become abusive, with the abuser becoming dependent on the drugs he or she is taking. Understanding why adolescents begin to take drugs and why they keep taking them is important so that effective drug abuse prevention programs can be developed.

Trends in Adolescent Alcohol and Drug Use

Every year the Institute for Social Research ☎ at the University of Michigan conducts a survey, called "Monitoring the Future: A Continuing Study of American Youth." The survey reveals the behavior and attitudes of nearly 50,000 students around the country. One dramatic finding that has emerged from the "Monitoring the Future" surveys was the decrease in illicit drug use by young Americans between about 1980 and 1992. Unfortunately however, a second dramatic finding was an increase in such use during the 1990s. After reaching a low of 27 percent in 1992, annual use among high-school seniors was back up to 41 percent in 2001. Lifetime use in 2001 was back to 54 per-

antisocial personality disorder condition in which people disregard the rights of others and violate these rights by acting in immoral, unethical, aggressive, or even criminal ways

depression state in which an individual feels intensely sad and hopeless; may have trouble eating, sleeping, and concentrating, and is no longer able to feel pleasure from previously enjoyable activities; in extreme cases, may lead an individual to think about or attempt suicide

abuse related to drug use, describes taking drugs that are illegal, or using prescription drugs in a way for which they were not prescribed

dependence psychological compulsion to use a substance for emotional and/or physical reasons

uppers slang term for amphetamines, drugs that act as stimulants of the central nervous system

downers slang term for drugs that act as depressants on the central nervous system (e.g., barbiturates)

☎ See *Organizations of Interest* at the back of Volume 1 for address, telephone, and URL.

ADOLESCENTS, DRUGS, AND ALCHOL USE

	8th Graders					10th Graders					12th Graders				
	1997	1998	1999	2000	2001	1997	1998	1999	2000	2001	1997	1998	1999	2000	2001
Any Illicit Drug Use															
lifetime	29.4	29	28.3	26.8	26.8	47.3	44.9	46.2	45.6	45.6	54.3	54.1	54.7	54	53.9
annual	22.1	21	20.5	19.5	19.5	38.5	35	35.9	36.4	37.2	42.4	41.4	42.1	40.9	41.4
30-day	14.6	12.1	12.2	11.9	11.7	23	21.5	22.1	22.5	22.7	26.2	25.6	25.9	24.9	25.7
Marijuana/Hashish															
lifetime	22.6	22.2	22	20.3	20.4	42.3	39.6	40.9	40.3	40.1	49.6	49.1	49.7	48.8	49
annual	17.7	16.9	16.5	15.6	15.4	34.8	31.1	32.1	32.2	32.7	38.5	37.5	37.8	36.5	37
30-day	10.2	9.7	9.7	9.1	9.2	20.5	18.7	19.4	19.7	19.8	23.7	22.8	23.1	21.6	22.4
daily	1.1	1.1	1.4	1.3	1.3	3.7	3.6	3.8	3.8	4.5	5.8	5.6	6	6	5.8
Inhalants															
lifetime	21	20.5	19.7	17.9	17.1	18.3	18.3	17	16.6	15.2	16.1	15.2	15.4	14.2	13
annual	11.8	11.7	10.3	9.4	9.1	8.7	8	7.2	7.3	6.6	6.7	6.2	5.6	5.9	4.5
30-day	5.6	4.8	5	4.5	4	3	2.9	2.6	2.6	2.4	2.5	2.3	2	2.2	1.7
Hallucinogens															
lifetime	5.4	4.9	4.8	4.6	4	10.5	9.8	9.7	8.9	7.8	15.1	14.1	13.7	13	12.8
annual	3.7	3.4	2.9	2.8	2.5	7.6	6.9	6.9	6.1	5.2	9.8	9	9.4	8.1	8.4
30-day	1.8	1.4	1.3	1.2	1.2	3.3	3.2	2.9	2.3	2.1	3.9	3.8	3.5	2.6	3.2
LSD															
lifetime	4.7	4.1	4.1	3.9	3.4	9.5	8.5	8.5	7.6	6.3	13.6	12.6	12.2	11.1	10.9
annual	3.2	2.8	2.4	2.4	2.2	6.7	5.9	6	5.1	4.1	8.4	7.6	8.1	6.6	6.6
30-day	1.5	1.1	1.1	1	1	2.8	2.7	2.3	1.6	1.5	3.1	3.2	2.7	1.6	2.3
Cocaine															
lifetime	4.4	4.6	4.7	4.5	4.3	7.1	7.2	7.7	6.9	5.7	8.7	9.3	9.8	8.6	8.2
annual	2.8	3.1	2.7	2.6	2.5	4.7	4.7	4.9	4.4	3.6	5.5	5.7	6.2	5	4.8
30-day	1.1	1.4	1.3	1.2	1.2	2	2.1	1.8	1.8	1.3	2.3	2.4	2.6	2.1	2.1
Crack Cocaine															
lifetime	2.7	3.2	3.1	3.1	3	3.6	3.9	4	3.7	3.1	3.9	4.4	4.6	3.9	3.7
annual	1.7	2.1	2.1	1.8	1.7	2.2	2.5	2.4	2.2	1.8	2.4	2.5	2.7	2.2	2.1
30-day	0.7	0.9	0.8	0.8	0.8	0.9	1.1	0.8	0.9	0.7	0.9	1	1.1	1	1.1
Heroin															
lifetime	2.1	2.3	2.3	1.9	1.7	2.1	2.3	2.3	2.2	1.7	2.1	2	2	2.4	1.8
annual	1.3	1.3	1.4	1.1	1	1.4	1.4	1.4	1.4	0.9	1.2	1	1.1	1.5	0.9
30-day	0.6	0.6	0.6	0.5	0.6	0.6	0.7	0.7	0.5	0.3	0.5	0.5	0.5	0.7	0.4
Tranquilizers															
lifetime	4.8	4.6	4.4	4.4	4.7	7.3	7.8	7.9	8	8.1	7.8	8.5	9.3	8.9	9.2
annual	2.9	2.6	2.5	2.6	3	4.9	5.1	5.4	5.6	5.9	4.7	5.5	5.8	5.7	6.5
30-day	1.2	1.2	1.1	1.4	1.6	2.2	2.2	2.2	2.5	2.9	1.8	2.4	2.5	2.6	3
Alcohol															
lifetime	53.8	52.5	52.1	51.7	50.5	72	69.8	70.6	71.4	70.1	81.7	81.4	80	80.3	79.7
annual	45.5	43.7	43.5	43.1	41.9	65.2	62.7	63.7	65.3	63.5	74.8	74.3	73.8	73.2	73.3
30-day	24.5	23	24	22.4	21.5	40.1	38.8	40	41	39	52.7	52	51	50	49.8
daily	0.8	0.9	1	0.8	0.9	1.7	1.9	1.9	1.8	1.9	3.9	3.9	3.4	2.9	3.6
Cigarettes (any use)															
lifetime	47.3	45.7	44.1	40.5	36.6	60.2	57.7	57.6	55.1	52.8	65.4	65.3	64.6	62.5	61
30-day	19.4	19.1	17.5	14.6	12.2	29.8	27.6	25.7	23.9	21.3	36.5	35.1	34.6	31.4	29.5
1/2 pack+/day	3.5	3.6	3.3	2.8	2.3	8.6	7.9	7.6	6.2	5.5	14.3	12.6	13.2	11.3	10.3
Smokeless Tobacco															
lifetime	16.8	15	14.4	12.8	11.7	26.3	22.7	20.4	19.1	19.5	25.3	26.2	23.4	23.1	19.7
30-day	5.5	4.6	4.5	4.2	4	8.9	7.5	6.5	6.1	6.9	9.7	8.9	8.4	7.6	7.8
Daily	1	1	0.9	0.9	1.2	2.2	2.2	1.5	1.9	2.2	4.4	3.2	2.9	3.2	2.8
Steroids															
lifetime	1.8	2.3	2.7	3	2.8	2	2	2.7	3.5	3.5	2.4	2.7	2.9	2.5	3.7
annual	1	1.2	1.7	1.7	1.6	1.2	1.2	0.7	2.2	2.1	1.4	1.7	1.8	1.7	2.4
30-day	0.5	0.5	0.7	0.8	0.7	0.7	0.6	0.9	1	0.9	1	1.1	0.9	0.8	1.3
MDMA															
lifetime	3.2	2.7	2.7	4.3	5.2	5.7	5.1	6	7.3	8	6.9	5.8	8	11	11.7
annual	2.3	1.8	1.7	3.1	3.5	3.9	3.3	4.4	5.4	6.2	4	3.6	5.6	8.2	9.2
30-day	1	0.9	0.8	1.4	1.8	1.3	1.3	1.8	2.6	2.6	1.6	1.5	2.5	3.6	2.8

Lifetime - use at least once during respondent's lifetime

Annual - use at least once during year preceding survey

30–Day - use at least once during month preceding survey

SOURCE: 2001 Monitoring the Future Study (MTF). The MTF survey is conducted by the University of Michigan's Institute for Social Research and is funded by the National Institutes of Health, <http://www.nida.nih.gov/Infofax/HSYouthtrends.html>.

Trends in drug use of 8th, 10th, and 12th graders shows modest changes from five years earlier.

cent from a low of 41 percent in 1992. The 2001 survey showed that overall drug use among American teens generally remained about the same as in 2000, after a slight decline in the late 1990s.

Increases during the 1990s were particularly sharp among 8th and 10th graders. No data are available before 1991, so longer-term trends are not known, but it is clear that there were significant increases between 1991 and 2001. Among 8th graders in 1991, 11 percent had used an illicit drug in the previous twelve months; that figure increased to 20 percent by 2001. Similarly, among 10th graders, annual use increased from 21 percent in 1991 to 37 percent in 2001.

Marijuana. Marijuana is the most frequently used illicit drug. In 2001, 37 percent of seniors—well over one in three—reported using marijuana in the past twelve months. Among 8th graders, annual marijuana use increased from 6.2 percent in 1991 to 15 percent in 2001 (peaking at 18 percent in 1996). Among 10th graders, annual marijuana use almost doubled between 1991 and 2001, from 17 percent to 33 percent (peaking at 35 percent in 1997).

Inhalants. Although not necessarily illicit drugs, inhalants are sometimes used illicitly for the purpose of getting high. This particular behavior is generally more often seen among younger students than among high-school seniors. In 2001, for example, 4.5 percent of 12th graders reported using inhalants to get high at least once in the past twelve months, compared to 6.6 percent of 10th graders, and 9.1 percent of 8th graders.

Alcohol. In 2001 nearly one-third (30 percent) of high-school seniors reported that they had had five or more drinks in a row at least once during the past two weeks. (Drinking five or more drinks in a row is enough to render the average teenager intoxicated.) The trend over the course of the 1990s was not encouraging, with levels of alcohol consumption increasing slightly over earlier levels. The trends in the 1990s for 8th and 10th graders were also not encouraging: In 2001 levels of heavy drinking were slightly higher than they were in 1991. For example, in 2001, 25 percent of 10th graders reported having had five or more drinks in a row in the past two weeks, compared to 23 percent of 10th graders in 1991.

Cocaine. The use of cocaine among adolescents also increased in the 1990s, and by 2001 annual cocaine use among high-school seniors reached 4.8 percent. In the 2001 survey, several illicit drugs showed a slight decline in use over the previous two years, including heroin (in forms that are not injected), LSD, powdered cocaine, and crack.

Crack cocaine first appeared in the early 1980s and became a significant factor among the illicit drugs in the mid-1980s. The use of crack cocaine increased during the 1990s, with 3.7 percent of 12th graders having tried it at least once, according to the 2001 survey. These numbers are below peak levels in the 1980s.

Other Drugs. There have also been significant increases in adolescents' use of anabolic steroids and the drug ecstasy. The 2001 report also noted that teen tobacco smoking continued to decline sharply, but was still well above rates of the early 1990s. Drugs that showed little change in use included amphetamines, tranquilizers, heroin, and the so-called "club drugs": Rohypnol, GHB, and ketamine.

The Reasons and Risk Factors for Drug Use

Many factors determine whether teenagers are likely to engage in harmful behaviors such as drug-taking.

Family Life. Researchers have investigated the influence of parents and home life on children's alcohol and drug use. A survey of 12,118 teenagers found that teenagers who felt close to their parents and siblings, teachers, and classmates were less likely to engage in risky behaviors. In another study, a large group of New Jersey adolescents was interviewed by phone at two different times, three years apart. Between 1979 and 1981, 1,380 subjects aged 12, 15, and 18 were interviewed. Three years later, 95 percent of them (1,308 subjects) were interviewed again. The interviews included topics of family harmony and closeness, parenting styles, and the attitudes and behaviors of parents. The greatest influence on whether younger children drank alcohol seemed to be the alcohol use and attitudes of the same gender parent. Older adolescents, though, were most strongly affected by the father's alcohol use. Children with hostile and emotionally cold parents were more likely to use drugs and alcohol than were those who described a warmer relationship with their parents.

In other research, 4,023 adolescents aged 12 to 17 years were interviewed by telephone about their own and their family members' substance use and their experiences of being victims of violence. Adolescents had a greater risk for substance abuse or dependence if they had been physically or sexually abused, or had family members with alcohol or drug-use problems.

Physical Factors. An adolescent who tries a particular type of drug is more likely to use that substance again if he or she enjoys the drug's effects. If the drug produces unpleasant effects, trying it again is less likely. Once an adolescent tries a drug and likes it, other factors de-

THE IMPACT OF ILLICIT DRUG USE

Using illicit drugs can harm the abuser's body, but can also hurt the user in other ways:

- The use of alcohol and other drugs is a major cause of teenager deaths, ranging from motor vehicle crashes to homicides to suicides.

- In the college environment, students with average grades of Ds or Fs drink three times as much as those who earn As.

- Nearly one in two college students who were victims of crimes said they were drinking or using other drugs when they were victimized.

- Sexually active teens who have more than five drinks are three times less likely to use condoms, and so risk becoming pregnant and/or infected by HIV and other sexually transmitted diseases.

termine whether he or she will continue to use it. Tolerance and withdrawal are two of the most important factors.

As the body becomes used to the effect of a drug, the person needs to take more of it to obtain the same effect. This is known as **tolerance**, and once tolerance to a drug develops, larger and larger doses are required. When the effect of a drug (such as heroin, nicotine, or caffeine) begins to wear off, the user may experience unpleasant symptoms. This is known as **withdrawal**. To avoid these withdrawal symptoms, a user may feel the need to take the drug on a regular basis.

Social Life. The social and emotional needs of adolescents also influence drug use. Teenagers looking for peer acceptance or wanting to appear "cool" might decide to try taking drugs, beginning a path toward continuing use. Teenagers also want to be seen more like adults, with the freedom to do what adults do. By using tobacco or alcohol—illegal for adolescents, yet both legal and socially acceptable for adults—the adolescent seeks an adult image. Adolescents are exposed to advertising on television and in magazines for beer, wine, and cigarettes that portrays drinking and smoking as desirable. They may want to emulate celebrities such as movie or pop stars who are seen smoking or drinking in the media. Once adolescents begin using drugs—for any of these reasons—they may find that they are unable to stop.

The Drug-Use Sequence

Using one drug often leads to the subsequent use of another. Typically, drug use begins with alcohol or cigarettes. The next drug of use is typically marijuana, and occasional drinking may develop into **problem drinking**. Next in the sequence are other illicit drugs. Cocaine use tends to follow marijuana use, with crack-cocaine use occurring after cocaine use. In other words, it is likely that someone who smokes crack has already tried tobacco, alcohol, marijuana, and cocaine. Many adolescents who use drugs in one category, however, do not necessarily progress to drug use in a higher category, and many stop before the drug use becomes a habit.

The use of alcohol and cigarettes typically—but not always—begins at an earlier age than does the use of illegal drugs. Adolescents who progress to illicit drugs, such as crack, generally begin smoking and drinking earlier than those who do not. Research indicates that a person who begins using drugs before the age of 15 is very likely to abuse drugs and alcohol as an adult.

Studies of adults show that regular adolescent drug use is connected to further drug use later in life. For example, there is a good

tolerance condition in which higher and higher doses of a drug or alcohol are needed to produce the effect or "high" experienced from the original dose

withdrawal group of physical and psychological symptoms that may occur when a person suddenly stops the use of a substance or reduces the dose of an addictive substance

problem drinking a behavior when a person's drinking disrupts her or his life and relationships, causing problems for the drinker

People who believe drugs are used in sequence point out that virtually no users of illicit drugs (e.g., marijuana, crack, cocaine, or heroin) are abstinent of cigarette and alcohol use. In 2000 a mere 2.7 percent of young adults who had used illicit drugs did *not* smoke cigarettes or drink alcohol.

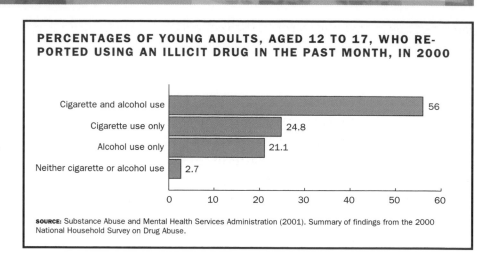

PERCENTAGES OF YOUNG ADULTS, AGED 12 TO 17, WHO REPORTED USING AN ILLICIT DRUG IN THE PAST MONTH, IN 2000

Cigarette and alcohol use — 56
Cigarette use only — 24.8
Alcohol use only — 21.1
Neither cigarette or alcohol use — 2.7

SOURCE: Substance Abuse and Mental Health Services Administration (2001). Summary of findings from the 2000 National Household Survey on Drug Abuse.

chance that an adolescent who smokes crack will become an adult who takes therapeutic drugs such as tranquilizers and sedatives. Studies of people participating in drug-treatment centers often reveal that these people not only need treatment for use of substances such as cocaine or heroin, but that they are also addicted to caffeine, tobacco, and/or alcohol—the very substances they first started using.

Adolescents who take drugs may move on to other drugs as they grow older. They may seek different drugs that cost less or are easier to obtain, or keep trying different drugs to get the effect that they want. Often, peers introduce each other to new substances. Multiple-drug use also occurs when an individual tries to counteract the effect of one drug with the effect of another. For example, cocaine may produce feelings of anxiety, so the user will then take tranquilizers to calm down.

Prevention Programs

Given our understanding of how drug use follows a sequence, prevention programs should try to reach adolescents before their first use of alcohol and cigarettes. Ideally, this would help prevent their later use of marijuana and other drugs. For adolescents who have already smoked marijuana, prevention programs must aim to reduce the chance that these adolescents will go on to try other drugs.

Educating young people about the dangers of drugs is an important tool in prevention. For example, teenage athletes sometimes take anabolic steroids to improve their performance on the field. A school-based series of seven weekly classes on the dangers of anabolic steroids appeared to help reduce anabolic-steroid use among 702 teenage athletes. The athletes also learned about safe alternatives to anabolic steroids. In another group of 804 athletes, who were simply given a pamphlet about anabolic steroids, the reduction of their levels of drug use was less successful.

The Consequences of Substance Abuse

Although drugs can sometimes make one feel good for a few minutes or hours, extensive research has shown that young people who abuse drugs or alcohol often suffer long-term, harmful consequences as a result. These harmful consequences are sometimes irreversible, and can negatively affect a person's health for the rest of her or his life. In some cases, even a single, one-time use of a drug (for example, ecstasy) can cause long-term—and perhaps permanent—damage to a young person's brain or other organs. Studies have also shown that, in general, teenagers who abuse drugs and/or alcohol are more likely than others to:

- have behavioral and academic problems at school
- be involved in criminal acts and traffic accidents
- become sexually active at earlier ages, have unprotected sex, and contract sexually transmitted diseases
- suffer from depression and other psychiatric disorders
- become victims of violent crimes
- be killed by drowning, fire, suicide, and homicide.

SEE ALSO ADDICTION: CONCEPTS AND DEFINITIONS; PREVENTION; PREVENTION PROGRAMS; RISK FACTORS FOR SUBSTANCE ABUSE; USERS.

Adult Children of Alcoholics (ACOA)

People over the age of 18 who have at least one biological parent with severe and repetitive life problems with alcohol are referred to as adult children of alcoholics. Because they have family and genetic ties to an alcoholic, these people carry an increased risk of severe alcohol problems themselves—from two to four times that of children of non-alcoholics. When children of alcoholics reach adolescence or adulthood, they might be slightly more likely to have problems with marijuana-type drugs or with stimulants (such as cocaine or amphetamines).

Some researchers have also observed that people whose childhood homes were disrupted by alcohol-related problems may have greater difficulties managing their adult lives. Research has indicated that

SOME STATISTICS ABOUT ALCOHOLISM

If you live or lived with an alcoholic, you are not alone:

- Seventy-six million Americans, about 43 percent of the U.S. adult population, have been exposed to alcoholism in their families.

- Almost one in five adult Americans (18 percent) lived with an alcoholic while growing up.

- Roughly one in eight American adult drinkers is an alcoholic or experiences problems due to the use of alcohol. The cost to society is estimated at more than $166 billion each year.

- There are an estimated 26.8 million children of alcoholics in the United States. Some research suggests that over 11 million are under the age of 18.

some adult children of alcoholics have problems with procrastination, with honesty, with forming close, trusting relationships, and with learning to have fun. Some children of alcoholics worked so hard throughout their childhoods to be the mature caregiver to their child-like, substance-abusing, dependent parent, that they find it impossible to stop acting as a caregiver. They are unable to make choices that benefit themselves, sacrificing instead to the often overwhelming and unreasonable needs of others.

Adult Children of Alcoholics ☎, or ACOA, is the formal name of a self-help group. People with at least one alcoholic parent can meet with others to have discussions, to share past and current experiences, and to offer support to each other. Those who join this voluntary organization usually feel impaired by their experiences and thus seek help in coping with their past and/or present problems.

In the fields of **psychology** and **psychiatry**, there is interest in tracing the origin of certain personality traits thought to be common among adult children of alcoholics. These traits may or may not come about because of specific alcohol-related experiences in the childhood home. They may instead stem from (1) the general childhood environment in which an individual was raised, (2) additional psychiatric conditions among the parents, or (3) general factors associated with a **disordered** childhood home.

Alcoholic parents leave a legacy that can affect their children well after those children have themselves become adults. Luckily, a number of groups exist to help these people go on to live healthy, happy, productive lives. SEE ALSO AL-ANON; ALATEEN; CODEPENDENCE; CONDUCT DISORDER.

☎ See *Organizations of Interest* at the back of Volume 1 for address, telephone, and URL.

psychology scientific study of mental processes and behaviors

psychiatry branch of medicine that deals with the study, treatment, and prevention of mental illness

disordered state characterized by chaotic, disorganized, or confused functioning; may refer to problems with a person's individual thought processes or problems within a system, such as a family

Advertising and the Alcohol Industry

The beverage alcohol industry includes companies that market beers and brews (malt liquors), wines and sparkling wines (such as champagne), and distilled spirits (e.g., whiskey, vodka, scotch, gin, rum, and flavored liquors). Businesses must obtain a special license to sell one or more of the above categories of products. For example, if a restaurant has only a beer and wine license, it cannot serve other types of alcoholic beverages.

In the United States, it is illegal to sell alcoholic beverages to minors, or those who are less than 21 years of age. Yet every day, thousands of minors buy beer and wine coolers with no questions asked by store clerks or owners. Even if a store refuses to sell to them, minors can often get around the law by finding an older friend to buy the alcohol for them. The illegal use of alcoholic beverages by teenagers creates a high level of concern on the part of health-care professionals, police, parents, and activist groups such as Mothers Against Drunk Driving ☎ and the Center for Science in the Public Interest.

☎ See *Organizations of Interest* at the back of Volume 1 for address, telephone, and URL.

The Advertising Problem

The high level of alcohol use by those under age 21 creates an advertising problem for the companies that market alcoholic beverages. How do you advertise to the 21 and over group and also appear not to target the under-21 group? Teenagers have a very strong desire to participate in activities they view as adult. This makes them **vulnerable** to anything they think would help them achieve that goal.

vulnerable at greater risk

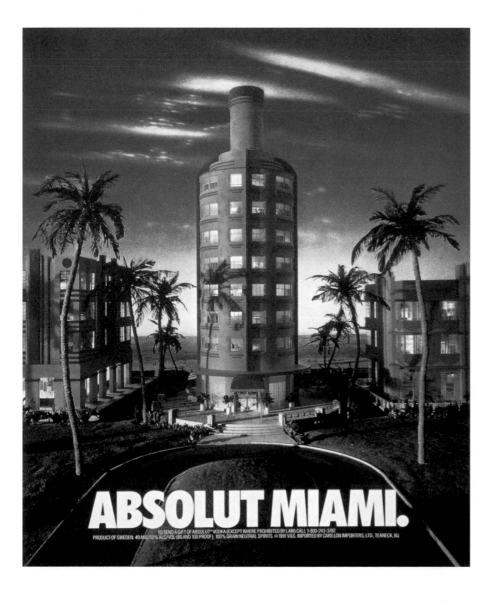

Absolut vodka advertisements have become a part of popular culture. The distinctive bottle shape appears in each ad with a descriptive word or theme tied to *Absolut,* suggesting an attractive identity for alcohol drinkers.

Critics accuse alcoholic-beverage companies of purposely making their advertising and promotional programs inviting to teenagers. The companies deny this, pointing with pride to public service messages such as "friends don't let friends drive drunk" or those that encourage drinkers to "know when to say when," "drink smart or don't start," "think when you drink," or "drink safely."

Who Minds the Store?

The U.S. Bureau of Alcohol, Tobacco, and Firearms (ATF) in the Department of the Treasury is responsible for overseeing the alcohol industry. Its rules discourage advertising claims that are **obscene** or misleading, as well as those that associate athletic ability with drinking. Alcoholic beverages sold in the United States must carry a warning on the container that states: "GOVERNMENT WARNING: (1) According to the Surgeon General, women should not drink alcoholic beverages during pregnancy because of the risk of birth defects. (2) Consumption of alcoholic beverages impairs your ability to drive a car or operate machinery, and may cause health problems."

The Federal Trade Commission (FTC) also reviews advertising, especially instances of false or misleading ads. But, with few exceptions, neither the ATF nor the FTC has been aggressive in challenging ads that appeal to young drinkers or ads that seem to encourage heavy drinking.

☎ See *Organizations of Interest* at the back of Volume 1 for address, telephone, and URL.

The Food and Drug Administration ☎ in the Department of Health and Human Services has no legal control over alcohol advertising, except for wines with less than 7 percent alcohol. Unlike drug companies, alcoholic beverage makers are not required to state the risks, consequences, or benefits of use on their labels or in advertising materials. Americans see ads that encourage people to drink, but the ads fail to provide information about the down side of drinking, especially excessive drinking.

What is Advertising?

Merriam-Webster's Collegiate Dictionary defines the verb "advertise" as "to call public attention to especially by emphasizing desirable qualities so as to arouse a desire to buy or patronize." The definition of the noun "advertising" includes the phrase "by paid announcements." Advertisers use television, radio, and print ads, billboards, signs and displays in stores where the product is sold, and, increasingly, sponsorship of special events such as music festivals, auto-, bicycle-, and boat racing, and other sports.

The Role of Advertising

Advertising is used as a major tool in marketing. When a company first introduces a new product, the goals generally are:

- To inform potential purchasers that a particular product is available and suggest why they might like to try this new product.

- To persuade people that they should go out and buy the product.

- To let people know where the product can be purchased.

- To reassure people who buy the product that they have made a wise choice in doing so.

Where more than one company has products in a given category, the goals generally become:

- To increase **market share** by taking business away from a competitive product.

- To increase the size of the market by **inducing** more people to start using the product. This can be done by increasing the product's appeal in certain ways. An alcoholic beverage advertisement tries to persuade viewers that using the product in the ad will make them feel more confident, more outgoing, more popular, more appealing to the opposite sex, and, in the case of minors, more adult.

- To increase the size of the market by inducing people to increase their use of the product(s). This can be done by tying the product to occasions such as spring break or a football game.

- To keep reassuring heavy drinkers that they are in good company by drinking the particular brand of beer or liquor being advertised. Since the 10 percent of those who drink most heavily account for about 50 percent of all alcohol consumed in the United States, this is a major **incentive** to advertise.

market share percentage of total sales of a product that is controlled by a company

induce to bring about or stimulate a particular reaction

incentive something, such as a reward, that encourages a specific action or behavior

The Connection between Advertising and Consumption

Alcohol advertisements are generally successful at making alcohol use seem desirable and enjoyable. Exposure to, or awareness of, advertising contributes to some increase in drinking, according to research reports. But researchers do not agree on just how much advertising contributes to heavier drinking. The amount of money a beer company spends on advertising does not **correlate**, for instance, with the amount of beer consumed. Advertising for wine and liquor has a more significant correlation with consumption.

correlate to link in a way that can be measured and predicted

The Beer Institute Advertising and Marketing Code

Critics often charge that beer industry advertising is targeted at minors. In response, companies point to the Beer Institute's Advertising

deflect to cause somebody to change what he or she usually does or plans to do

and Marketing Code, a set of guidelines created voluntarily by the industry. The beer industry's goal may be to ensure appropriate advertising, or it may be to create a positive image that will **deflect** criticism. A copy of the entire code is available from the Beer Institute or the Internet. Here are a few of the guidelines:

- Beer advertising and marketing materials should portray beer in a responsible manner.
- Brewers are committed to the policy of responsible advertising and marketing directed to persons of legal purchase age.
- Beer advertising and marketing materials are intended for adults of legal purchase age who choose to drink.
- Beer advertising and marketing activities should not associate or portray beer drinking before or during activities in situations which require a high degree of alertness or coordination.
- Beer advertising and marketing materials should not refer to any intoxicating effect that the product may produce.

The Distilled Spirits Council of the United States has a Code of Good Practice for Distilled Spirits Advertising and Marketing that is similar to that of the Beer Institute and Anheuser-Busch has a College Marketing Guide. One of its guidelines states that "Anheuser-Busch will limit its event sponsorship and promotion on campus to licensed retail establishments and those activities open to the general public, where most of the audience is reasonably expected to be above the legal purchase age."

Limitations of Voluntary Beer Industry Advertising Codes. The beer industry's voluntary advertising codes are written to prevent restrictions on advertising. In addition, voluntary codes are not legally enforceable. Most of the statements give the industry a lot of leeway in ads. For example, the Anheuser-Busch code specifies that advertising is intended to be used "where most of the audience is reasonably expected to be above the legal purchase age." The word "most" is the key: even if almost half the audience is below the legal purchase age, the code permits such advertising. SEE ALSO ADVERTISING AND THE TOBACCO INDUSTRY; COSTS OF SUBSTANCE ABUSE AND DEPENDENCE, ECONOMIC; TOBACCO: INDUSTRY.

Advertising and the Tobacco Industry

Tobacco companies spend more than $5 billion annually to advertise and promote cigarettes and other tobacco products. The companies

COMPARISON OF ADVERTISING TO BRAND PREFERENCE IN ADOLESCENTS AND ADULTS

Cigarette maker	Dollars spent on advertising (in millions)	Percent of adolescents who said this was their favorite brand	Percent of adults who said this was their favorite brand
Marlboro	$75	60.00%	23.50%
Camel	$43	13.30%	3.90%
Newport	$35	12.70%	4.80%
Kool	$21	1.20%	3.00%
Winston	$17	1.20%	6.70%

SOURCE: 1993 TAPS II, The Maxwell Consumer Report 1994, Ad & Summary 1993.
<http://www.cdc.gov/tobacco/research_data/advcoadv/brndtbl.htm>.

In the early 1990s Marlboro was reportedly the most popular brand of cigarettes among adolescents, and was the brand that spent the most on advertising.

claim that the purpose of their advertising is simply to provide information and to influence brand selection among current smokers, although only about 10 percent of smokers switch brands in any one year. Every year more than one million adult smokers stop smoking and almost a half-million other adult smokers die from smoking-related diseases. Therefore the tobacco companies must recruit an average of 3,300 new young smokers every day to replace those who die or stop smoking. Tobacco companies argue that smoking is an adult habit and that adult smokers choose to smoke. However, medical research has shown that cigarette addiction almost always begins before the age of 18. Adults who smoke started as children and could not quit.

Government **regulates** the advertising of **pharmaceuticals**, alcoholic beverages, and tobacco. But restrictions on the tobacco industry have been few. The basic regulations state that companies (1) cannot use paid advertising on television or radio, (2) cannot claim what they cannot prove (for example, that low-tar cigarettes are less hazardous to health), and (3) must include one of four warnings on cigarette packages and ads.

regulate bring under the control of law or authorized agency

pharmaceuticals legal drugs that are usually used for medical reasons

The fact that warning labels are printed on a pack of cigarettes has been successfully used by the tobacco companies as a defense against tobacco victims' lawsuits. This situation changed in 1997 and early 1998, when Florida, Minnesota, Mississippi, and Texas reached an agreement with the major tobacco companies and won **compensation** for the effects of smoking on their health-care expenses. On November 23, 1998, the major tobacco companies entered into a multibillion-dollar agreement with the other forty-six states. The Master Settlement Agreement settled lawsuits brought by the states and some organizations that wanted the tobacco companies to pay them back for costs related to the effect of smoking on public health. Under this agreement, the states and tobacco companies jointly

compensation amount of money or something else given to pay for loss, damage, or work done

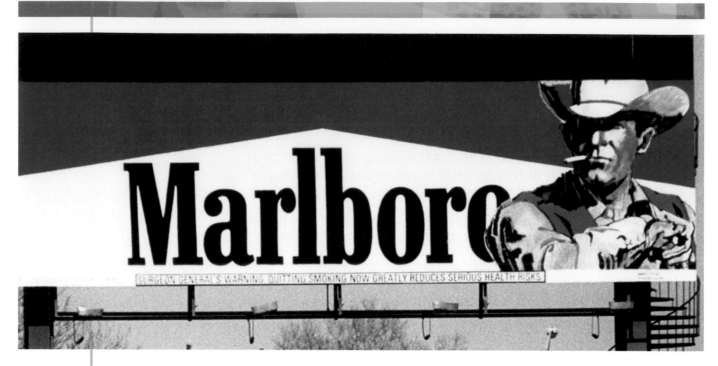

SURGEON GENERAL'S WARNING: QUITTING SMOKING NOW GREATLY REDUCES SERIOUS HEALTH RISKS

The Marlboro man—an attractive, physically fit, and athletic model—reinforces a positive image of smoking.

agreed on three major goals: (1) to try to reduce youth smoking, (2) to create new public health initiatives, and (3) to establish important new rules the tobacco companies must follow when doing business. In Florida a two-year education effort and ad campaign begun after the agreement was followed by a decrease in the number of teen smokers. After this campaign middle-school smoking was reduced by more than half, and smoking among high-school students was lowered by 24 percent.

Regulations on Tobacco Promotion

The Master Settlement Agreement changed the way cigarette companies can market, advertise, and promote their cigarettes. These are some of the rules:

- No participating manufacturer may take any action, directly or indirectly, to target youth in the advertising, promotion, or marketing of its products. No action can be taken whose main purpose is to initiate, maintain, or increase youth smoking.

- Billboards, stadium signs, and transit signs advertising tobacco are banned. Stores selling tobacco may have signs up to fourteen square feet inside or outside their stores.

- The use of cartoon characters in advertising, promoting, packaging, or labeling of tobacco products is banned. This does not cover the standard Camel cigarettes **logo**, a simple drawing of a camel. The Marlboro man and other human characters can continue to be used. By the early 1990s, "Joe Camel," used by RJR Nabisco to advertise the Camel brand, had become the

logo identifying symbol (as for advertising) that a company uses as a way of gaining recognition

center of the most effective advertising campaign ever created to influence the values and behavior of young people. The cartoon symbol had boosted Camel's share of the teenage market from next to nothing to almost 35 percent in just three years. The Master Settlement Agreement prohibits RJR Nabisco from using this character in any future advertising.

- Participating manufacturers and others licensed by them may no longer market, distribute, offer or sell, or license any clothing or merchandise bearing a tobacco brand name.

- Free product sampling is banned anywhere, except for a facility or enclosed space where the operator can ensure that no minors are present.

- No use of a tobacco-brand name as part of the name of a stadium is allowed.

- Cigarette manufacturers should advertise and promote their products only to adult smokers and will support the enactment and enforcement of state laws prohibiting the sales of cigarettes to persons under 18 years of age.

Rules applying specifically to advertisements are as follows:

- Cigarette advertising will not appear in publications directed primarily at those under 21 years of age, including school, college, or university media (such as athletic, theatrical, or other programs), comic books or comic supplements.

- No one depicted in cigarette advertising will be or appear to be under 25 years of age.

- Cigarette advertising will not suggest that smoking helps a person socially or that smoking can help people achieve distinction, success, or sexual attraction.

- Cigarette advertising will not show anyone who is or has been well known as an athlete to be a smoker. It will not show any smoker participating in, or obviously just having participated in, a physical activity requiring stamina or athletic conditioning beyond that of normal recreation.

- Sports or other celebrities who would have special appeal to persons under 21 will not be used to give **testimonials** about smoking.

testimonial statement that backs up a claim or supports a fact

The Effectiveness of Regulations

It is important to note that the tobacco companies have always found ways to get around restrictions. For example, once billboard advertising was banned, the companies simply increased their level of advertising in magazines, many of which are read by teenagers. In a survey, for example, 73 percent of teens (aged 12–17) reported see-

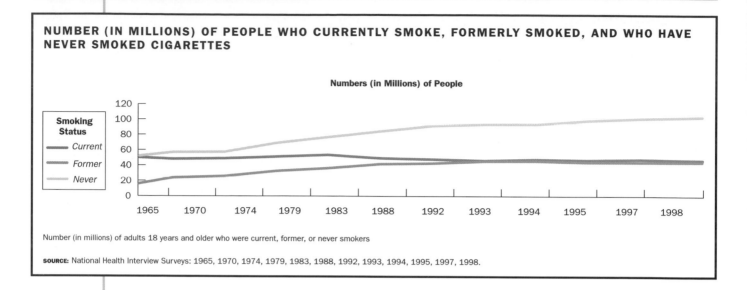

NUMBER (IN MILLIONS) OF PEOPLE WHO CURRENTLY SMOKE, FORMERLY SMOKED, AND WHO HAVE NEVER SMOKED CIGARETTES

Numbers (in Millions) of People

Smoking Status
—— Current
—— Former
—— Never

Number (in millions) of adults 18 years and older who were current, former, or never smokers

SOURCE: National Health Interview Surveys: 1965, 1970, 1974, 1979, 1983, 1988, 1992, 1993, 1994, 1995, 1997, 1998.

The number of people who report never smoking has doubled since 1965, numbers that coincide with the increased awareness of the health hazards of smoking and nicotine.

nicotine alkaloid derived from the tobacco plant that is responsible for smoking's addictive effects

dependent someone who has a psychological compulsion to use a substance for emotional and/or physical reasons

withdrawal group of physical and psychological symptoms that may occur when a person suddenly stops the use of a substance or reduces the dose of an addictive substance

ing tobacco advertising in the previous two weeks compared to only 33 percent of adults.

The same survey also revealed that 77 percent of teens said it was easy for people under the age of 18 to buy cigarettes and other tobacco products. Many displays of cigarettes in convenience stores are at waist level, making them available to children. Campaigns to restrict access to cigarettes by youths under the age of 18 have not been very successful.

In his memoirs, former Surgeon General C. Everett Koop said this about the tobacco industry: "After studying in depth the health hazards of smoking, I was dumbfounded—and furious. How could the tobacco industry trivialize extraordinarily important public-health information: the connection between smoking and heart disease, lung and other cancers, and a dozen or more debilitating and expensive diseases? The answer was—it just did."

Understanding the Smoking Habit

Almost all smokers started before the age of 21. Most begin smoking before the age of 18, and many before the age of 14. Young people who learn to inhale the cigarette smoke and experience the mood-altering effects from the inhaled **nicotine** quickly become **dependent** on cigarettes. Having developed a nicotine dependence, they find they must continue smoking to avoid the unpleasant side effects of nicotine **withdrawal**. The younger people are when they begin smoking, the more dependent they seem to become—and the sooner they start to experience smoking-related health problems. Six years of research at the National Center on Addiction and Substance Abuse at Columbia University revealed that a person who gets to the age of 21

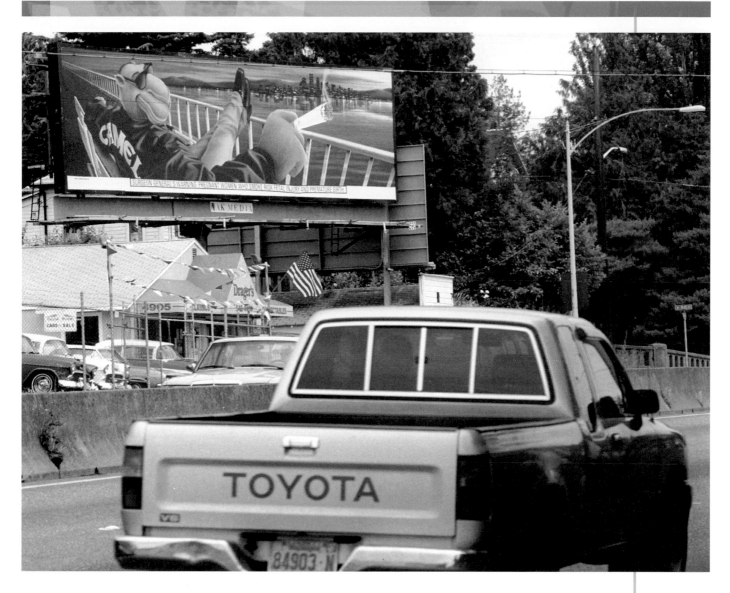

without smoking, using illegal drugs, or abusing alcohol is virtually certain never to do so.

A survey conducted by the U.S. Department of Health and Human Services among high school students who smoked half a pack of cigarettes a day found that 53 percent had tried to quit but could not. When asked whether they would be smoking five years later, only 5 percent said they would be—but eight years later, 75 percent were still smoking.

The cartoon advertisement character "Joe Camel" appeared cool when he smoked cigarettes. Found to be appealing to children, Joe Camel has since been retired by Camel cigarettes.

The Purpose of Cigarette Advertising

The tobacco companies have become masters at using advertising and promotional programs to help them accomplish several major objectives:

1. To reassure current smokers that smoking is not necessarily harmful. Thousands of studies show the adverse health effects

of smoking. The warning labels on cigarette packages themselves make this clear. Yet until a landmark legal case in Florida in 2000, when a jury found that cigarettes are in fact deadly and addictive, the tobacco industry continued to claim that no one had yet proven that smoking causes health problems.

2. To associate smoking with enjoyment. In their ads, tobacco companies show healthy young people enjoying parties, dancing, sporting events, picnics at the beach, sailing, and so on. The ads imply that if you smoke, you too will have the kind of good times enjoyed by the smokers in the ads.

3. To associate smoking with other risk-taking activities. Ads for cigarettes often show people in such risky activities as ballooning, mountain climbing, sky diving, and motorcycle riding. This is the industry's way of saying: Go ahead and take a risk by smoking—you are capable of deciding how much risk you want to take. The tobacco companies are betting that most young people do not think any bad effects of smoking will ever happen to them.

4. To associate cigarette smoking with becoming an adult. Teenagers want to be seen as adults. They want to be free to make their own decisions, without anyone telling them what they can and cannot do. The tobacco companies understand this. They stress that smoking is an adult habit—that only adults have the right to choose whether or not to smoke. So the simple act of smoking cigarettes becomes the perfect way for a teenager to show the world that he or she is an adult.

5. To associate cigarette smoking with attractiveness. Many ads for cigarettes imply that if you smoke, you will also be attractive to members of the opposite sex. In fact, surveys of young adults show that most people prefer to date nonsmokers.

6. To associate smoking with women's rights. For years the advertising theme for Virginia Slims cigarettes was "You've come a long way baby." Women were supposed to feel that along with women's liberation came the freedom to smoke. What the ads did not say is that women who smoke like men will die like men who smoke. In the 1990s lung cancer became the number-one cancer found in women, exceeding the incidence of breast cancer.

7. To show that smoking is an essential part of our society. The sheer number of cigarette ads—on billboards, on t-shirts, on signs at ballgames—along with movies in which actors are seen smoking leaves the impression that smoking is socially accept-

able by the majority of people. The message is that everybody is doing it.

9. To gain **legitimacy**. Tobacco companies spend millions of dollars to support educational programs, arts organizations, historical commemorations, and other popular endeavors. In this way, they try to borrow a positive image from the event or program they sponsor.

SEE ALSO ADVERTISING AND THE ALCOHOL INDUSTRY; TOBACCO: HISTORY OF; TOBACCO: INDUSTRY.

legitimacy meeting or conforming to legal or recognized standards

AIDS *See Substance Abuse and AIDS*

Al-Anon

Al-Anon ☎ is a fellowship for family members and friends of alcoholics. Although separate from Alcoholics Anonymous (AA) ☎, Al-Anon uses many of the same strategies, beliefs, and philosophies in its efforts to help families of alcoholics cope with the confusing and disturbing experiences of living with or being close to an active alcoholic. Al-Anon grew out of AA as a way to include families in a separate but similar organization, and thus also teach them about the beliefs and practices of AA. As AA expanded and more alcoholics became recovering ones, many close relatives realized that the lessons AA taught could help them solve some of their own personal problems. The AA strategy known as the Twelve Step program worked for them, even though they themselves were not alcoholics. In 2001 there were 24,389 Al-Anon groups worldwide, as well as 2,350 Alateen ☎ groups of children of alcoholics.

☎ See *Organizations of Interest* at the back of Volume 1 for address, telephone, and URL.

Al-Anon's Strategy

Al-Anon tries to direct its members' attention away from the alcoholic in their lives. Instead, Al-Anon members learn to focus on their own behavior and emotions. In many ways, the personalities of people living closely with an active alcoholic resemble those of the alcoholics. Alcoholics attempt to control their drinking by sheer force of their individual will. They are in **denial** as to their need for help. Similarly, family members attempt to control the feelings and behaviors of the alcoholic in their midst by simple force of personal will. Often, the family members are in denial, too, and do not see that they need help coping. Family members often become codependent—as obsessed with the alcoholic's behavior as the alcoholic is with the bottle.

denial psychological state in which a person ignores obvious facts and continues to deny the existence of a particular problem or situation

resent to feel anger, bitterness or ill will towards someone or something

For example, the alcoholic's spouse or partner may have attempted many times to control the drinking, with no success. The spouse may plead for the alcoholic to stop, but except for brief periods, those pleas are rejected. Or the alcoholic may promise to stop, yet fail to keep that promise. Often, while the alcoholic continues to drink and enjoy the effects of intoxication, the spouse or other caretaker must take over and do all the work of running the household, caring for the children, and working steadily to earn a living. If the alcoholic enters a treatment center and begins to show signs of improvement, the spouse may **resent** it deeply, since it appears that strangers have been able to do more in a short period than all the partner's efforts over the years. The partners and relatives of alcoholics often feel that they have not been wise enough, or determined enough, or superhuman enough, to get the alcoholics in their lives to stop drinking.

Al-Anon introduces the Twelve Steps of AA into the lives of family members as a way to reduce resentment and anger and to help them stop the controlling behavior they often display. AA's first step is: "We admitted we were powerless over alcohol—that our lives had become unmanageable." Al-Anon's version of AA's first step is: "We admit we are powerless to control an alcoholic relative, that we are not self-sufficient." Al-Anon groups tell family members they must admit that it is a waste of time to try to control what is in fact beyond their control. It is then no longer necessary for them to deny that their efforts at control are useless. They feel relieved of an enormous burden and sense of guilt.

Al-Anon tries to help families recover from the terrible effects of living with someone who is out of control. Al-Anon members work together to support each other, and to give each other strength. Ultimately, Al-Anon tries to teach family members that they can never successfully take responsibility for anyone else's behavior, and that they should never consider themselves the cause for anyone's choice to drink. Al-Anon encourages family members to separate themselves emotionally from their loved one's drinking problems, but to learn how to safely love that person. Family members are reassured that they can create a happy, successful life for themselves despite the choices that their alcoholic loved one is making for herself or himself. The Twelve Step strategy allows the family members to accept outsider treatment and to welcome its possible success. SEE ALSO ADULT CHILDREN OF ALCOHOLICS (ACOA); ALATEEN; ALCOHOLICS ANONYMOUS (AA); CODEPENDENCE; FAMILIES AND DRUG USE; TREATMENT TYPES: AN OVERVIEW.

Alateen

Alateen☎ is a division of the Al-Anon Family Group, which administers self-help groups for adult family members of drinkers. Alateen members are typically teenagers whose lives are being affected by someone else's drinking problem. Alateen members range in age from 12 to 18, with an average age of 14. Some Alateen groups welcome younger children between the ages of 10 and 12. Most Alateen members attend because one or both parents are problem drinkers, although some Alateen members attend because of a drinking brother or sister.

Alateen began in the late 1950s with a teenager who was attending Alcoholics Anonymous (AA)☎ and Al-Anon☎ meetings with his parents. His father had just gotten sober in AA and his mother was an active member of Al-Anon. The teenager felt that the **Twelve Steps** of AA were helping him. His mother suggested that he start a group for teenagers and pattern it after Al-Anon. The young man found five other teenage children of alcoholic parents and, while the adult groups met upstairs, he got them together downstairs.

As other teenagers came forward from Al-Anon groups, the idea spread. As of 2001, 2,350 Alateen groups are meeting worldwide. These groups are an important and integral part of the Al-Anon Family Group. They are coordinated from the Al-Anon Family Group Headquarters in New York City and tied closely to its public-information programs. Alateen groups meet in churches and schools, often in the same building as Al-Anon but in a different room. An active, adult member of Al-Anon usually serves as a sponsor. Also, members of Alateen can choose a personal sponsor from other Alateen members or from Al-Anon members.

Alateen enables its members to share their experiences openly and find ways to cope with the problem of living closely with an alcoholic parent or other relative. Typically the teen is obsessed with trying to control the drinking relative's behavior. He or she may be in **denial** as to the severity of the drinking problem. Through meetings, members learn that they can change their own thinking about that relative but that they cannot control his or her drinking. Scolding, tears, or persuasion are useless. Members also learn that they did not cause the problem drinking and have nothing to feel guilty for. As Al-Anon explains the goals of Alateen meetings, the teens must "learn to take care of themselves whether the alcoholic stops or not." In the last step of the AA Twelve-Step program, members declare: ". . .we tried to carry this message to alcoholics." Alateen changes this to: ". . .we tried to carry this message to others."

☎ See *Organizations of Interest* at the back of Volume 1 for address, telephone, and URL.

Twelve Steps program for remaining sober developed by Alcoholics Anonymous; adopted by many other groups, such as Narcotics Anonymous

denial psychological state in which a person ignores obvious facts and continues to deny the existence of a particular problem or situation

Along with the Twelve Steps, Alateen adapts and applies AA's Twelve Traditions to the conduct of their groups. For example, members remain anonymous by not using their last names. This helps maintain privacy and reduces competitiveness among members. Alateen uses the strategy of AA to help teens deal with anger, feelings of guilt, and denial. Newcomers gain hope as they bond with other teenagers similarly coping with their parents' and other relatives' drinking problems. Children are encouraged to learn how to remove themselves from the emotional turmoil of the drinker's problems but still love that person. Alateen teaches that everybody, regardless of the bad choices other people in their lives may be making, is in control of his or her own life, and can create a happy, healthy, successful life for himself or herself. SEE ALSO ADULT CHILDREN OF ALCOHOLICS (ACOA); AL-ANON; ALCOHOLICS ANONYMOUS (AA); CODEPENDENCE; FAMILIES AND DRUG USE; TREATMENT TYPES: AN OVERVIEW.

Alcohol- and Drug-Free Housing

Alcohol- and drug-free housing is for people who choose to live in an environment that is free of alcohol and/or drugs. Often, people who have recently left a rehabilitation facility will try to find alcohol- and drug-free housing to move into while they continue to work on remaining sober and free of drug use.

Alcohol- and drug-free housing units do not have structured meeting, therapy, or treatment programs. They are simply places where residents have agreed to follow three simple rules: (1) They must remain alcohol- and drug-free. (2) They must pay their rent on time. (3) They must abide by the landlord-tenant agreement. SEE ALSO TREATMENT: HISTORY OF, IN THE UNITED STATES.

Alcohol: Chemistry

fermentation controlled process in which an organic compound is enzymatically transformed

Alcohol occurs naturally when fruits, vegetables, and grains exposed to bacteria in the air undergo the process of **fermentation**. People can create and speed up the conditions for fermentation to produce ethyl alcohol, also called ethanol. Pure ethanol is not drinkable but is an ingredient of alcoholic beverages, such as beer, wine, and liquors. The concentration of ethanol in beer is approximately 4 to 5 percent; in wine it is 11 to 12 percent; and in most liquors it is 40 to 50 percent. Also, alcoholic beverages are often diluted by water before they are consumed.

The Effects of Alcohol on the Body

Ethanol acts as a **depressant** on the central nervous system, which is made up of the brain and spinal cord. This means it slows brain and nervous system function. It produces **sedation** and even sleep at higher doses. When people drink a moderate amount of ethanol, they may feel an initial stimulation or rush of energy. But soon after that first phase, alcohol decreases memory, the ability to concentrate, quickness of reaction, and judgment.

When a person drinks a beverage that has alcohol in it, the ethanol is absorbed from the stomach by simple diffusion into the bloodstream. Strong drinks with a higher percentage of alcohol are absorbed more quickly, while beer and wine are absorbed more slowly. Food slows the absorption process. Peak **blood alcohol concentration** occurs within thirty to ninety minutes of drinking—earlier on an empty stomach and later on a full stomach. Once absorbed, ethanol spreads throughout the parts of the body that contain water, going wherever water goes.

Recent evidence suggests that low or moderate amounts of ethanol (one to two drinks per day) can indirectly reduce the risk of heart attacks. The doses must be low enough to avoid liver damage. Scientists believe that this beneficial effect occurs because alcohol raises the level of a certain type of cholesterol in the blood. This cholesterol slows the development of **arteriosclerosis**, often the cause of heart attacks.

Tolerance, Dependence, and Abuse

Tolerance develops to a drug when the dose must be increased to achieve the effect of the original dose. Tolerance to ethanol can occur in just a few weeks or may take years, depending on how much and how consistently a person drinks. Like tolerance, dependence on ethanol can develop after only a few weeks of consistent drinking. When a dependent person stops drinking, he or she experiences withdrawal symptoms. These symptoms include the "shakes," hallucinations, nausea, vomiting, diarrhea, fever, sweating, and sometimes convulsions. Several days after the last drink, an individual sometimes goes through a severe phase of withdrawal called the delirium tremens. Symptoms of this last phase of withdrawal include confusion, disorientation, and vivid hallucinations. SEE ALSO ACCIDENTS AND INJURIES FROM ALCOHOL; ALCOHOL: COMPLICATIONS OF PROBLEM DRINKING; ALCOHOL: WITHDRAWAL; ALCOHOL TREATMENT: BEHAVIORAL APPROACHES; ALCOHOL TREATMENT: MEDICATIONS; BLOOD ALCOHOL CONCENTRATION.

depressant chemical that slows down or decreases functioning; often used to describe agents that slow the functioning of the central nervous system; such agents are sometimes used to relieve insomnia, anxiety, irritability, and tension

sedation process of calming someone by administering a medication that reduces excitement; often called a tranquilizer

blood alcohol concentration (BAC) amount of alcohol in the bloodstream, expressed as the grams of alcohol per deciliter of blood; as BAC increases, the drinker experiences more psychological and physical effects

arteriosclerosis hardening of the arteries

Alcohol: Complications of Problem Drinking

Alcohol is a legal drug for adults over 21 years of age. Yet drinking large amounts of alcohol over long periods can cause many medical complications. There is almost no organ system that alcohol does not damage. Alcohol affects how cells function throughout the body and the brain. Some effects of alcohol occur immediately, while others occur only after many years of heavy drinking.

The Liver

The liver is the largest internal organ of the human body and its functions are essential to life. The human liver has a remarkable resilience and capacity to recover after injury or illness. But this is true only up to a certain point. If illness pushes a person's liver beyond its ability to perform, she or he will die.

The liver performs many complex functions and is justly called the laboratory of the human body. Its most important functions include: (1) helping process and store nutrients, including fats, sugars, proteins, and vitamins; (2) producing substances necessary for blood clotting and healthy immune function; (3) filtering and cleansing the blood of various substances that are poisonous if allowed to accumulate; and (4) providing quick bursts of energy when needed. Many diseases can seriously damage the liver and interfere with its important functions. Taken in large quantities over a long period of time, alcohol can be directly poisonous to liver cells. Alcoholism is one of the most serious ways in which permanent liver damage can occur.

The number of deaths from liver damage caused by alcoholism is very high. Chronic heavy drinking can damage the liver in several ways:

Alcoholic Fatty Liver. Fat accumulation in the liver occurs in the majority of heavy drinkers. The liver cells become loaded with bubbles of fat. This condition may present no symptoms, but in an examination of the abdomen, a doctor may notice that the liver is enlarged. A **biopsy** reveals the presence of fat in the liver cells. In most cases, a fatty liver does not affect the patient's health. However, it is an early warning of further liver damage if the person continues to drink. This condition can be reversed if the patient stops drinking.

Alcoholic Hepatitis. The word "hepatitis" means liver inflammation, or swelling. While hepatitis can be due to an infection (such as hepatitis A, hepatitis B, and hepatitis C), it can also occur when the

biopsy procedure in which body tissue, cells, or fluids are removed for examination in a laboratory

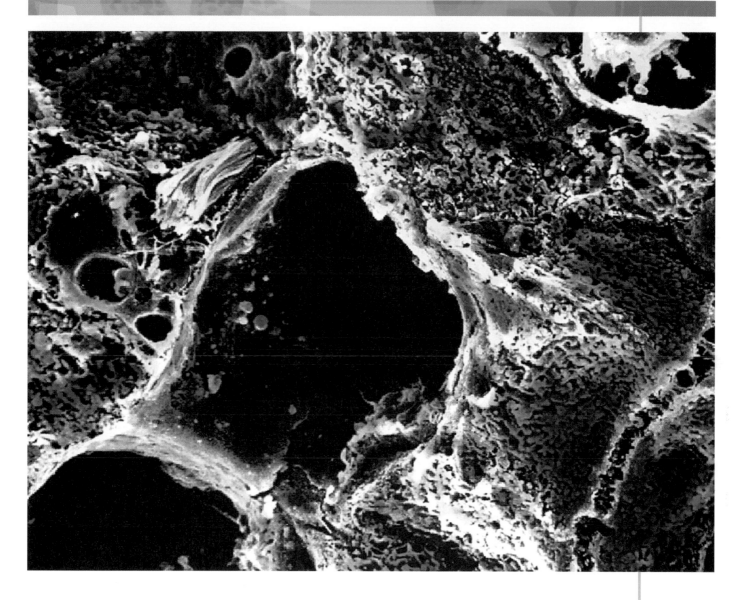

liver becomes inflamed due to damage from alcohol. Alcoholic hepatitis is a potentially more serious form of alcoholic liver disease, in which there is an accumulation of white blood cells and the death of some liver cells. The liver becomes less able to cleanse the blood of toxins. Some patients with alcoholic hepatitis experience no symptoms. Others may have a swollen and painful liver, fever, and mental disturbance. People with alcoholic hepatitis often become jaundiced; that is, the whites of their eyes and their skin become yellow, due to **bile** leaking into the bloodstream. Repeated episodes of drinking and alcoholic hepatitis can lead to the last stage of alcoholic liver disease—cirrhosis.

Alcoholic Cirrhosis. Once a liver becomes cirrhotic, the liver cannot become normal again. Damaged liver tissue is replaced by scar tissue that cannot perform any of the liver's normal functions. Scar

About 5 to 25 percent of alcoholics get cirrhosis, which is one of the leading causes of all deaths. This is a micrograph of a cirrhotic liver.

bile digestive substance made in the liver

tissue interferes with blood circulation in the liver and increases the pressure in the blood vessels. Increased blood pressure in these blood vessels makes them prone to bursting, leading to major hemorrhage (uncontrollable bleeding). Cirrhosis can be fatal. Although a number of other conditions can also cause cirrhosis, alcoholism is by far its most common cause.

Mental Disorders

In addition to its effects on the body, heavy drinking can also have negative effects on a person's mental health. Alcoholism is associated with several mental disorders.

antisocial personality disorder condition in which people disregard the rights of others and violate these rights by acting in immoral, unethical, aggressive, or even criminal ways

1. People with **antisocial personality disorder** (APD) often have problems with alcoholism as well. In fact, alcoholics are 21 times as likely to also fulfill the criteria for diagnosing antisocial personality disorder. People with APD often disregard and repeatedly violate the rights of others. A person with APD may engage in bullying, violence, vandalism, and lying, and show no remorse for these actions. As much as 2 percent of the male population of the United States are diagnosed as having both APD and alcoholism. Antisocial alcoholics generally begin problem drinking at an early age, have a family history of alcoholism, and have symptoms of other psychiatric disturbances, such as drug abuse, depression, and suicide attempts.

depression state in which an individual feels intensely sad and hopeless; may have trouble eating, sleeping, and concentrating, and is no longer able to feel pleasure from previously enjoyable activities; in extreme cases, may lead an individual to think about or attempt suicide

2. Alcoholism is sometimes linked to **depression**. Heavy drinkers are more likely to suffer from depression than are people who do not abuse alcohol. The relationship between alcohol use and depression is complex. Like the old question, "Which came first, the chicken or the egg?," experts continue to explore whether using alcohol can cause or increase feelings of depression, or whether a person with depression drinks alcohol to relieve symptoms of depression he or she is already experiencing. (The use of alcohol to try to get rid of troublesome symptoms is sometimes referred to as self-medication.)

3. Alcohol has long been used to relieve anxiety, a feeling of nervousness and fear that strikes nearly everyone at various times in their lives. Some individuals are diagnosed with anxiety disorders, which include generalized anxiety disorder, panic disorder, and phobias. For these people, anxiety overwhelms their ability to function normally. They may feel that alcohol provides temporary relief from some of their symptoms. Alcohol, however, can in fact contribute to anxiety disorders. Many individuals with these anxiety disorders are also alcoholics. Unfortunately, while alcohol may relieve symptoms of anxiety in

some people and at some times, it also can greatly increase the symptoms of anxiety, particularly during the period when the effects of the alcohol are beginning to wear off.

4. Adolescents and adults with **attention-deficit/hyperactivity disorder** (ADHD) have higher rates of drug abuse and alcoholism. Again, researchers are unclear why this is the case. Do some people have differences in brain chemistry that cause them to have symptoms of both ADHD and substance abuse? Or do people with ADHD use alcohol to self-medicate, that is, to relieve some of the symptoms of ADHD?

5. Alcohol is involved in at least 50 percent of completed suicides (i.e., suicide attempts that actually result in death). Studies of completed suicides show that, prior to the suicide, some people may have confused and conflicted feelings about going through with the act. Alcohol or substance abuse may become the weight that tips the scale toward suicide.

6. Chronic alcoholism can cause **delirium** and **dementia**. Abrupt withdrawal from alcohol can cause delirium tremens. When someone drinks alcohol regularly, for a long time, it begins to destroy brain cells. If the liver also becomes damaged and unable to remove certain poisons from the bloodstream, these poisons may circulate into the brain, further damaging it. Delirium is an on-again-off-again condition in which a person is confused, forgetful, and "out of it." Dementia is a permanent condition in which an individual no longer has good

attention-deficit/ hyperactivity disorder ADHD is a long-term condition characterized by excessive, ongoing hyperactivity (overactivity, restlessness, fidgeting), distractibility, and impulsivity; distractibility refers to heightened sensitivity to irrelevant sights and sounds, making some simple tasks difficult to complete

delirium mental disturbance marked by confusion, disordered speech, and sometimes hallucinations

dementia disease characterized by progressive loss of memory and the ability to learn and think

---

DIRECT AND INDIRECT HEALTH COMPLICATIONS DUE TO ALCOHOL

Primary Causes of Deaths Directly Due to Alcohol

Brain diseases (alcoholic psychoses, alcoholic polyneuropathy)	388
Alcoholism (alcohol dependence syndrome and nondependent abuse of alcohol)	6,005
Heart disease (alcoholic cardiomyopathy)	878
Stomach inflammation (alcoholic gastritis)	90
Liver scarring (alcoholic cirrhosis)	11,868
Alcohol poisoning (excessive blood level of alcohol, accidental poisoning)	213
Total	19,442

Secondary Causes of Death Directly Due to Alcohol

Lung diseases (respiratory tuberculosis, pneumonia and influenza)	4,022
Cancers (malignant neoplasm of lip, cavity, pharynx, esophagus, stomach, and/or liver)	17,411
Heart disease (cerebrovascular disease, hypertension)	10,401
Diabetes mellitus	2,423
Liver diseases (chronic hepatitis, cirrhosis of liver, biliary cirrhosis, chronic liver damage, and portal hypertension)	6,387
Diseases of esophagus, stomach, and duodenum	892
Diseases of the pancreas (acute pancreatitis, chronic pancreatitis)	1,033
Total	42,569
Combined Total	**62,011**

SOURCE: Analysis by The Lewin Group based on data from the National Institute on Alcohol Abuse and Alcoholism. <http://www.nida.nih.gov/EconomicCosts/Table5_3.html>.

One study found that more than 62,000 people died from diseases caused by alcoholism in a single year.

control over his or her behavior, thoughts, and ability to remember, understand, and learn. Delirium tremens is a condition that occurs specifically around the time that someone stops using alcohol. Because the person's brain has become dependent on the presence of alcohol in order to function, abruptly cutting off the presence of alcohol can make the individual temporarily confused, agitated, and shaky.

The Central Nervous System

depressant chemical that slows down or decreases functioning; often used to describe agents that slow the functioning of the central nervous system; such agents are sometimes used to relieve insomnia, anxiety, irritability, and tension

Alcohol is a **depressant** of the central nervous system, which is made up of the brain and spinal cord. Because of these depressant effects, a **blood alcohol concentration (BAC)** above the legal limit (for adults over 21, in most states, the limit is 0.08 grams of alcohol per deciliter of blood) typically impairs a person's ability to drive and operate machinery. Even relatively low BACs can affect hand-eye coordination, selective attention (for example, concentrating on making a turn rather than watching other cars speed by), and decision making. Intoxication can increase risk-taking, aggressive, or dangerous behaviors because of a loosening of inhibitions. As the amount the person drinks increases, he or she loses the ability to evaluate the consequences of his or her actions. As a result, intoxication is frequently associated with severe injuries, including traumatic brain injuries, and is a common cause of fatal motor vehicle accidents and violent incidents.

blood alcohol concentration (BAC) amount of alcohol in the bloodstream, expressed as the grams of alcohol per deciliter of blood; as BAC goes up, the drinker experiences more psychological and physical effects

A binge of heavy drinking can lead to memory lapses or alcoholic blackouts, in which the individual is unable to remember events that took place while he or she was drunk. Drinking below the legal limit of intoxication can also affect a person's ability to remember new information. Studies of the brain structures of chronic alcoholics reveal an **atrophy** of the cortex and low brain weight. Some studies even show loss of cerebral tissue in moderate drinkers.

atrophy condition that involves a shrinking of size or wasting away of tissue or a body part

The Cardiovascular System

Alcoholism can cause serious damage to the heart muscle. Alcoholics who have a history of heart problems often have high blood pressure and arrythmias (abnormal heart rhythms). In alcoholics who have had at least one episode of heart failure, alcohol can lead to further heart failure. The symptoms of heart failure—such as weakness, fatigue, blood clots, and abnormal heartbeat—generally disappear if the person stops drinking. Even small amounts of alcohol affect the cardiovascular system. When nonalcoholics drink alcohol, the alcohol causes the heart to pump less blood per contraction. This is one of alcohol's depressant effects.

The Endocrine and Reproductive System

The body communicates with itself through two different systems: the nervous system and the endocrine system. The nervous system handles communications that are important for thinking and for controlling the immediate actions of our muscles. The nervous system communicates directly to the target cells through nerve cells. In contrast, the endocrine system uses chemical messengers called hormones. Hormones flow in the bloodstream to handle more long-term communications, such as controlling growth and sexual differences. Examples of hormones are insulin, estrogen, and testosterone.

Research has shown that alcohol causes problems in hormonal function in chronic heavy drinkers. Chronic heavy drinking prevents the release of hormones necessary for sexual functioning. Male alcoholics commonly experience impotence, a decrease in sperm count or complete absence of sperm, infertility, and decreased sex drive. In young females, alcohol abuse can cause amenorrhea (absence of menstruation) and can prevent ovulation. Women who drink heavily for many years may experience early menopause. During pregnancy, alcoholism increases the risk of spontaneous abortion (miscarriage). Babies born to alcoholic mothers may have fetal alcohol syndrome (FAS), a condition in which children have facial abnormalities and problems with growth and development. Alcohol's suppression of the sex hormone progesterone may be related to the development of FAS.

The Immune System

Alcohol can interfere with the functioning of the body's immune system, the system that fights off infection. Chronic drinking decreases the body's resistance to infections, particularly those caused by bacteria. For example, alcoholics are at increased risk of pockets of infection in the lungs (known as abscesses), tuberculosis, and infections of the lining of the abdomen (called peritonitis).

Increasing evidence suggests that chronic drinking not only damages the body's defenses against bacteria but also against cancer cells. A strong association exists between alcohol use and cancers of the esophagus, pharynx (in the throat), and mouth. Chronic heavy drinkers have more cases of esophageal cancer than the general population. The risk increases as alcohol consumption increases. There is no evidence that alcohol itself is a carcinogen, that is, a cancer-causing substance. However, alcohol appears to increase the carcinogenic effects of other chemicals, such as those in tobacco. The cancers with which alcohol is most closely associated are also cancers associated with smoking.

This relationship suggests that alcohol enhances the carcinogenic effects of smoking.

Nutrition

The body needs energy for its actions, protein to build and maintain cells, and a variety of **micronutrients** to support function. People who drink heavily often eat less than is necessary for health. Some heavy drinkers take in as much as 50 percent of their daily calorie needs as alcohol. As a result, they do not consume enough essential nutrients, protein, carbohydrate, and fat. Their bodies are deprived of the energy intake and materials needed to build tissues.

Alcohol interferes with nutrition by affecting digestion and the way the body uses, stores, and excretes nutrients. Alcohol prevents nutrients from breaking down into substances the body can use. It also slows the absorption of nutrients by damaging cells in the stomach and intestines, and interferes with the transport of some micronutrients into the blood from digested foods.

Alcohol also affects blood sugar levels. An undernourished person who drinks alcohol can develop hypoglycemia. Hypoglycemia, or decreased blood sugar, can cause serious injury even if it is only temporary. When there is no food to supply energy, the sugar that is stored in the body decreases. As a result, the brain and other organs do not get the amounts of glucose (sugar) needed for energy and proper functioning.

Chronic heavy drinking causes deficiencies—inadequate amounts—of vitamins A, E, and D. Vitamin D deficiency can cause bone loss; vitamin A deficiency can cause night blindness; deficiencies of vitamins A, C, D, E, K, and B can interfere with wound healing and cell functions. Deficiencies of various vitamins can cause damage to the brain and nervous system.

The Health Risks of Drinking Alcohol

Many people have a casual attitude toward drinking, but it is important to understand the real health and safety risks that alcohol presents. Small amounts of alcohol can temporarily affect normal functioning in body and brain. Heavy drinking can have serious, permanent consequences. Understanding that alcohol can have both short- and long-term health effects can help people make informed choices about their drinking habits. SEE ALSO ACCIDENTS AND INJURIES FROM ALCOHOL; ALCOHOL: CHEMISTRY; ALCOHOL: POISONING; ALCOHOL: PSYCHOLOGICAL CONSEQUENCES OF CHRONIC ABUSE.

micronutrients nutrients that the body requires, although often in small amounts, including vitamins and minerals

Alcohol: History of Drinking

Over the course of human history, alcohol has played a role in religion, economics, sex, politics, and many other aspects of societies around the world. Its role has varied from culture to culture, and has also changed over time within cultures. A complex array of customs, attitudes, beliefs, and values surround the use—or avoidance—of alcohol.

The way people feel about their alcohol consumption may have little to do with its actual impact on the human body. In much of France and Italy, for example, people think of wine as a food. Many Scandinavians and Germans think of beer in much the same way. In the United States many people who regularly drink beer in large quantities do not think of themselves as using alcohol. The following brief review of the history of drinking looks at the various roles that alcohol has played in different societies.

In Ancient Times

Throughout history, people have viewed alcohol as a substance that nourishes and gives comfort. Many societies and cultures have even thought that alcohol possesses supernatural powers. According to the Bible, one of the first things Noah did after the great flood was plant a vineyard (Genesis 9:21). Many myths and religious beliefs reflect the importance of alcohol. The ancient Egyptians believed that the great god Osiris taught them how to make beer, a substance that had great religious as well as nutritional value for them. Beer was buried in royal tombs and offered to the deities. Greeks drank wine as a form of worship. The Greeks believed wine had been given to them by the god Dionysus. In Roman times, the god Bacchus was thought to be both the originator of wine and always present within it. The Aztecs believed that the goddess Mayahuel taught them how to make a mild beer from the sap of the century plant. Even to this day, beer continues to be important in the diet of many Indians.

Early wines and beers were quite different from the drinks we know in the twenty-first century. Until as recently as 1700, most wines and beers were dark, dense with sediments, and extremely uneven in quality. Home-brewed beers tended to be highly nutritious but lasted only a few days before going sour. Homemade wines had relatively little in the way of vitamins or minerals but could last a long time if adequately sealed.

Although it is impossible to say exactly where or when *Homo sapiens* first sampled alcohol, chemical analysis of the residues found in pots dating from 3500 B.C.E. shows that wine was already being made

The ancient Greeks believed that the god Dionysus, often depicted with lion characteristics, gave them wine. Pottery such as this lion's head rhyton, or drinking pitcher, was used to serve alcohol.

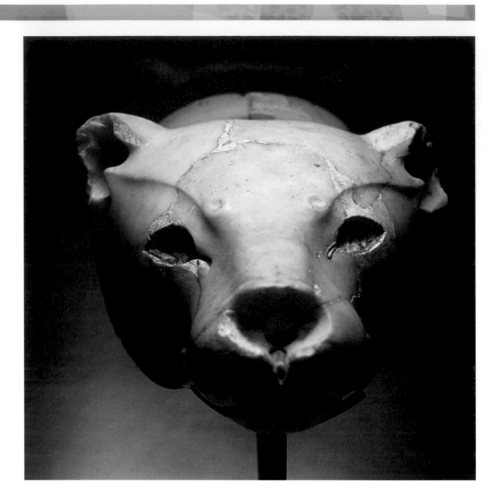

from grapes in Mesopotamia (now Iraq). This discovery makes alcohol almost as old as farming. In fact, beer and bread were first produced at the same place at about the same time from the same ingredients. We know little about the gradual process by which people learned to control fermentation, to blend drinks, or to store and ship them in ways that kept them from souring. However, by studying the different styles of wine vessels from various regions, we have learned about how goods were transported from one region to another during ancient times.

It was the custom of the ancient Greeks to dilute wine with water and to drink it only after meals. This kept them sober, compared to neighboring populations, who often sought drunkenness through beer as a transcendental state of altered consciousness. Certainly the Greeks and Romans drank heavily at religious orgies honoring their gods. Alexander the Great (356 B.C.E.–325 B.C.E.), who conquered most of the known world in his time, was famous for his constant drunkenness.

The religious practices of the Hebrews in about 500 B.C.E. differed greatly from previous practices of other cultures. They drank wine in sacred family rituals, but the Hebrews placed an overall emphasis on temperance, or drinking in only moderate amounts and at certain times. This pattern persists into the twenty-first century and often marks drinking by religious Jews as different from that of their neighbors. Early Christians, many of whom had been Jews, praised the healthful and social benefits of wine while condemning drunkenness. The Bible makes many positive references to drinking. Jesus' choice of wine to symbolize his blood continues into the twenty-first century in the solemn rite of the Eucharist, or Holy Communion, a central practice in many Christian churches.

Although little is known about ancient Africa, mild fermented home brews (such as banana beer) were commonplace there, just as they were in Latin America. In Asia, we know most about China, where as early as 2000 B.C.E. grain-based beer and wine were used in ceremonies, offered to the gods, and included in royal burials. Clearly, drink and drinking had highly positive meanings for early peoples, as they do now for many non-Western societies.

From 1000 to 1500

Christianity and Islam spread rapidly during the Middle Ages. Also during this time, people began to come together as national groups. The cultures of these emerging nations differed from each other, and each culture had preferences for certain drinks and ways of drinking. For peasants and craftspeople, home-brewed beer was a major part of the diet. Nobles criticized excessive drinking by poor people, but they themselves enjoyed a rich array of food and drink. In towns and villages, taverns became important social centers, often condemned by the wealthy as damaging to religion, political stability, and the family.

During this period, hops, which enhanced both the flavor and durability of beer, were introduced. In Italy and France wine became even more popular, both in the diet and as a product to be traded. The Arabs had known how to **distill** spirits (such as whiskey, brandy, and other drinks that today are often called hard liquor) since about 800. In Europe, a small group of religious leaders, physicians, and alchemists controlled that technology until about 1200. The spirits they produced as beverages were sold as a luxury item and for use as medicine.

Among populations across northern Africa and much of Asia, drinking and drunkenness were celebrated as ways to alter consciousness. However, as the teachings of Islam, Buddha, and Confucius spread, most Africans and Asians became **temperate** and sometimes **abstinent**. China and India both went through periods of prohibition, during which alcohol use was forbidden. In the Hindu

distill to separate alcohol from fermenting juices

temperate to be moderate in the use of alcohol

abstinent describing someone who completely avoids something, such as a drug or alcohol

religion, some castes, or social classes, drank liquor as a sacred rite. Others looked down on drinking.

During the Renaissance, European exploration of the seas expanded. Europeans came into contact with civilizations and tribal peoples who had long occupied North America, Central America, and South America. Alcoholic beverages appear to have been totally unknown north of Mexico, although a vast variety of beers and other fermented brews were important in Mexico as foods, as offerings to the gods, and as direct ways to achieve religious ecstasy.

From 1500 to 1800

The Protestant Reformation affected ways of life throughout Europe. One such change was the belief that drunkenness as a form of celebrating was wrong. The faithful frowned upon long-term heavy drinking. Even so, public drinking establishments became important town meeting places, where workers could catch up on the news, gossip, and play games. The aristocracy increasingly drank **brandies**, and champagne was introduced as a luxury beverage, as were various cordials and liqueurs. Brewing and wine making grew into major businesses as technology and quality controls improved.

brandies liquor distilled from wines

Throughout Latin America and parts of North America, the Spanish and Portuguese *conquistadors* (conquerors) found that indigenous peoples already had home brews that were important to them for food, medicine, and religious purposes. For the Aztecs of Mexico, beer offered a significant portion of their nutritional intake, but drunkenness was allowed only for priests and old men. The Yaqui (in what is now Arizona) made a wine from cactus as part of their rain ceremony. Spanish and Portuguese colonial authorities tried to impose laws and regulations on drinking and producing alcohol, but they enforced these laws inconsistently. As merchants from various countries competed for trade with the various Native American groups of North America, liquor quickly became an important item.

In the colonies that later became the United States, rum—distilled from West Indies sugar production—became an important item in international trade. In the Triangle Trade, captive black Africans were shipped to the West Indies for sale as slaves. Many worked on plantations there, producing not only refined sugar, a sweet and valuable new food, but also molasses, much of which was shipped to New England. Distillers there turned molasses into rum, which was in turn shipped to West Africa, where it could be traded for more slaves.

During the American Revolution (1775–1783), however, that trade triangle was interrupted and North Americans shifted to pro-

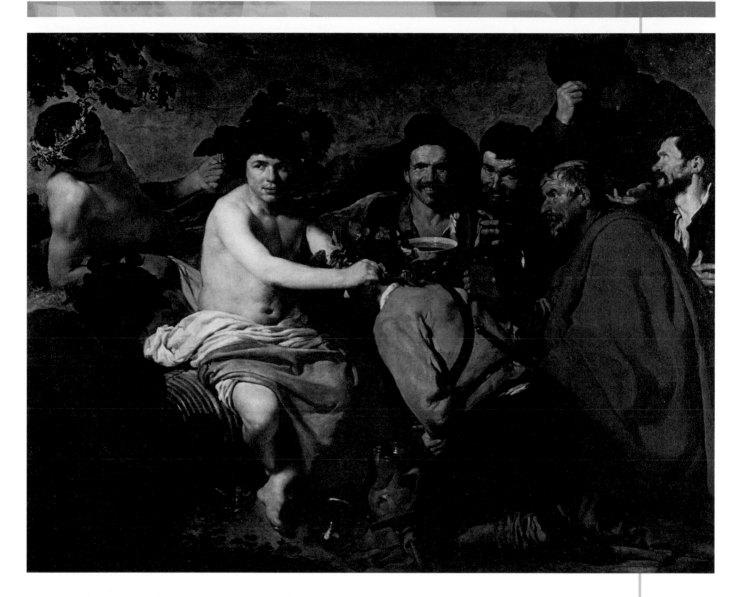

ducing whiskey. Farmers east of the Mississippi River, along what was then the frontier, were eager to make money from their surplus corn by distilling it into whiskey. In 1790 a federal tax was imposed on whiskey to help pay off the debt owed by the new United States. The producing farmers were so angry about the new tax that they joined forces to oppose it. Their protest, known as the Whiskey Rebellion of 1794, forced the new federal government to call up the militia (federal troops) for the first time to put down the opposition. At about the same time, Benjamin Rush, a noted physician and signer of the Declaration of Independence, started a campaign against long-term heavy drinking, asserting that it was damaging to one's health.

Because of the Protestant Reformation, drunkenness was frowned upon throughout Europe. A 1629 painting by Diego Rodríguez de Silva y Velázquez reveals drunkards in a drinking establishment.

The 1800s

Throughout Europe during the Industrial Revolution, beer, wine, and distilled liquor became important products. Businesses and industries sold their products to countries around the world. As a new middle class emerged with more time and money to spend, drinking became a valued leisure activity. For many it provided a release from the strict atmosphere of the workplace.

At this time alcohol began to lose much of its religious importance. Some Protestant groups and Catholic priests believed it led to crime, family disruption, unemployment, and other social problems. Some doctors and scholars also linked long-term heavy drinking with disease, although liquor remained an important part of medicine for certain purposes. Many medicines were formulated using herbs steeped in alcohol. In fact, alcohol was the base of most patent medicines marketed for every possible ill imaginable. Even babies were the target of these medicines, which were used to soothe colicky infants. Little was known about how or why drinking created problems for some people but not for others.

Early in the 1800s a wave of religious activity, including concern over the use of alcohol, swept over the United States. By 1850 a dozen states had banned the production of alcohol. These local prohibition laws were eventually overturned when religious intensity calmed. After the Civil War (1861–1865), the public became fascinated with hard-drinking cowboys, miners, lumberjacks, and other colorful characters of the expanding frontier. Wealth became an important sign of social status as the United States expanded westward. Certain public drinking establishments conveyed social status or importance by serving only people of a particular economic class.

New opposition to alcohol developed toward the end of the 1800s. Protestants in northern states such as New York and Massachusetts saw the large numbers of immigrants, many of them Catholic, as trouble. These new Catholic immigrants competed for jobs and threatened the control Protestants had long had over politics, government, and mainstream values. The Protestants looked down on the new immigrants' drinking habits, calling instead for "clean living." Native American populations, in the meantime, were being displaced from their land and in some cases wiped out. The stereotype of the drunken Indian began to appear in novels and news accounts. In reality, many Indians remained abstinent.

The Twentieth Century

The twentieth century brought many significant changes to daily life. Some of these innovations, such as **pasteurization**, mass production, commercial canning and bottling, and rapid transport, improved the conditions for producing and selling alcohol. Also at this time, new

pasteurization at a certain temperature and prolonged exposure, the destruction of objectionable organisms in a substance (e.g., milk) without substantially altering its chemical composition

ideas emerged about the government's role in protecting public health and social welfare. These ideas resulted in our current expectations that the state should set rules on drinking and the sale of alcohol.

In the United States, a combination of religious objections to drinking and unproven medical claims about its dangers resulted in the nationwide prohibition of alcohol in 1919. The Eighteenth Amendment to the Constitution forbade commercial sales of alcohol but said nothing about drinking or possession. At first there was relatively little home production of alcohol and a low incidence of smuggling. But illegal sources eventually appeared. Those who distilled liquor illegally were called moonshiners, and those who smuggled it within the United States or from abroad were bootleggers. Speakeasies, or secret bars and cocktail lounges, sprang up in cities and towns, and drinking became even more fashionable than before prohibition. Some business owners became immensely wealthy from dealing in alcohol. The government, meanwhile, was suffering from the loss of income from taxes on alcohol.

Then came the stock-market crash in 1929, followed by massive unemployment, a crisis in agriculture, and worldwide economic depression. Americans became angry about prohibition, and some of the same influential people who had demanded it now called for it to end. The Twenty-first Amendment, the first and only repeal to affect the U.S. Constitution, ended federal prohibition in 1933. Specific regulations about retail sales were left up to the states. Many states remained officially dry, meaning no liquor could be sold within state lines. Others allowed counties or towns to decide for themselves whether they would permit alcohol.

U.S. consumption of all alcoholic beverages increased gradually from the end of prohibition until the early 1980s, with a marked increase following World War II (1939–1945). In the mid-twentieth century, a group of people suffering from alcohol addiction formed Alcoholics Anonymous (AA). ☎ AA has grown to be an international fellowship of individuals whose main purpose is to keep from drinking. Also mid-century, scientists started studying the effects of alcohol, and our knowledge has grown rapidly. The public has come to view alcoholism as a disease rather than as a moral problem.

☎ **See** *Organizations of Interest* **at the back of Volume 1 for address, telephone, and URL.**

Around 1980, sales of spirits started dropping and have continued to do so. A few years later, wine sales leveled off and have since gradually fallen; beer sales also appear to have passed their peak even more recently. These reductions occurred despite increased advertising. A general belief in a healthy lifestyle—stressing physical exercise and a good diet—may account for the drop in alcohol consumption.

Conclusion

Research has shown a relationship between the amount of alcohol people drink and a broad range of alcohol-related problems, including domestic violence, child neglect, social violence, psychiatric illness, physical illness, and traffic fatalities. It is important to remember, however, that those who enjoy moderate drinking have little in common with those who insist on drinking heavily. Alcohol can be a safe and enjoyable part of life when people understand not only the effects of alcohol but also what they expect to get from their drinking. SEE ALSO ALCOHOL: CHEMISTRY; ALCOHOLICS ANONYMOUS (AA); BEERS AND BREWS; TEMPERANCE MOVEMENT; TREATMENT: HISTORY OF, IN THE UNITED STATES.

Alcohol: Poisoning

The image of a drunken individual may not immediately come to mind when one hears the term "drug overdose." Yet the sad reality is that 20,000 individuals die from alcohol-induced causes, and 30,000 young people require immediate medical treatment for acute alcohol poisoning each year in the United States.

How Does Alcohol Poisoning Occur?

depressant chemical that slows down or decreases functioning; often used to describe agents that slow the functioning of the central nervous system; such agents are sometimes used to relieve insomnia, anxiety, irritability, and tension

Alcohol is a **depressant** of the central nervous system, which is made up of the brain and spinal cord. It produces different behaviors, emotions, and physical effects as it acts upon specific parts of the brain. First affected is the cerebrum, which controls such functions as recognition, vision, reasoning, and emotion. Low amounts of alcohol reduce inhibitions and affect judgment. For example, someone who is often quiet and reserved may become loud, outspoken, and more dramatic. Others may become depressed, withdrawn, even distressed and tearful. Later, as alcohol levels rise, vision, movement, and speech become impaired. When alcohol depresses the next brain area, the cerebellum, problems with coordination, reflexes, and balance occur.

The last portion of the brain to be affected is the medulla, which controls basic survival functions such as respiration (breathing) and heartbeat. When a person has consumed so much alcohol that the medulla is affected, his or her brain's ability to control respiration and heart rate becomes severely diminished. The heart rate can drop and breathing may stop, which will lead to a coma and then death.

How Much Alcohol is Lethal?

Most authorities agree that a lethal dose of alcohol is about 0.40 percent, or about five times the 0.08 legal limit of many states. Death from alcohol poisoning may occur at much lower levels, however, especially with inexperienced drinkers. For a 120-pound individual, it would only take about nine to ten drinks in an hour to reach the lethal level.

It is important to note that the liver can only oxidize or "clear" about one ounce (approximately one drink) of alcohol an hour. Depending on an individual's stomach contents, the amount consumed, and how quickly the individual drinks, it may be as much as thirty to ninety minutes after drinking ceases before an individual reaches his or her highest level of intoxication. Because this occurs whether the person is conscious or passed out, it is critical that someone who is semiconscious or unconscious be evaluated constantly.

Recognizing the Symptoms and Knowing How to Respond

The symptoms of alcohol poisoning include:

- vomiting
- passing out
- having difficulty waking up
- slow, shallow breathing
- cool, pale, or clammy skin

It is extremely dangerous to assume that someone showing the signs of alcohol poisoning will just sleep it off. These steps should be taken:

1. Check to see if the person can be awakened. Call his or her name or pinch the skin—he or she should have a reaction. (Remember, alcohol numbs the nerves so pinching the skin will help you gauge how far along in the overdose the person is.)

2. Turn the person onto his or her side so that the person does not choke on his or her own vomit.

3. Check skin color and temperature. If the skin is pale or bluish, or cold or clammy, call 911 immediately. The person is not getting enough oxygen.

4. Check the person's breathing. If the person is breathing less than twelve times per minute, or stops breathing for periods of ten seconds or more, call 911.

Remember that these are just some of the potential signs of acute alcohol poisoning. A person may have one or all of these signs. If the person cannot be awakened, the situation is serious. If you are at all concerned that someone has alcohol poisoning, do not hesitate to get help. You should not worry about whether it is a false alarm— remember that you are acting out of concern for your friend. Worrying about how your friend will respond tomorrow should not prevent you from getting help when needed. Make sure you and your friend have the next day to talk it over. SEE ALSO ACCIDENTS AND INJURIES FROM ALCOHOL; ALCOHOL: CHEMISTRY; ALCOHOL: COMPLICATIONS OF PROBLEM DRINKING.

Alcohol: Psychological Consequences of Chronic Abuse

Chronic alcohol abuse—heavy drinking over a long period—can seriously damage a person's well-being, not only physically but mentally. A chronic drinker may lose the ability to pay attention and concentrate. He or she may become anxious and depressed, and behave in ways that pose risks to health and safety.

Long-term heavy drinking can also lead to impaired cognitive abilities. This means that the long-term heavy drinker of alcohol may not be able to think clearly about complex issues or concentrate in order to solve problems. These impairments include:

- Visual-spatial deficits: difficulties with recognizing actual distances between objects or with depth perception
- Language (verbal) impairments: confusing or mispronouncing previously known words, or having difficulty expressing ideas
- Memory impairments (alcoholic amnestic syndrome): the inability to recall words, names, or previously familiar basic ideas. Also a reduced capacity to take in and retain new information
- Alcoholic dementia (in a small fraction of chronic alcohol abusers): syndrome in which the alcoholic suffers problems in almost every area of thinking, feeling, remembering, and behaving

These impairments may come about because of the harmful lifestyle of alcoholics. For example, the poor eating habits of alcoholics lead to vitamin deficiencies, which can affect mental functioning. Heavy drinkers often suffer from head trauma caused by accidents, falls, and fights. Head injuries can also damage the brain's ability to function normally.

Chronic heavy drinking often results in poor performance in work or school and inappropriate social behavior. Heavy drinkers often lose the support of family and friends, some of whom may be moderate drinkers. As conflict and disapproval increases at home and at work, many heavy drinkers, especially women, feel like they are losing control over their lives. This loss of control often expresses itself as **depression**. To get relief from depression, the person may drink even more. Unfortunately, since this "cure" usually has little success, the person falls into a vicious cycle of drinking. Research on suicide suggests that chronic alcohol abuse is involved in 20 to 36 percent of reported cases.

Researchers are not certain if the chronic drinking results in depression, or if the depression already existed and is made worse by drinking. However, for most alcoholics who undergo detoxification (ending all alcohol consumption), depressive symptoms improve within weeks. This suggests that, for many, the toxic effects of alcohol led to the depressive symptoms.

A common problem among men who abuse alcohol is **aggression**. Young men who are chronic alcohol abusers may already have a tendency to act aggressively or violently. The toxic effects of alcohol appear to increase that behavior. SEE ALSO ACCIDENTS AND INJURIES FROM ALCOHOL; ALCOHOL: COMPLICATIONS OF PROBLEM DRINKING; RESEARCH; VIOLENCE AND DRUG AND ALCOHOL USE.

depression state in which an individual feels intensely sad and hopeless; may have trouble eating, sleeping, and concentrating, and is no longer able to feel pleasure from previously enjoyable activities; in extreme cases, may lead an individual to think about or attempt suicide

aggression hostile and destructive behavior, especially caused by frustration; may include violence or physical threat or injury directed toward another

Alcohol: Withdrawal

Alcohol acts as a **depressant** on the central nervous system (the brain and spinal cord). It also has a depressant effect on the peripheral nervous system (the nerves throughout the rest of the body). Long-term, heavy drinking often leads to physical dependence on alcohol, a condition in which a person's body cannot function normally without the presence of alcohol. A person who is dependent on alcohol and who then suddenly stops drinking goes through a painful and potentially life-threatening withdrawal syndrome as the body adjusts to the absence of alcohol. The goals of treatment of alcoholic withdrawal syndrome are to relieve discomfort and to prevent medical complications. Treatment of withdrawal sometimes involves medications. While alcohol withdrawal requires careful medical attention, getting through this phase does not mean that an individual has received treatment for alcoholism itself. After the immediate problems associated with withdrawal from regular use of alcohol have passed, an alcoholic person will still need to undergo intensive (and, some would say, lifelong) treatment for their addiction to alcohol.

depressant chemical that slows down or decreases functioning; often used to describe agents that slow the functioning of the central nervous system; such agents are sometimes used to relieve insomnia, anxiety, irritability, and tension

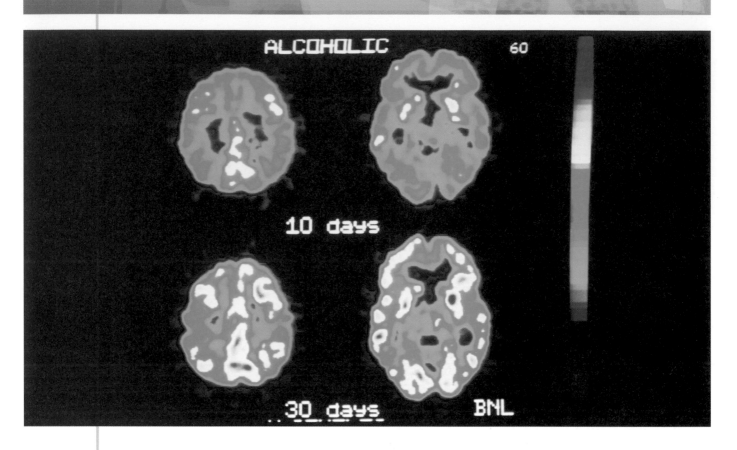

ALCOHOLIC   60

10 days

30 days   BNL

Alcohol is a depressant, which means it decreases the activity of the brain and the spinal column. These PET scans show the effects of heavy alcohol-drinking on the brain (top) and, once the person stops drinking alcohol, the increased nerve cell activity (bottom).

intoxicated state in which a person's physical or mental control has been diminished

blood alcohol concentration (BAC) amount of alcohol in the bloodstream, expressed as the grams of alcohol per deciliter of blood; as BAC goes up, the drinker experiences more psychological and physical effects

People who have not previously drunk alcohol, or who drink lightly, may occasionally drink enough alcohol to become **intoxicated**. When no longer intoxicated, these drinkers can also experience a withdrawal syndrome, commonly called a hangover. The symptoms reflect the fall in **blood alcohol concentration (BAC)**—as the person's BAC falls, the symptoms worsen. These symptoms include insomnia (inability to sleep), headache, and nausea. Usually no treatment is required, and there are no serious consequences of this withdrawal. However, the withdrawal syndrome following long-term, heavy drinking is a much more serious disorder that can last from months to years.

Some people who are dependent on alcohol who want to stop drinking must go through a process of **detoxification**. This process usually takes fifteen to twenty years. The typical person admitted to detoxification clinics or hospitals is about 42 years old. (People as young as 20 and as old as 80 also sometimes need detoxification.) The withdrawal syndrome seen in people requiring detoxification ranges from mild discomfort to a potentially life-threatening disorder. The severity of the withdrawal syndrome depends both on the amount of alcohol the person typically drinks and the length of time over which the person has been drinking.

People have different patterns of drinking. Some drinkers consume alcohol in a binge pattern, drinking large amounts of alcohol in a short span of time. Others drink in a more consistent, long-term pattern. The amount of time for alcohol addiction to develop differs from person to person. One drinker may take two or three years to become dependent, another fifteen years, and yet another forty years. A person who has previously experienced significant alcohol-withdrawal symptoms may be at higher risk for developing repeat symptoms. Other factors that may be involved in the severity of the withdrawal syndrome include age, nutrition, and presence of other physical disorders or illness (for example, inflammation of the pancreas or an infection such as pneumonia).

detoxification
process of removing a poisonous, intoxicating, or addictive substance from the body

The Symptoms of Alcohol Withdrawal

As alcohol is eliminated from the body, symptoms and signs of alcohol withdrawal appear in direct relation to the decreasing amounts. Many alcoholics require a drink in the morning to "steady the nerves" and calm their anxiety. The following are some of the more common symptoms of alcohol withdrawal: anxiety, agitation, restlessness, insomnia, feeling shaky inside, loss of appetite, nausea, changes in sensory perception (skin feels itchy, ordinary sounds seem louder than usual, average light seems startlingly bright), headache, and heart palpitations. Common physical signs include vomiting, sweating, increase in heart rate, increase in blood pressure, tremor (shakiness of hands and sometimes face, eyelids, and tongue), and seizures.

In a more severe case of withdrawal, the above symptoms and signs become more intense. The person may have hallucinations (feeling, hearing, or seeing things that are not there) and become confused and disoriented. This most severe phase of withdrawal is called delirium tremens. After a person stops drinking, the more common and milder symptoms usually peak twelve to twenty-four hours later and for the most part disappear after forty-eight hours. More severe withdrawal symptoms usually peak seventy-two to ninety-six hours after the person stops drinking, and are potentially, though rarely, life-threatening. Fewer than 5 percent of people withdrawing from alcohol develop a severe reaction. With appropriate drug treatment, even fewer develop a major withdrawal reaction. Under ideal circumstances, for example, under close monitoring in a hospital, there should be almost no deaths from withdrawal syndrome on its own.

Treatment of Alcohol Withdrawal

Health-care professionals supervising a patient with alcohol withdrawal syndrome may recommend over-the-counter medicines and sometimes prescription medicines. An important over-the-counter medicine for treatment of alcohol withdrawal is the B vitamin thi-

benzodiazepine drug developed in the 1960s as a safer alternative to barbiturates; most frequently used as a sleeping pill or an anti-anxiety medication

amine. Alcoholics are commonly lacking in thiamine, and this deficiency can cause brain damage. The alcoholic also requires extra fluids (to avoid dehydration) and carefully managed nutrition (many alcoholics suffer from malnutrition). The patient should sleep and rest in a dark quiet room, with comfort and reassurance from medical personnel. Some patients will require more intensive care.

Over 100 prescription drugs have been suggested as useful in the treatment of alcohol withdrawal syndrome, but very few studies have been conducted on their effectiveness. The drugs of choice are the longer-acting **benzodiazepines**, especially diazepam (Valium), as well as chlordiazepoxide (Librium), lorazepam (Ativan), and oxazepam (Serax). Occasionally doctors prescribe a long-acting barbiturate such as phenobarbital. Many patients do very well with no drug therapy.

Prescription-drug treatment given before most withdrawal symptoms have occurred can prevent discomfort and possibly more severe withdrawal symptoms. However, for some patients it is an unnecessary treatment. When prescription-drug treatment is given after symptoms appear, doctors can calculate a more appropriate dose of the medication according to the individual patient's needs. However, patients may experience unnecessary discomfort before the drug therapy is begun. In addition, they may develop inappropriate drug-seeking behavior. (Occasionally, individuals with a tendency to become cross-addicted to substances in addition to alcohol may exaggerate reports of their symptoms in an effort to receive prescription drugs.)

Benzodiazepines can prevent the complications of serious withdrawal, such as seizures, hallucinations, and irregular heartbeat. In general, high doses of benzodiazepines are provided early in treatment, to cover the patient for the time of severe withdrawal (usually twenty-four to forty-eight hours). Some patients require very large doses of a drug (for example, several hundred milligrams of diazepam) to suppress symptoms. Patients with histories of withdrawal seizures (convulsions) or those who have epilepsy are always treated to prevent seizures, usually with benzodiazepines and with other drugs to fight convulsions. Patients who develop hallucinations are given a **neuroleptic** or **antipsychotic drug** (in addition to benzodiazepines). Typical drugs from this class include haloperidol (Haldol), and chlorpromazine (Thorazine).

neuroleptic one of a class of antipsychotic drugs, including major tranquilizers used in the treatment of psychoses such as schizophrenia

antipsychotic drug drug that reduces psychotic behavior; often has negative long-term side effects

Conclusion

Alcohol withdrawal syndrome is a set of symptoms and signs that occur when a person goes through alcohol detoxification. Symptoms occur as the nervous system adapts to the absence of alcohol in the body. In most cases, these signs and symptoms are a source of mild discomfort and disappear after a short period. Occasionally, more severe withdrawal symptoms occur, or patients have other complications (for example, seizures). Under these circumstances, appropriate drug treatment is required to relieve symptoms and to prevent further complications.

Helping someone withdraw from alcohol is only the first step in the process of treating alcoholism. Even while withdrawal is being accomplished, an individual should be starting to receive treatment for his or her addiction. While alcohol withdrawal may be achieved within days to weeks, treating alcoholism is a long-term, sometimes lifelong, process. SEE ALSO ALCOHOL: CHEMISTRY; ALCOHOL TREATMENT: BEHAVIORAL APPROACHES; ALCOHOL TREATMENT: MEDICATIONS; BLOOD ALCOHOL CONCENTRATION; DIAGNOSIS OF DRUG AND ALCOHOL ABUSE: AN OVERVIEW; TOLERANCE AND PHYSICAL DEPENDENCE.

Alcohol Treatment: Behavioral Approaches

Imagine that every time you see a red traffic light you get angry. You begin to grit your teeth, curse, and generally become abusive toward everyone riding in the car with you. You know that this response will not change the fact that you will have to wait in traffic until the light changes. And getting angry with other people will not change anything, except that you may lose a few friends and develop an ulcer or high blood pressure in the process. To change this response, or any other kind of unhealthy, undesirable behavior, you might use **behavioral therapy**. For many years, behavioral treatments or therapy has been used to help people who abuse alcohol. In the nineteenth century, Benjamin Rush, often thought of as the founder of American psychiatry, described a variety of psychological cures for long-term drunkenness. Modern research studies show that behavioral treatments can be effective for alcohol problems. Also, combining behavioral and prescription-drug treatment often produces good results.

behavioral therapy form of therapy whose main focus is to change certain behaviors instead of uncovering unconscious conflicts or problems

Why Use Behavioral Approaches?

The success or failure of any type of treatment is measured by whether and how much a person continues to drink. Many psychological factors influence a person's drinking behavior: beliefs and expectations, the examples of friends and family, the customs for drinking within one's society or social circle, emotions, family dynamics, and the

Alcoholics Anonymous participants are sometimes awarded key-chain medallions for extended lengths of sobriety. This medallion reminds its keeper to enjoy life one day at a time.

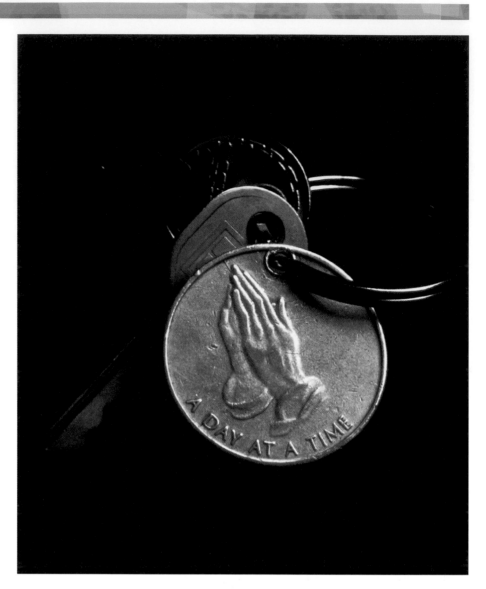

positive and negative consequences of drinking. Treatments that address these factors directly, then, might be expected to help a person overcome alcohol problems. In fact, dozens of studies since the 1960s show the long-term success of behavioral treatments. Typically, they are more effective than treatment using medications.

Behavioral treatment can also prevent relapse, or a return to drinking behavior after treatment. Relapse is less likely when people have a stable relationship, a job, the support of friends, personal coping skills, and self-confidence. Behavioral methods can anticipate the challenges people will face in these aspects of their lives and give them the skills needed to cope.

Goals and Methods

Sometimes the goal of behavioral treatment is total and permanent abstinence: giving up drinking for the rest of a person's lifetime.

Sometimes the goal is to reduce drinking to a level that will no longer threaten a person's physical or emotional health. The goals of treatment may also include other important dimensions besides drinking—to get and hold a job, to have a happier marriage and family life, to learn how to deal with anger, and to find new ways of having fun that do not involve drinking. To reach these goals, behavioral therapy makes use of several methods.

Teaching New Skills. People who drink often do so in an attempt to cope with their problems. People may drink to relax or loosen up, to get to sleep, to feel better, to enhance sexuality, to build courage, or to forget painful memories. But alcohol rarely helps people to deal with emotional and relationship problems. In the long run, it often makes such problems worse. When a person relies on drinking to cope, that person is termed psychologically dependent on alcohol.

One behavioral approach, sometimes called broad-spectrum treatment, directly addresses this problem by teaching people new skills to cope with their problems. In social-skills training, people learn how to express their feelings appropriately, ask for things they are uncomfortable about, make their emotional needs known in their relationships, refuse drinks, and carry on rewarding conversations without drinking. Stress-management training teaches people how to relax and deal with stressful life situations without using alcohol or drugs.

Self-Control Training. Self-control training teaches people how to manage their own behavior. They learn how to do the following:

- set clear goals for behavior change
- keep records of their drinking behavior and urges to drink
- reward themselves for progress toward goals
- make changes in the way they drink
- identify high-risk situations where the temptation to drink is strong
- learn strategies for coping with those high-risk situations

Self-control training is often used to help people reduce their drinking to a moderate level that does not cause problems. But it can also be used when total abstinence is the goal. This method is particularly helpful for less severe problem drinkers. It is also more effective than educational lectures for drunk-driving offenders.

Marital Therapy. Problem drinking commonly affects the drinker's partner in negative ways. Treatment that involves the husband or wife of a problem drinker can help both partners. A husband or wife

ALCOHOL IN FICTION

Drug and alcohol abuse can turn academic and athletic success into failure. In his novel, *Imitate the Tiger* (1996), Jan Cheripko wrote about a young adult in a detoxification program (a recovery program), and in a series of flashbacks shows how alcohol turned a football star into a dropout and his long road back.

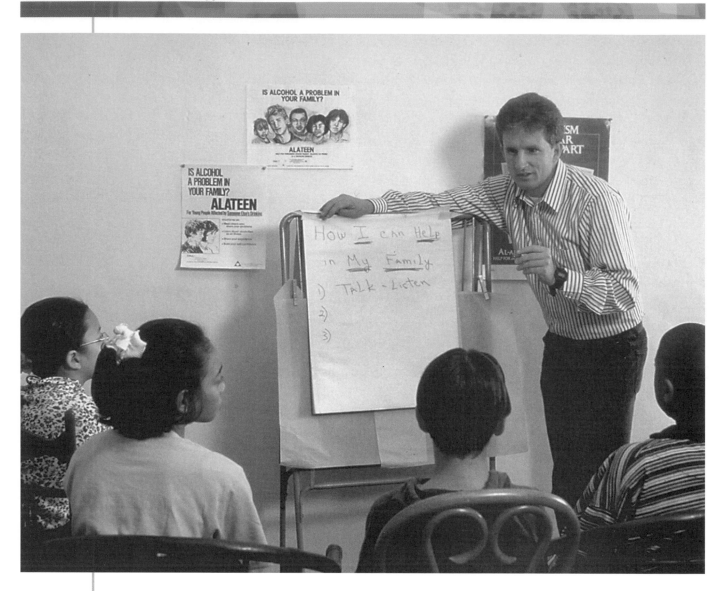

A counselor talks to a group of teenagers during an Alateen meeting.

can help to clarify problems and suggest ways that the drinker can change the problem behavior. Marital distress can be an important factor in problem drinking, so direct treatment of marital problems can help to prevent relapse. Research indicates that problem drinkers treated together with a spouse do better than those treated individually.

Aversion Therapy. In another treatment method, drinking is paired with unpleasant images and experiences. For example, the taste of alcohol may be paired with foul odors or with unpleasant experiences in the person's imagination. Whenever the person has a drink, he or she will be reminded of those unpleasant images and sensations. Eventually the person loses the desire for alcohol and drinks less. The person develops an aversion to drinking, which means that the taste and even the thought of alcohol become unpleasant. Aversion therapy may be especially useful for drinkers who continue to feel a strong **craving** for alcohol.

Psychotherapy. Many kinds of psychotherapy have been tried with alcohol abusers. The goal of psychotherapy is generally to gain insight into the unconscious causes of drinking. This type of therapy has been largely unsuccessful. Group psychotherapy also has a poor track record in the treatment of problem drinking.

Changing the Environment. Yet another behavioral approach aims to change the motivations for drinking by changing the environment of drinking. The goal here is to eliminate consequences of drinking that a person might find rewarding. For example, if a person often visits the same bar and drinks to feel part of the crowd there, a counselor might recommend that the person find a new place or a new way to socialize. The person is encouraged to find alternative ways to have rewarding experiences.

Brief Motivational Counseling. Researchers have discovered that some treatments consisting of only one to three sessions were as effective as longer and more complex treatment regimens. In this approach, a doctor or therapist makes a thorough assessment of a patient's drinking problem and presents feedback of findings to the patient. The doctor then offers clear advice to change, stressing the importance of personal responsibility and **optimism**. The key seems to be to trigger a decision and commitment to change. Through this brief and simple process, problem drinkers acquire the motivation to change their drinking behavior. People frequently proceed to change their drinking on their own without further professional help. In fact, the personal motivation to change is so important that other treatment approaches that skip over this first step may fail.

Conclusion

It is unlikely that research will ever identify a single superior treatment for alcohol abuse. Drinking and alcohol-related problems are far too complex. Yet the number of approaches that have been successful is a cause for real optimism. The chances that an individual will find an effective approach are good. The most successful treatment strategies will match the method to the individual based on his or her characteristics. SEE ALSO ALATEEN; AL-ANON; ALCOHOL TREATMENT: MEDICATIONS; ALCOHOLICS ANONYMOUS (AA); DIAGNOSIS OF DRUG AND ALCOHOL ABUSE: AN OVERVIEW; TREATMENT: HISTORY OF, IN THE UNITED STATES; TREATMENT PROGRAMS, CENTERS, AND ORGANIZATIONS: A HISTORICAL PERSPECTIVE; TREATMENT TYPES: AN OVERVIEW.

craving powerful, often uncontrollable desire for drugs and/or alcohol

optimism positive outlook

Alcohol Treatment: Medications

Treating alcoholism with medications is an ongoing field of research, with scientists seeking answers to many questions. Research suggests that behavioral treatments—a course of action designed to teach an individual how to change his or her unhealthy behavior—can be effective for alcohol problems. The best treatment may be a combination of behavioral and prescription-drug treatment.

There are four main categories of medications that are either currently available or are still being tested for the treatment of alcoholism and alcohol abuse:

- drugs that increase a person's sensitivity to alcohol
- drugs that directly reduce drinking behavior
- drugs that improve mental processes in patients with impairments (damage) caused by alcohol
- drugs that treat **psychiatric** problems a person may have in addition to alcoholism

Drugs That Increase Sensitivity to Alcohol

Some drugs used to treat alcoholism produce a very unpleasant reaction when the person who takes them also drinks alcohol. In other words, the person's sensitivity to alcohol's effects increases. For example, drinking a small amount of alcohol might now upset a person's stomach and cause nausea. As a result, the drugs help to prevent the alcoholic from drinking.

Currently, the most widely used medication in this category is disulfiram (Antabuse), which has been in use for about fifty years. An alcoholic who takes disulfiram and also drinks alcohol will experience the following symptoms: facial flushing, tachycardia (rapid heartbeat), heart palpitations, indigestion, lowered blood pressure, headaches, nausea, and vomiting. The severity of that reaction depends on the amount of alcohol and disulfiram in the blood. The dose of disulfiram depends on the needs of each patient. High doses can produce side effects such as **sedation**, **lethargy**, **depression**, and toxic hepatitis (a liver disease). Some patients have died as a result of a severe reaction to the combination of disulfiram and alcohol in their bodies.

Drugs That Reduce Drinking Behavior

The development of medications to reduce drinking behavior is an important and exciting area of alcohol research. Researchers have studied the interactions among several brain chemicals, including the serotonin, opioid, and dopamine systems. Medications have been de-

psychiatric relating to the branch of medicine that deals with the study, treatment, and prevention of mental illness

sedation process of calming someone by administering a medication that reduces excitement; often called a tranquilizer

lethargy state of being slowed down, sluggish, very drowsy; lacking all energy or drive

depression state in which an individual feels intensely sad and hopeless; may also have trouble eating, sleeping, and concentrating, and is no longer able to feel pleasure from previously enjoyable activities; in extreme cases, may lead an individual to think about or attempt suicide

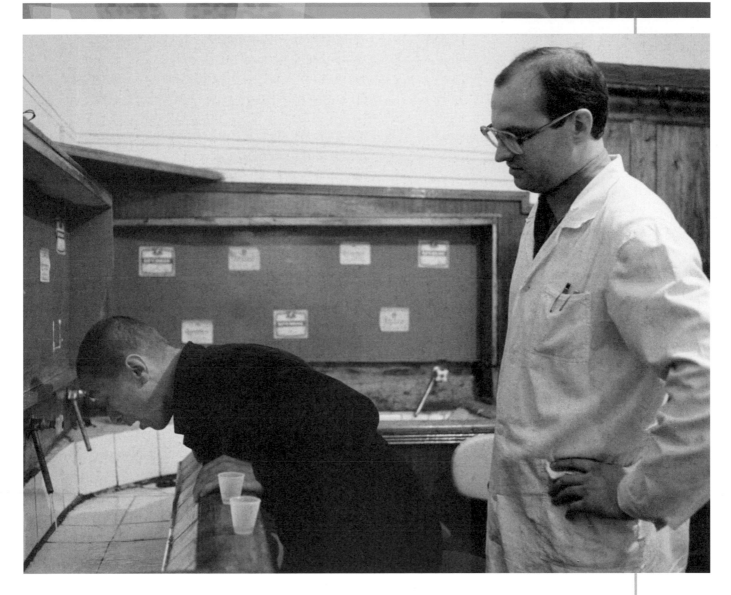

veloped to change the way these chemical systems work. The result of these changes is to reduce a person's drinking behavior.

Medications That Affect the Serotonin System. Research suggests that the **neurotransmitter** serotonin is associated with alcoholism. Alcoholics appear to have less serotonin than nonalcoholics. Drugs known as selective serotonin reuptake inhibitors (SSRIs), such as fluoxetine (Prozac), fluvoxamine (Luvox), citalopram (Celexa), and viqualine seem to be modestly effective in reducing alcohol consumption. SSRIs act by helping to increase the amount of the brain chemical serotonin available to nerve cells (neurons). Scientists do not fully understand why these medications can help decrease a person's alcohol use. It may be that higher levels of serotonin interfere with some of the sense of reward that some individuals feel when drinking alcohol. Although SSRIs are sometimes used to help alcoholics

A Russian doctor watches a young prisoner react to Antabuse, a drug that increases a person's sensitivity to alcohol. A person taking this medication feels sick and may throw up if he or she drinks beverages with alcohol.

neurotransmitter chemical messenger used by nerve cells to communicate with other nerve cells

decrease their alcohol intake, these medications are more useful for other psychiatric disorders, such as depression and anxiety. When used for alcoholism, the results have been modest—individuals tend to decrease their alcohol intake by about 25 percent.

Medications That Affect the Dopamine System. Dopamine is another brain chemical that influences drinking behavior. Scientists believe that dopamine plays a major role in the effects of alcohol (as well as other drugs) that make people want to drink repeatedly. Research is under way to test the effectiveness of drugs that increase brain dopamine levels to reduce drinking. In studies conducted on rats bred to prefer alcohol, medications such as bromocriptine, GBR 12909, and amphetamine reduced alcohol intake. In studies involving humans, bromocriptine reduced alcohol **craving** and drinking in severe alcoholics.

Medications That Affect the Endogenous Opioid System. Studies have shown that a chemical system within the body called the endogenous opioid system also plays a role in drinking behavior. Endogenous opioids are compounds that the body produces naturally, such as endorphins and enkephalins. These substances have opium-like or morphine-like properties, including masking pain and increasing feelings of pleasure. Alcohol is thought to increase the availability of endogenous opioids in the brain, causing drinkers to have positive feelings, and reinforcing their desire to drink more.

Naltrexone (Trexan) and naloxone are two drugs that block the effects of alcohol on endogenous opioid availability in the brain. Several studies show that use of these drugs can cause a decrease in drinking. Alcoholics treated with naltrexone have fewer drinking days, fewer **relapses**, and reduced craving for alcohol. In addition, naltrexone appears to cause few side effects. Interestingly, alcoholics treated with naltrexone who did have one or two drinks were less likely to continue drinking. This is important, since some alcoholics appear to lose control of drinking after one or two drinks.

Drugs That Improve Mental Processes

Heavy drinking over many years can lead to damage of many essential mental processes, including abstract thinking, problem solving, and memory. The two most common diseases affecting mental processes in alcoholics are alcoholic amnestic disorder (Wernicke-Korsakoff syndrome) and alcoholic dementia. Alcoholic amnestic disorder causes severe memory problems. Alcoholic dementia causes difficulties in short-term and long-term memory, abstract thinking, intellectual abilities, and judgment.

craving powerful, often uncontrollable desire for drugs and/or alcohol

relapse term used in substance abuse treatment and recovery that refers to an addict's return to substance use and abuse following a period of abstinence or sobriety

Little research has been conducted with medications to treat these conditions. Some areas of drug research may overlap with research on drugs that directly reduce drinking. For example, serotonin-uptake inhibitors have shown some promise in improving learning and memory. In one study with the serotonin-uptake inhibitor fluvoxamine, patients suffering from alcohol amnestic disorder had improved memory, but patients with alcoholic dementia did not. In general, treatment of alcoholics with these conditions has little success.

Drugs to Treat Psychiatric Disorders in Combination with Alcoholism

People with alcoholism may also be diagnosed with other psychiatric problems, including anxiety, depression, **antisocial personality disorder**, panic disorders, and phobias (fears). Part of the problem in treatment is to determine if the psychiatric disorder developed before alcoholism, or after (as a result of) alcoholism.

Several studies have been conducted with medications used to treat depression. Alcoholism and depression often go together, and depressed alcoholics have high rates of relapse. Depression is often treated with medications called tricyclic antidepressants (desipramine, imipramine, amitriptyline, and doxepin). Whether they can successfully treat alcoholics with depression is still unknown. Furthermore, because mixing tricyclic antidepressants with alcohol can cause adverse effects, depression and alcoholism might be more safely treated with one of the SSRI antidepressants.

Many individuals who abuse alcohol also suffer from **anxiety disorders**. Buspirone, a medication commonly used to treat anxiety, has shown potential in reducing alcohol consumption. One study reported that buspirone diminished alcohol craving and reduced anxiety. Another

antisocial personality disorder condition in which people disregard the rights of others and violate these rights by acting in immoral, unethical, aggressive, or even criminal ways

anxiety disorder condition in which a person feels uncontrollable angst and worry, often without any specific cause

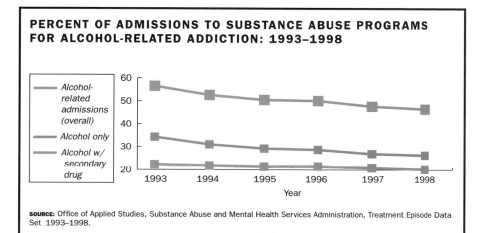

PERCENT OF ADMISSIONS TO SUBSTANCE ABUSE PROGRAMS FOR ALCOHOL-RELATED ADDICTION: 1993–1998

- Alcohol-related admissions (overall)
- Alcohol only
- Alcohol w/ secondary drug

SOURCE: Office of Applied Studies, Substance Abuse and Mental Health Services Administration, Treatment Episode Data Set 1993–1998.

Rising awareness and prevention campaigns may be factors in the overall drop in the number of people admitted into substance abuse programs who list alcohol as their primary drug of abuse.

study found buspirone to be more effective with alcoholics suffering from high anxiety than those with low levels of anxiety. A third study on more severe alcoholic patients found no effect. Further research is needed before this drug's effectiveness can be accurately evaluated.

Future Outlook

New medications that may decrease drinking, prevent relapse, and restore damaged mental processes in alcoholics continue to be developed. In the future, alcoholism treatment may combine these new medications with other types of therapy, including behavioral therapy. As research reveals the mechanisms responsible for alcohol craving, drinking behavior, and psychiatric disorders such as depression and anxiety, better medications may be developed to cope with these problems. Treating alcoholism with medications is an area of research with many avenues to pursue. SEE ALSO ALCOHOL: CHEMISTRY; ALCOHOL: COMPLICATIONS OF PROBLEM DRINKING; ALCOHOL TREATMENT: BEHAVIORAL APPROACHES; BRAIN CHEMISTRY; BRAIN STRUCTURES; TREATMENT TYPES: AN OVERVIEW.

Alcoholics Anonymous (AA)

☎ **See** *Organizations of Interest* at the back of Volume 1 for address, telephone, and URL.

sober in relation to drugs and alcohol, state in which someone is not under the influence of drugs or alcohol

abstinent describing someone who completely avoids something, such as a drug or alcohol

Alcoholics Anonymous ☎ is a fellowship of problem drinkers, both men and women, who voluntarily join because they want to stop drinking and remain **sober**. It was started in the United States in the 1930s. Since then, it has been maintained by alcohol-troubled people who had themselves "hit bottom" and discovered that the troubles associated with their drinking far outweighed any pleasures it might provide. AA does not offer professional guidance such as counseling or therapy. The key to AA is the support members give each other.

AA is not the only hope for alcoholics; nor is it everything they need. Even so, thousands of alcoholics in the United States and many other countries have become **abstinent** by following its program and attending meetings. AA has never attempted to keep formal membership lists, so it is difficult to get completely accurate figures on total membership at any given time. However, in 2001 there were an estimated 2.1 million members worldwide, with over 51,000 groups in the United States and over 100,000 groups worldwide.

The Twelve Steps of Alcoholics Anonymous

AA's program for remaining sober is called the Twelve Steps. The goal of AA is to have members come to accept and live according to

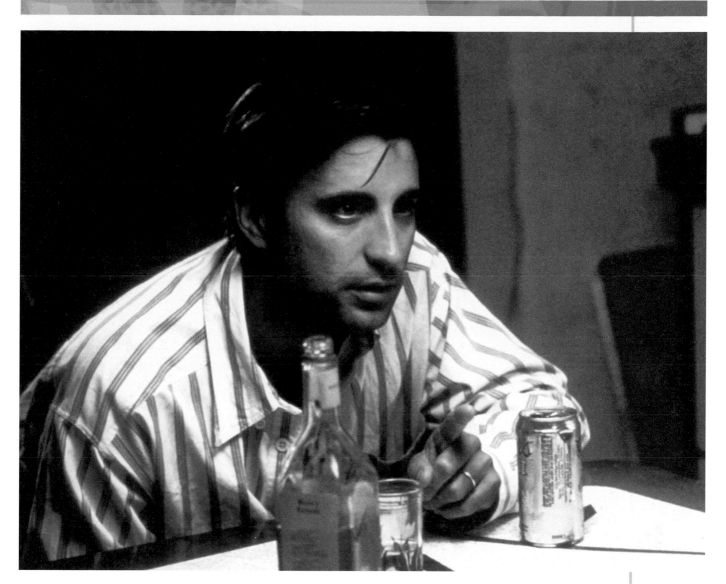

the beliefs of all Twelve Steps, which build upon each other. A paraphrase of the Twelve Steps follows. Members of AA agree that:

1. They are powerless over alcohol—that their lives have become unmanageable.

2. They believe that a power greater than themselves can restore them to sanity.

3. They must turn their will and lives over to the care of God *as they understand God.*

4. They must make a searching and fearless moral inventory of themselves, examining where they have failed or not behaved toward themselves or others as they should.

5. They will admit to God, to themselves, and to another human being the exact nature of our their wrongs.

In the 1994 film *When A Man Loves A Woman,* Andy Garcia played Michael Green, a husband dealing with his wife's habitual drinking. The movie told a painful story illustrating the intervention often necessary to relieve alcohol addiction.

6. They are entirely ready to have God remove all these defects of character.

7. They must humbly ask God to remove their shortcomings.

8. They must make a list of all persons they have harmed, and become willing to make up for wrongs they have done.

9. They will make direct amends to these people wherever possible, except when to do so would injure them or others.

10. They will continue to examine their behavior and to admit promptly when they are wrong or behaved improperly.

11. They will seek through prayer and meditation to improve their conscious contact with God *as they understand God*, praying only for knowledge of God's will and the power to carry it out.

12. Having had a spiritual awakening as the result of these steps, they try to carry this message to other alcoholics and to practice these principles in all their affairs.

The steps are based on the experiences members have had in becoming and staying sober. At meetings both open to the public and "closed" (for members only), members closely examine the Twelve Steps and candidly tell about their drinking histories—their AA stories. Members describe for each other how the AA program has helped them to stay sober.

An AA group comes into being when two or more alcoholics join together to practice the AA program. There are no dues or fees for membership; AA is self-supporting and is not associated with any religious sect or denomination, political group, or other organization. It does not support or oppose any causes. AA is not set up as a centralized organization, although it does put out a monthly magazine, the *Grapevine*. Its board of trustees, consisting of fourteen alcoholic and seven nonalcoholic members, meets four times a year.

The Process of Joining AA

The typical AA member, or affiliate, has had a long and usually severe history of alcoholism. Certain events in an alcoholic's life set the stage for the person's interest in joining, or affiliating, with AA: Usually, he or she has heard positive comments about AA. Long-time drinking friendships have faded, but the drinker has formed a habit of sharing troubles with others. Quitting through sheer willpower seems impossible. Finally, if the alcoholic has also decided that drinking is causing many more problems than it is giving pleasure, the person is likely to attend an AA meeting.

Once the drinker has made a decision to follow the AA program, five phases follow: (1) first-stepping, (2) making a commitment, (3) accepting one's problem, (4) telling one's story, and (5) doing twelfth-step work.

First-stepping involves the initial contact with AA. The person goes to orientation meetings to learn about the group's ideas about alcoholism as a disease. He or she learns step one in the twelve-step program, an admission that the person feels powerless around or over alcohol. When a problem drinker is willing to say the words, "I admit that I am powerless over alcohol . . . and that my life has become unmanageable because of it," he or she has completed step one. An AA guide will then become the newcomer's sponsor and try to help the member reach the second stage, commitment. The AA group acts quickly to ensure that the newcomer will affiliate, challenging the newcomer to attend "ninety meetings in ninety days." The group seeks to keep a close watch over the newcomer, gently forcing the person to give up other commitments and spend a significant share of time with AA program affiliates or taking part in AA activities.

In the third phase, acceptance of a drinking problem begins with the phrase, "I'm Chris X and I'm an alcoholic." Throughout the initial weeks and months, the group presses newcomers, sometimes gently but sometimes forcefully, to realize that they are alcoholics. Accepting that one is an alcoholic can occur immediately or after a long process.

In the fourth phase, the group encourages newcomers to tell their stories to the entire group at an open meeting. Telling one's story to the public is an act of commitment that demonstrates one is a genuine AA member, and members greet this act with applause and congratulations.

In the final phase, the person must perform the program's twelfth step, a promise to remain in the process of recovery: "Having had a spiritual awakening as a result of these Steps, we tried to carry this message to alcoholics, and to practice these principles in all our affairs." One of AA's basic philosophies is that alcoholism is not a disease from which people can recover once and for all. Instead, they are always in the process of recovering. To remain sober, then, a member must remain active in AA and carry the program to those who are still active alcoholics. By doing twelfth-step work, members reinforce their membership and their new definition of themselves as recovering alcoholics.

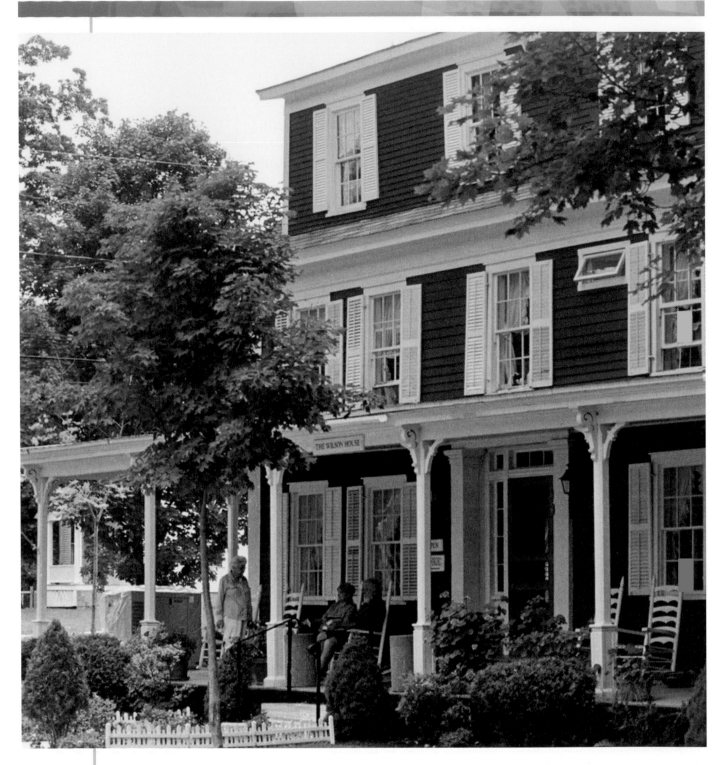

The birthplace of Alcoholics Anonymous co-founder Bill Wilson, known as the Wilson House (East Dorset, Vermont), now serves as an inn and a gathering place for AA participants.

While in the process of affiliation, some recovering AA members have a relapse into drinking. This relapse is called "slipping." Most AA members respond to another's slipping with sympathy and understanding, feelings that strengthen group solidarity. Seeing another person slip also strengthens recovering members' resolve to remain abstinent.

Criticism of AA

Critics of AA argue that the program is not a successful treatment for general populations of alcoholics. They say that only certain kinds of alcoholics benefit from the Twelve Steps—members must have a particular emotional makeup and a readiness for the treatment strategy. Those who do not fit comfortably into the AA world may slip—and slipping makes them feel that they cannot regain control. As a result, critics say that AA can hurt the chances for some alcoholics to remain sober. Others claim that AA rejects scientific research that contradicts its own beliefs about alcoholism. Finally, some critics point out that the AA commitment may interfere with other serious commitments in a person's life, such as work and family.

Adaptation of AA to Other Disorders

Despite the criticisms that have been directed against AA, its format and beliefs have helped many individuals, and the AA program has been applied to a wide variety of other addictions and behavior disorders. Narcotics Anonymous (NA)☎ applies the AA pattern to narcotic drug addicts. Marijuana Anonymous☎ uses a twelve-step system to help marijuana users learn to abstain. AA's beliefs and strategies have also been adapted to help people with gambling, eating, and excessive buying disorders. Al-Anon☎ family groups and Alateen☎ groups have adapted AA's philosophy to family, children, and friends of problem drinkers. Veteran AA members point to these other programs as evidence that AA's influence goes well beyond its impact on AA members. They argue that this widespread adaptation to other disorders demonstrates the essential value and appeal of the AA program. SEE ALSO AL-ANON; ALATEEN; ALCOHOL TREATMENT: BEHAVIORAL APPROACHES; ALCOHOL TREATMENT: MEDICATIONS; TREATMENT TYPES: AN OVERVIEW.

☎ See *Organizations of Interest* at the back of Volume 1 for address, telephone, and URL.

Alcoholism: Abstinence versus Controlled Drinking

What should be the goal for an alcoholic? Should it be complete and total **abstinence** from alcohol, or can an alcoholic learn to use alcohol in moderate, controlled ways? The Alcoholics Anonymous☎ organization states that the goal of treatment for those who are dependent on alcohol must be total, complete, and permanent abstinence from alcohol. Most therapists who treat alcoholism in the United States agree. They reject controlled drinking—drinking moderate but never excessive amounts—as a goal of treatment, believing

abstinence complete avoidance of something, such as the use of drugs or alcoholic beverages

that such a goal is harmful to the alcoholic. An alcoholic, in this view, cannot control his or her drinking. Controlled-drinking therapy is widely available in Europe, however, and some in the United States argue that controlled drinking is in fact a reasonable and realistic goal. SEE ALSO ALCOHOL TREATMENT: BEHAVIORAL APPROACHES; ALCOHOLICS ANONYMOUS (AA).

Allergies to Alcohol and Drugs

Alcohol, opiates, barbiturates, and some street drugs have been reported to cause allergic reactions.

Types of Reactions

The symptoms and signs of immediate hypersensitivity reactions are hives, wheezing, swelling of face and lips, or full-blown anaphylaxis, a combination of all the above symptoms plus a dangerous drop in blood pressure. Abdominal pain and irregular heartbeat may also occur with anaphylaxis. Allergies to bee stings or penicillin cause similar reactions.

Symptoms of delayed hypersensitivity reactions include skin rashes, which may be red, itchy, or blistered. Also, the lymph nodes can become enlarged and nodules (small lumps) may appear in the skin or in organs. Poison ivy and cosmetic allergies cause symptoms of this type.

Alcohol

True allergic reactions to alcohol (ethanol) are rare. A person who appears to have an allergic reaction to an alcoholic beverage is usually reacting to other chemicals in the beverage, such as yeasts, metabisulfite, papain, or dyes. Some people get hives after drinking alcohol, and some people of Asian background have a high risk of developing hives from contact with alcohol.

Opiates, Barbiturates, and Street Drugs

Morphine, an opiate, can cause hives in some people. Anaphylaxis may also occur with either morphine or codeine. Heroin may cause some people to wheeze. Patients who have anaphylactic reactions to local anesthesia during surgery often are reacting to the preservative methylparaben rather than to the opiate itself. Numerous reports exist of anaphylactic reactions following the use of barbiturates, which are given to lower a patient's anxiety before surgery. Skin rashes also occur frequently following barbiturate usage.

Street drugs have been reported to cause asthma symptoms (shortness of breath, wheezing) and/or anaphylaxis. Drug users who smoke cocaine or who inject heroin experience wheezing. This may occur more often in patients who have a previous history of asthma. The asthma may persist after the subjects have stopped smoking cocaine. Pulmonary edema (fluid in the lungs) may also occur with freebasing, a way of preparing pure cocaine so that it can be smoked. Marijuana does not appear to increase the incidence of either asthma or anaphylaxis.

Because it is hard to predict how severe an allergic reaction may become, someone who develops allergic symptoms should immediately contact his or her healthcare provider, or go immediately to a hospital emergency department. SEE ALSO ALCOHOL: COMPLICATIONS; COMPLICATIONS FROM INJECTING DRUGS.

Amantadine *See Cocaine Treatments: Medications*

Amobarbital *See Barbiturates*

stimulant drug that increases activity temporarily; often used to describe drugs that excite the brain and central nervous system

Amphetamine

Amphetamine was first synthesized, or made, in a laboratory in 1887. However, scientists did not know of its effects as a **stimulant** on the central nervous system (the brain and spinal cord) until the early 1930s. In the 1880s cocaine projects were introduced as risk free. In the same way, the medical profession promoted amphetamine as an effective cure for a wide range of ills without any risk of addiction. Doctors recommended it to treat alcohol hangovers, depression, and vomiting during pregnancy, and to help patients lose weight. Public interest grew in this supposed miracle drug, which was inexpensive, easy to obtain, and had long-lasting effects. Beginning in the 1930s, amphetamines became drugs of abuse.

Drugs created from amphetamine, such as methamphetamine, became available for therapeutic uses in both oral (to be taken by mouth) and intravenous (to be injected) form. Despite occasional bad reactions, Americans—college students, athletes, truck drivers, and housewives—took enormous quantities of amphetamines in the 1940s and 1950s. The medical community still did not recognize the drugs' abuse potential, that is, the likelihood that they would be abused. Dur-

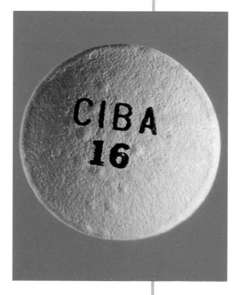

Most amphetamine drugs are taken orally or swallowed, in the form of pills.

illicit something illegal or something used in an illegal manner

ing World War II, the U.S., British, German, and Japanese militaries provided amphetamines, including methamphetamine, to soldiers in combat in order to counteract fatigue, to increase alertness during battle and night watches, to increase endurance, and to elevate mood. Approximately 200 million Benzedrine (amphetamine) tablets were dispensed to the U.S. Armed Forces during World War II. In fact, much of the research on the effects of the amphetamines on performance was carried out on enlisted personnel during this period.

Since 1945, amphetamines and cocaine have each at different times been the most popular **illicit** stimulant. The first major amphetamine epidemic in the United States peaked in the mid-1960s. Approximately 13.5 percent of the university population in 1969 had used amphetamines at least once. By 1978, amphetamine use declined substantially as cocaine use increased. In the early 1990s, use of amphetamines began to rise again, peaking around 1997, then declined slightly before leveling off. The major amphetamine of concern in the United States in the 1990s was methamphetamine, with pockets of "ice" (smoked methamphetamine) abuse. In 2001 use of methamphetamine continued to increase, although the rate of increase appeared to be gradually slowing.

Amphetamines are now controlled under Schedule II of the Controlled Substances Act. Substances in Schedule II—including the stimulants amphetamine, methamphetamine, cocaine, methylphenidate, and phenmetrazine—have a high potential for abuse but also have accepted medical uses in the United States.

Biological Responses

The amphetamines act by increasing concentrations of brain chemicals known as neurotransmitters. The two main neurotransmitters, dopamine and norepinephrine, accumulate in the spaces between brain cells, known as the neuronal synapse. Amphetamines increase the release of dopamine and norepinephrine and block their absorption of uptake into brain cells. Cocaine also blocks uptake of these transmitters but does not increase their release. Amphetamine continues to act in the body for about ten hours, compared to one hour for cocaine and five hours for methamphetamine.

Amphetamines increase heart rate, respiration, and blood pressure. High doses can cause cardiac arrhythmias (irregular heartbeat). In addition, the amphetamines help suppress rapid eye movement sleep—the stage of sleep associated with dreaming—and total sleep. A single moderate dose of amphetamine generally produces the following effects in humans:

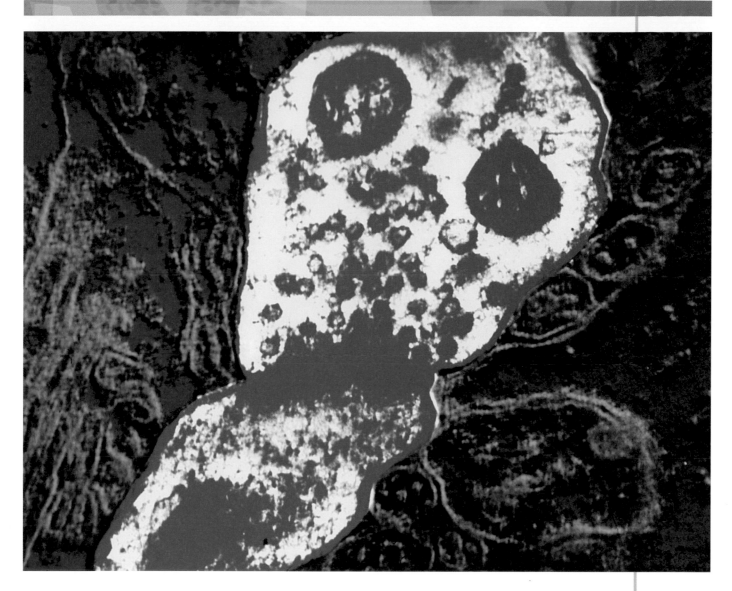

- an increase in activity and talkativeness

- **euphoria** and a general sense of well-being

- decrease in food intake

- decrease in fatigue

Higher doses can produce repetitive motor activity. This means that the user performs a particular action repeatedly, such as tapping his or her fingers or jiggling limbs uncontrollably. Very high doses can lead to convulsions, coma, and death.

Medical Uses

Doctors frequently prescribe amphetamines to treat narcolepsy, obesity, and attention deficit disorder.

Amphetamine use will cause an excessive amount of neurotransmitters to gather in the synapse between neurons, disrupting the communication between brain cells.

euphoria state of intense, giddy happiness and well-being, sometimes occurring baselessly and out of sync with an individual's life situation

tolerance condition in which higher and higher doses of a drug or alcohol are needed to produce the effect or "high" experienced from the original dose

Narcolepsy. People with narcolepsy have sudden attacks of sleep. In large doses over long periods of time, amphetamines can generally prevent these attacks. Interestingly, few narcolepsy patients develop **tolerance** to the effects of these drugs, and most stay on the same dose for years.

Obesity. Because amphetamines are extremely effective appetite suppressants, doctors prescribe them extensively to treat obesity. However, many patients rapidly develop tolerance to the appetite-suppressant effects. After several weeks of use, the patient must take a higher dose to achieve the same effect achieved with the initial dose. Taking high doses over long periods of time can result in toxic side effects: insomnia, irritability, increased heart rate and blood pressure, and tremulousness (shaking). Therefore, these drugs should be taken only for relatively short periods of time (four to six weeks).

Studies show that amphetamines are not effective at helping a person maintain weight loss. Rapid weight gain occurs when he or she stops taking them. The lack of long-term effectiveness, along with the dependence-producing effects of amphetamines, makes them a poor choice for maintaining weight loss.

Attention-Deficit/Hyperactivity Disorder. For children with attention-deficit/hyperactivity disorder, amphetamines (such as Ritalin) can dramatically reduce restlessness and distractibility and lengthen attention span. Those who support the use of amphetamines for this disorder recommend limiting the dose and the duration of treatment to prevent side effects.

The Effects on Behavior

According to research reports, amphetamines do not directly enhance performance. Scientists believe that amphetamines' other effects, such as reducing fatigue or boredom and increasing alertness, are the cause of any improvements in performance.

Trained athletes experience only very small improvements in performance when taking amphetamines. However, studies suggest that even these very small changes can result in the 1 to 2 percent improvement that makes the difference in a close athletic competition. As a result, some athletes take stimulants before athletic events, particularly those calling for strenuous activity over long periods, such as bicycle racing. But taking amphetamines for this purpose presents serious risks, including hyperthermia (elevated body temperature), collapse, and even death.

Amphetamines can produce changes in a person's moods. Users report increased self-confidence, elation, euphoria, friendliness, and generally positive feelings. However, users who take repeated doses develop tolerance to these mood-elevating effects. The user must take increasingly larger amounts of amphetamine to achieve the same effect. Thus the mood-elevating effect is closely related to abuse.

Experienced stimulant users, given a variety of stimulant drugs, often cannot tell the difference between one drug or another. Cocaine, amphetamine, methamphetamine, and methlyphenidate all appear to have similar effects. The major difference is in how long the drugs' effects last.

Side Effects

A major side effect of long-term amphetamine use in humans is a **psychosis** that resembles **schizophrenia**. In one study, volunteers with no histories of psychosis took an amphetamine drug for one to five days. Five of the six subjects developed **paranoid** psychosis, which cleared when the drug was discontinued. Unless the user continues to take the drug, the psychosis usually ends within a week, although it is possible that symptoms will keep occurring. The symptoms of amphetamine psychosis include feelings of being persecuted, hyperactivity and excitation, hallucinations—seeing and hearing things that are not real—and changes in body image.

Amphetamine abusers taking repeated doses of the drug can develop repetitive behavior patterns that continue for hours at a time. These can take the form of constant cleaning, taking apart small appliances over and over again, or picking at wounds. Stopping amphetamine use after long-term high doses generally results in loss of energy, depression, and abnormal sleep patterns. These symptoms may be due to the long-term lack of sleep and reduced food intake typical of chronic use.

Animals given unlimited access to amphetamine will self-administer it repeatedly. Most will continue self-administration until they die. Animals maintained on high doses of amphetamines develop tolerance to many of the damaging effects. They also develop irreversible damage in some parts of the brain, including long-lasting **depletion** of dopamine.

Abuse

Amphetamines, like other stimulants, are generally abused in binges. People take the drug repeatedly for some period of time—usually every three or four hours for three or four days. Then, during a crash

---

THE SIGNS OF AMPHETAMINE USE

Here are some signs that may indicate that someone you know could be using amphetamines:

- Dilated pupils

- Dry mouth and nose

- Frequent lip licking

- Excessive activity, difficulty sitting still, lack of interest in food or sleep

- Irritability, moodiness, and/or nervousness

psychosis mental disorder in which an individual loses contact with reality and may have delusions (i.e., unshakable false beliefs) or hallucinations (i.e., the experience of seeing, hearing, feeling, smelling, or tasting things that are not actually present)

schizophrenia psychotic disorder in which people lose the ability to function normally, experience severe personality changes, and suffer from a variety of symptoms, including confusion, disordered thinking, paranoia, hallucinations, emotional numbness, and speech problems

paranoid someone who is excessively or irrationally suspicious

depletion state of being used up or emptied

period, the user sleeps, eats, and takes no drug at all. As tolerance develops, the user takes higher doses. Stopping amphetamine use suddenly usually results in depression. Mood generally returns to normal within a week, although craving for the drug can last for months. There is little evidence for the development of **physical dependence** to the amphetamines. Although some experts view the crash—with low energy, depression, exhaustion, and increased appetite—that can follow the amphetamine binge as a **withdrawal** syndrome, others believe that the symptoms can also be related to the effects of chronic stimulant use. In other words, during the binge, users have not slept or eaten much, resulting in depression, exhaustion, and hunger when the binge ends.

Treatment of Amphetamine Abuse

As with cocaine abuse, the most promising forms of treatment for amphetamine abuse include behavioral therapy, prevention of relapse (return to drug use), rehabilitation (for example, vocational, educational, and social-skills training), and psychotherapy. Few studies have tested medications for amphetamine abuse. Those that have been done report no success in preventing a return to amphetamine use. SEE ALSO ATTENTION-DEFICIT/HYPERACTIVITY DISORDER; RITALIN; SPEED.

physical dependence condition that may occur after prolonged use of a particular drug or alcohol, in which the user's body cannot function normally without the presence of the substance; when the substance is not used or the dose is decreased, the user experiences uncomfortable physical symptoms

withdrawal group of physical and psychological symptoms that may occur when a person suddenly stops the use of a substance or reduces the dose of an addictive substance

Anabolic Steroids

synthetic something produced artificially

Anabolic steroids are **synthetic** versions of the naturally occurring male sex hormone, testosterone. They have two main effects: they build muscle size and strength, and they bring about male characteristics in the body. Testosterone causes male characteristics to appear during puberty in boys, including enlargement of the penis, hair growth on the face and pubic area, muscular development, and deepened voice. Females also produce natural testosterone, but ordinarily in much smaller amounts than males.

Although anabolic steroids are sometimes referred to simply as steroids, they are in fact only one kind of steroid. They are not to be confused with corticosteroids, such as prednisone and cortisone, which are commonly used to treat illnesses such as arthritis, colitis, and asthma. Street or slang terms for anabolic steroids include "roids" and "juice."

Bodybuilders and Olympic athletes began using these drugs in the middle of the twentieth century. In 1998 a study reported that 6.6

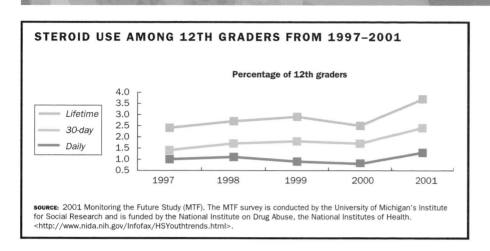

STEROID USE AMONG 12TH GRADERS FROM 1997–2001

Percentage of 12th graders

Lifetime
30-day
Daily

SOURCE: 2001 Monitoring the Future Study (MTF). The MTF survey is conducted by the University of Michigan's Institute for Social Research and is funded by the National Institute on Drug Abuse, the National Institutes of Health. <http://www.nida.nih.gov/Infofax/HSYouthtrends.html>.

In every category for frequency of use, more 12th graders used anabolic steroids in 2001 than in previous years.

percent of American male high-school seniors had tried anabolic steroids. This study made it clear that elite athletes were not the only ones taking these drugs. By 1991 anabolic steroids were added by federal law to a list of controlled substances that are recognized to have value as prescribed medicines but also have a potential for abuse. Some synthetic anabolic steroids are neither regulated by the Food and Drug Administration nor listed as controlled substances in the United States and have been sold over the counter as nutritional supplements in the United States since 1994.

Medical Uses of Anabolic Steroids

Anabolic steroids are prescribed by physicians to treat a variety of medical conditions. The most accepted use is for treating boys and men unable to produce normal levels of their own testosterone, a condition known as testosterone **deficiency** or hypogonadism. Anabolic steroids are also used to treat:

- a rare skin condition called hereditary angioedema
- certain forms of anemia (deficiency of red blood cells)
- advanced breast cancer
- endometriosis (a painful condition in females in which tissue usually found only in the uterus develops in other body parts)
- osteoporosis, a condition in which bone loss occurs
- **impotency** and low sexual desire
- as a male birth control pill
- Acquired Immune Deficiency Syndrome (AIDS) to stimulate appetite, weight gain, strength, and improvements in mood

deficiency having too little of a necessary vitamin or mineral

impotency condition in which one is unable to get or maintain an erection

Nonmedical Uses of Anabolic Steroids

Nonmedically, anabolic steroids are used to enhance athletic performance, physical appearance, and fighting ability. Because society

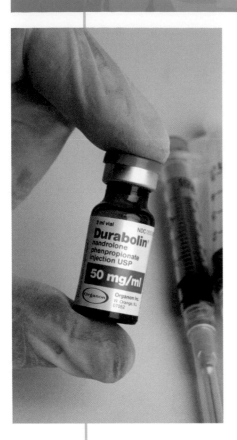

Anabolic steroids, such as DurabolinAt (shown here), build size and strength. At several of the most recent Olympics, the abuse of steroids to improve athletic performance has become a concern.

aesthete one who has a deep appreciation for beauty, especially in the arts or nature

euphoric to experience a state of intense, giddy happiness and well-being, sometimes occurring baselessly and out of sync with the circumstances

tends to reward people who look physically fit and attractive with many benefits and recognition, some individuals see anabolic steroids as a means to those benefits. There are three groups of users:

1. The athlete group aims to win at any cost. The athlete also believes, sometimes correctly, that the competitor is using anabolic steroids. The athlete seeks to attain the glory of victory, social recognition and popularity, and financial rewards such as college scholarships or major league contracts.

2. The **aesthete** group aims to create a beautiful body, as if to make the body into a work of art. Aesthetes may be competitive bodybuilders, or aspiring models, actors, or dancers. They put their bodies on display to obtain admiration and financial rewards.

3. The fighter group seeks to enhance the ability to fight or intimidate. They include body guards, security guards, prison guards, police, soldiers, bouncers, and gang members. These people depend on fighting for their very survival.

Whether anabolic steroids actually work to improve performance and appearance has been debated. Invariably, users believe they do, but some studies have failed to confirm this view.

The Consequences of Anabolic Steroid Use

Anabolic steroids have been associated with a variety of dangerous effects. In some cases anabolic steroids have even been fatal. Reported deaths in nonmedical users have occurred from liver disease, cancer, heart attacks, strokes, and suicide. Clearly, anyone using anabolic steroids should have his or her health monitored by a physician.

Psychiatric Effects. A serious, life-threatening consequence has been violent aggression toward other people. Previously mild-mannered individuals have committed murder and lesser assaults while taking anabolic steroids. Although such incidents are uncommon, most studies have found that high doses of anabolic steroids increase feelings and thoughts of aggressiveness. "Roid rage" is a slang expression used to describe the aggressive feelings, thoughts, and behaviors the drugs can produce.

Anabolic steroids can induce mood swings. Users commonly report that they feel energetic, confident, and even **euphoric** during a cycle of use. They may have a decreased need for sleep or find it difficult to sleep because of their high energy level. Such feelings may give way to feeling down, depressed, irritable, and tired between cycles of use. The appetite may also swing widely. During on cycles, huge quantities of food may be consumed to support the body's requirements for muscle growth and energy. During off cycles, appetite may diminish.

Psychosis, an even more dangerous consequence, means that a person cannot distinguish between what is real and what is not. For example, a psychotic person may believe that other people intend harm when no real threat exists, or that an impossible, life-threatening stunt can be performed without difficulty. Such false beliefs are called delusions. Most psychiatric effects of anabolic steroids tend to disappear soon after use is discontinued, although a depressed mood may last for several months.

Effects on the Liver. Anabolic steroids can affect the liver in various ways. Those available in pill form are more toxic to the liver than injectable forms of the drug. Most commonly, anabolic steroids cause the liver to release extra amounts of enzymes into the bloodstream. The liver enzymes usually return to normal levels when anabolic steroids are stopped. The liver also releases a substance called bilirubin, which in high amounts can cause the skin and the whites of the eyes to turn yellow (a condition called jaundice). Medical as well as nonmedical users can develop jaundice, a dangerous condition if left untreated. Jaundice can also signal other dangerous conditions of the liver, such as hepatitis. Liver tumors have been reported, some of them cancerous. Although more than half of the tumors disappeared when anabolic steroids were stopped, others resulted in death.

Effects on the Heart. Anabolic steroids can cause a decrease in a form of cholesterol known as good cholesterol. This effect in turn can increase the risk of heart attacks. When anabolic steroids are stopped, cholesterol levels return to normal. Studies have shown that anabolic steroids can cause small increases in blood pressure, also a risk factor for heart attacks and strokes. As a result of strenuous exercise, many athletes develop an enlarged heart that is not harmful. Some, but not all studies, however, suggest that drug users can develop an enlargement of the heart that *is* harmful.

Sexual Side Effects. Anabolic steroids can alter the levels of several sex-related hormones in the body, resulting in many adverse effects. In males, the **prostate gland** can enlarge, making it difficult to urinate; the testicles may shrink; and **sterility** can occur. These effects are, with few exceptions, reversible when anabolic steroids are stopped.

Male users can also develop enlarged breast tissue. Testosterone is changed in the body to estrogen, the female hormone, and thus the

prostate gland located near the bladder and urethra in men; it secretes the fluid that contains sperm

sterility condition in which one is unable to conceive a child

clitoris small erectile organ in females at front part of the vulva

male anabolic steroid user has more estrogen than is normal. Painful lumps in the male breast may persist after stopping anabolic steroids, and they sometimes require surgical removal. Females, however, may undergo shrinkage of their breasts, as a response to higher amounts of male hormone than normal. Menstrual periods become irregular and sterility can occur in females as well. Anabolic steroid use in females may cause the voice to deepen and the **clitoris** to enlarge. These effects do not always reverse after stopping anabolic steroids. Women may also develop excessive hair growth in typically masculine patterns, such as on the chest and face. Finally, both males and females may experience increases and decreases in their desire for sex.

Other Effects. In children of both sexes before the onset of puberty, anabolic steroids can bring on the characteristics of male puberty. They can also cause the bones to stop growing prematurely, which can result in shorter adult heights than would otherwise occur. Anabolic steroid use can cause premature baldness in some individuals, and it can cause acne. The condition called sleep apnea (which causes people to stop breathing for short intervals during sleep) is worsened by taking anabolic steroids, as are tics, or muscle twitches, in those who already suffer from them.

Patterns of Illegal Anabolic Steroid Use

Anabolic steroids are commonly smuggled from countries where they are obtained over the counter without a prescription, and then sold illegally in the United States. Dealers and users typically connect in weight-lifting gyms. Users report that anabolic steroids are relatively easy to obtain.

Steroids can be taken as pills, through skin patches, and by injection. Injection occurs into large muscle groups (buttocks, thigh, or shoulder) or under the skin, but not into veins. Cases of AIDS have been reported in steroid users due to needle sharing. Illicit users (those who use the drugs illegally) typically consume 10 to 100 times the amounts ordinarily prescribed for medical purposes. The actual dose cannot always be determined, however, because drugs purchased on the illegal market do not always contain what the labels indicate. Law-enforcement officials have confiscated vials contaminated with bacteria.

Anabolic steroid users often use other drugs in order to:

- manage the unpleasant steroid side effects
- increase body-building effect
- avoid detection by urine testing

These drugs may themselves cause a range of side effects.

The Addictive Potential of Anabolic Steroids

As with other drugs of abuse, dependence on anabolic steroids occurs when a user reports several of the following symptoms:

- inability to stop or cut down use

- taking more drugs than intended

- continued use despite having negative effects

- tolerance, or needing more of a drug to get the same effect that was previously obtained with smaller doses

- withdrawal, or the uncomfortable effects experienced when use of the drug is stopped

As noted, many of the undesirable effects go away when anabolic steroids are stopped. However, stopping steroids may cause other symptoms to begin, such as depressed mood, fatigue, loss of appetite, difficulty sleeping, restlessness, decreased sex drive, headaches, muscle aches, and a desire for more anabolic steroids. The depression can become so severe that suicidal thoughts occur. The risk of suicide described previously is thought to be highest during the withdrawal period.

Studies indicate that between 14 percent and 57 percent of nonmedical users develop dependence on anabolic steroids, primarily in terms of the muscle-altering effects rather than the mood-altering effects. Some researchers have questioned whether anabolic steroids produce dependence at all, because most definitions of dependence require that drugs be taken primarily for their mood-altering effects. SEE ALSO ADDICTION: CONCEPTS AND DEFINITIONS; ADOLESCENTS, DRUG AND ALCOHOL USE; COMPLICATIONS FROM INJECTING DRUGS; TOLERANCE AND PHYSICAL DEPENDENCE.

Analgesic

Analgesics are drugs used to control pain without producing loss of consciousness. Unlike anesthetics, which block all sensation, analgesics do not affect sensations other than pain. Mild analgesics, such as aspirin (e.g., Bayer, Bufferin), acetaminophen (Tylenol), and ibuprofen (Advil), work throughout the body at the source of pain. Researchers think acetaminophen may work at the nerve endings, dulling the sensation of pain. Ibuprofen and other nonsteroidal anti-inflammatory agents interfere with the production of pain-causing chemicals. Opiate analgesics, such as codeine and morphine, work within the central nervous system (the brain and spinal cord). Opiates work not by relieving the underlying reason for pain, but by changing the way the individual perceives pain. People who take opiates can become addicted to them, so these drugs require a doctor's prescription. SEE ALSO OPIATE AND OPIOID DRUG ABUSE.

Anhedonia

Anhedonia is a condition in which someone cannot experience pleasure or positive emotions. Anhedonia is often a symptom of depression and can also occur with other diseases, such as thyroid disease, multiple sclerosis, Parkinson's disease, migraine, brain tumors, and epilepsy. Anhedonia can be a side effect of some medications, particularly those for treating high blood pressure. Some researchers also believe that crack users experience severe anhedonia, following a binge. In an attempt to relieve this anhedonia, they are driven to use more crack. SEE ALSO CRACK.

Anorectic *See Appetite Suppressant*

Anorexia *See Eating Disorders*

Antidepressant

Antidepressants are a diverse group of drugs used to treat symptoms of depression. The term "depression" describes several psychiatric disorders in which a person has abnormal moods. Everyone has moods—silly, happy, angry, sad. Most people, no matter what mood they happen to be in, are able to follow their daily routines and meet obligations at school, at work, and with their families. Sometimes a person has moods, often of anger or sadness, that are extremely powerful. Often these moods, not the person, determine behavior. Very strong moods can prevent a person from completing work or lead to clashes with others. When this happens regularly, the moods are considered abnormal.

Antidepressants can also be useful for treating anxiety, panic disorders, and chronic pain. They are not helpful for short-term depressed moods that are part of everyday life or for the normal period of grief that follows loss of a loved one. Antidepressants include tricyclics (such as Tofranil and Aventyl), monoamine oxidase inhibitors

(Nardil, Marplan), lithium (Eskalith, Lithonate), nontricyclics, and selective serotonin-reuptake inhibitors (Prozac, Paxil, Zoloft). SEE ALSO ALCOHOL TREATMENT: MEDICATIONS; PERSONALITY DISORDER.

Antidote

An antidote is a medication or treatment that acts against a poison or its effects. An antidote may work by reducing the amount of poison that is absorbed from the stomach, or by blocking the absorption entirely. Some antidotes counteract a poison's effects directly. For example, an antidote can work by neutralizing an acid. Some antidotes work by blocking a poison at its receptor site in the brain. For example, a medication called naloxone blocks opiates such as heroin at its receptors, preventing death from heroin overdose. Many cities have a telephone poison hotline, where information on antidotes is given. In case of drug overdose or poisoning, call for expert medical help immediately by dialing 911. SEE ALSO HEROIN; HEROIN TREATMENT: MEDICATIONS.

Antipsychotic

Antipsychotic drugs (also called neuroleptic drugs) are used to treat schizophrenia and other acute psychotic illnesses. Antipsychotics include phenothiazines (such as Thorazine) and butyrophenones (such as Haldol). Some symptoms, such as hallucinations, often improve when a patient is treated with antipsychotics. However, these drugs are less effective for treating certain other symptoms, such as withdrawal (when a person avoids social contact). Side effects of these drugs may include drowsiness, slowed movements, muscle spasms, and weight gain. SEE ALSO NEUROLEPTIC.

Antisocial Personality

Antisocial personality disorder (APD) is a condition in which people disregard the rights of others and violate those rights by acting in aggressive, irritating, and even criminal ways. APD begins in childhood and early adolescence. People with APD engage in bullying, vandalism, violence, and lying, and they do not feel guilt or regret for their actions. Two-thirds of those diagnosed with APD are male.

The causes of APD are not known, but low levels of serotonin, a brain chemical, may be one factor. Problems with the functioning of dopamine, another brain chemical, may also play a role. APD patients often have antisocial relatives, with substance abuse, divorce, and child abuse common in the family.

A large percentage of alcohol and drug abusers suffer from APD. For some, the abuse of alcohol or drugs causes the antisocial behaviors. For other abusers, substance abuse is just one expression of a wide range of antisocial behaviors.

Alcoholism

A child who exhibits antisocial behavior problems is at greater risk for alcoholism later in life. Alcoholism in people with APD is usually more severe and of longer duration than in people without APD. The onset of symptoms of alcoholism in those with APD usually occurs earlier, at age 20, compared to nearly age 30 for those without APD. APD alcoholics do not respond as well to treatment, relapsing much earlier than alcoholics without APD. While males with APD have a shortened life expectancy, the disorder tends to get better with age or at least to stabilize.

Research reports suggest that alcoholism complicated by APD is more **heritable** than non-APD alcoholism. In a Swedish adoption study, for adopted sons whose biological fathers had APD and alcoholism, the risk of alcoholism was nine times that of adopted sons whose biological fathers did not have APD.

Other Problems

Females with APD frequently develop eating disorders as well as substance abuse disorders. Most of these patients have **bulimia nervosa** rather than **anorexia nervosa**. Treatment of an eating disorder generally takes longer in women with APD than in those without it.

AIDS presents other dangers for substance abusers with APD. Males with APD have a high rate of risky behaviors related to HIV infection. These behaviors include using intravenous (injected) drugs, sharing needles, having sex with multiple partners, and engaging in anal sex.

Most patients diagnosed with APD improve over time with treatment. The most beneficial forms of therapy for APD appear to be group and family therapies rather than individual psychotherapy or medications. SEE ALSO ADDICTIVE PERSONALITY; ALCOHOL: PSYCHOLOGICAL CONSEQUENCES OF CHRONIC ABUSE; CHILDHOOD BEHAVIOR

heritable trait that is passed on from parents to offspring

bulimia nervosa literally means "ox hunger"; an eating disorder characterized by compulsive overeating and then efforts to purge the body of the excess food, through self-induced vomiting, laxative abuse, or the use of diuretic medicines (pills to rid the body of water)

anorexia nervosa eating disorder characterized by an intense and irrational fear of gaining weight; results in abnormal and unhealthy eating patterns, malnutrition, and severe weight loss

AND LATER DRUG USE; CONDUCT DISORDER; RISK FACTORS FOR SUBSTANCE ABUSE.

Anxiety

Anxiety refers to an unpleasant, but normal, emotional state. If you are suffering from anxiety, you may feel nervous or fearful. You may even notice physical symptoms such as shortness of breath, sweating, and diarrhea. Anxiety is also a specific category of psychiatric disorder. In this case, the feelings and physical symptoms of anxiety overwhelm your ability to function normally. Specific anxiety disorders include generalized anxiety disorder, panic disorder, social or other phobias, post-traumatic stress disorder, and obsessive-compulsive disorder.

Alcohol, caffeine, and stimulant drugs such as amphetamines can contribute to feelings of anxiety. Some people with severe anxiety may drink alcohol or take nonprescribed **sedative-hypnotics** (such as Valium) in an attempt to relieve their symptoms, but these substances may worsen the condition. SEE ALSO ALCOHOL: COMPLICATIONS OF PROBLEM DRINKING; PRESCRIPTION DRUG ABUSE; RISK FACTORS FOR SUBSTANCE ABUSE; SEDATIVE AND SEDATIVE-HYPNOTIC DRUGS.

sedative-hypnotic drug that has a calming and relaxing effect; "hypnotics" induce sleep

Aphrodisiac

An aphrodisiac is a substance that causes someone to feel sexually aroused or that enhances sexual performance. Many foods, such as oysters, have a long-standing reputation as aphrodisiacs. Another common belief is that alcohol is an aphrodisiac, but in fact alcohol (a depressant) decreases sexual responsiveness in both men and women. Some drugs of abuse also have reputations as aphrodisiacs, including cocaine, marijuana, MDMA or "ecstasy," and amyl nitrite (an inhalant, often called poppers). To the contrary, the use of these drugs can lead to a loss of sexual desire, excitement, and capability.

Appetite Suppressant

An appetite suppressant is a substance that causes a person to consume less food. Appetite suppressants are also known as anorectics. Appetite suppressants can be substances that are purposely used or

antidepressant medication used for the treatment and prevention of depression

AIDS stands for **a**cquired **i**mmuno**d**eficiency **s**yndrome, the disease caused by the human immunodeficiency virus (HIV); in severe cases it is characterized by the profound weakening of the body's immune system

psychosis mental disorder in which an individual loses contact with reality and may have delusions (i.e., unshakable false beliefs) or hallucinations (i.e., the experience of seeing, hearing, feeling, smelling, or tasting things that are not actually present)

prescribed to decrease appetite. These include: phentermine (Adipex), sibutramine (Meridia) and some **antidepressants**. Appetite suppressants can also be herbal preparations, usually containing ephedra, which are claimed to aid in weight loss. Some medications have appetite suppression as a side effect. These include medicines given for attention-deficit/hyperactivity disorder, such as Ritalin, Adderall, and Dexedrine; some chemotherapy drugs used to treat cancer; some drugs used to treat HIV/**AIDS**; and some medicines used for thyroid conditions. Some drugs of abuse also have appetite suppression as a side effect (such as cocaine and amphetamines or speed).

Some prescription weight-loss medications have been banned. The medications fenfluramine (Pondimin) and dexfenfluramine (Redux) were often given along with phentermine in a combination called Fen-Phen or Dex-Phen. Both fenfluramine and dexfenfluramine were found to cause serious heart problems. Phentermine alone is still used for weight loss for extremely overweight (morbidly obese) individuals.

Herbal supplements containing ephedra (sometimes called ma Huang) have also received much attention in the news. Many people do not realize that a substance can be herbal but still have potentially life-threatening side effects. Dangerous side effects from preparations that contain ephedra include feelings of nervousness and anxiety, racing heart, high blood pressure, sleep problems, **psychosis**, seizures, heart attack, stroke, and even death. The Food and Drug Administration has issued a warning about ephedra-containing preparations. SEE ALSO AMPHETAMINE; EATING DISORDERS; HERBAL SUPPLEMENTS; NICOTINE.

Asset Forfeiture

When a person commits a crime, one of the punishments may be asset forfeiture. The criminal must give up (forfeit) money or property (assets) without compensation. Prosecutors can file civil lawsuits asking a court for permission to take property from a criminal defendant that was either used in the crime or was obtained through a criminal act. Since the 1970s, federal asset forfeiture laws have been used against drug dealers.

By 2000, however, many in Congress and the legal community were calling for reform, as these laws have often resulted in harsh and unfair outcomes for innocent third parties. In response, Congress enacted an "innocent owner defense" in civil drug forfeiture cases. For example, if the owner of a car innocently allows another person to borrow it and that person commits a drug offense in the car, the owner can offer this defense and retain the car. Congress also passed the Civil Asset Forfeiture Reform Act of 2000, requiring federal prosecutors to show a more substantial connection between the property and the crime. In 2001 assets worth over $439 million were seized as part of the U.S. Department of Justice Asset Forfeiture Program. SEE ALSO LAW AND POLICY: MODERN ENFORCEMENT, PROSECUTION, AND SENTENCING.

Attention-Deficit/Hyperactivity Disorder

Attention-deficit/hyperactivity disorder (ADHD) is a condition that affects an individual's self-control, causing problems with attention span, impulse control, and activity level. ADHD causes difficulty with concentration, persistence, and attention span. Although many individuals with ADHD often find it difficult to concentrate on the task at hand, some experts argue that the term "attention *deficit*" is somewhat misleading. Instead, they suggest that persons with ADHD actually have difficulty controlling or regulating their attention in general.

For example, they may find it very hard not to pay attention to irrelevant, distracting stimuli in their environment, such as noises or the mere presence of others. At other times, however, they may be so absorbed in what they are doing—especially if it is an activity in which they are very interested—that they do not notice anything else, such as a teacher calling on them. This kind of focus (or "hyperfocus") is also a sign of poor attention regulation, and it, too, may be part of ADHD.

Signs of ADHD

Youths with ADHD show an extremely high level of activity in many situations. The high level of activity becomes most apparent when a low level of activity is called for, such as in a classroom where children are asked to focus on particular tasks. ADHD children typically are **impulsive**, restless, and easily distracted. For example, they may repeatedly leave their desk or work area to wander about, checking out what is going on in other parts of the classroom.

The ability to control impulses is also affected in children with ADHD. Some children and adolescents act out or display their feelings, frustrations, and emotional conflicts more than others. In a typical classroom, the child who acts out is one who consistently

---

POSSIBLE SIGNS OF ATTENTION-DEFICIT/ HYPERACTIVITY DISORDER

Everybody has problems staying focused at one time or another, but Attention-Deficit/Hyperactivity Disorder is an ongoing inability to concentrate. Below are some signs that a person may have a more serious problem and should consult a professional:

1. Difficulty sustaining attention.

2. Frequently distracted and unfocused during activities and school.

3. Failing to follow instructions and to finish schoolwork or chores.

4. Organizing is challenging.

5. Losing things often— particularly supplies, homework, papers, etc.

6. Physically restless, fidgeting, hating to wait in line.

7. Always needing to be "on the go."

8. Trouble playing quietly or cooperating within a group.

9. Reacting impulsively.

impulsive acting before thinking through the consequences of the action blurts out his or her first reactions without waiting to be called upon or recognizing that others may be speaking. When the behavior of acting out becomes severe and out of control of the individual, these youths may be diagnosed with ADHD. Some people use the term "attention deficit disorder" (or ADD for short) instead of ADHD, while others may refer to ADHD without the hyperactive component as ADD.

Diagnosing ADHD

Experts often do not agree on how to diagnose ADHD. Some believe the criteria for judging whether a child or adult has ADHD are too vague. Most of them do agree, however, that a doctor should not diagnose a child with ADHD based only on one short office visit. According to guidelines set by the American Psychiatric Association, some hyperactive, impulsive, or inattentive symptoms must have been present before age 7, last for at least six months, and not be the consequence of an overall problem in the child's development. In addition, the behavior must be causing problems in at least two different settings (for example, in the classroom and at home) for this diagnosis to be assigned.

Who Has ADHD? Approximately 9 percent of boys and 3 percent of girls in the general population qualify for a diagnosis of ADHD. Boys and girls tend to show different symptoms, with girls being somewhat older than boys at the time of first diagnosis. Girls usually have more mood changes, fears, and social withdrawal than boys but are less aggressive and impulsive. There is some disagreement regarding the likelihood that a child with ADHD will also have the disorder as an adult, with estimates ranging between 30 and 80 percent. In general, hyperactive symptoms tend to decrease with age, but the attention problems are often carried over into adulthood.

Comorbid Disorders. Up to 60 percent of children with ADHD also have some **comorbid** disorders, including **conduct disorder**, **oppositional defiant disorder**, and anxiety disorders. Adults with a history of ADHD may experience other disorders, the most common being substance abuse and depression. Youths with ADHD do not always have these disorders later on, but they are at increased risk for these outcomes.

Treating ADHD

Several methods have been used successfully for treating ADHD, including the use of medications, behavioral treatments, and a combination of both.

comorbid two or more disorders that occur at the same time in a person

conduct disorder condition in which a child or adolescent exhibits behavioral and emotional problems, often finding it difficult to follow rules and behaving in a manner that violates the rights of others and society

oppositional defiant disorder psychiatric condition in which a person repeatedly shows a pattern of negative, hostile, disobedient, and/or defiant behavior, without serious violation of the rights of others

Medication. Drugs known as **psychostimulants** are helpful for approximately 75 percent of ADHD children and adults. The most commonly used medications are methylphenidate (Ritalin), amphetamine and dextroamphetamine (Adderall), and pemoline (Cylert). Some antidepressants are also effective in many cases. More than a hundred research studies have shown that these medications are useful for reducing problem behaviors of ADHD.

Although psychostimulants have been found to be effective for ADHD, some concerns have been raised regarding a possible connection between their long-term use and the development of **addiction**. The results of scientific research into this question have been mixed. One study has found a connection between stimulant medication treatment in ADHD youths and later adult **dependence** on cocaine and tobacco. But the results of several other studies indicate that stimulant medication may actually reduce the risk of substance abuse for young people with ADHD. In one study, for example, children who had been given stimulant medication for their ADHD had lower rates of marijuana, cocaine, and alcohol abuse when they grew up, compared to children with ADHD who had not received medication.

Lifestyle. A healthy lifestyle should be encouraged for all children with ADHD. This includes a regular schedule of bedtime, meals, homework, and recreation. Nutrition is important; however, contrary to popular belief, there is no substantive evidence linking diet or food allergies to ADHD. There is also no scientific evidence indicating that a special diet or some nutritional supplements can help relieve the symptoms of ADHD.

Environmental Changes. Structuring the environment so that there are few distractions is an important step. In the home, distracting stimulation from radio or television should be kept to a minimum, especially while the youth is doing homework. In the classroom, the teacher should consider the best seat location for an ADHD child, so that he or she is not distracted by other students and has fewer opportunities to be disruptive.

Behavior Modification. A youth with ADHD can be trained to control inappropriate impulses and to improve his or her behavior. This can be achieved by the use of various behavior modification techniques, which involve rewarding desirable behavior and providing negative consequences for inappropriate behavior. For example, when a parent catches a child doing something good (completing homework or going to bed on time, for instance), the child would be praised

psychostimulant medication that is prescribed to control hyperactive and impulsive behaviors

addiction state in which the body requires the presence of a particular substance to function normally; without the substance, predictable withdrawal symptoms are experienced

dependence psychological compulsion to use a substance for emotional and/or physical reasons

and given some reward (points or tokens that could later be converted into extra privileges, such as going to a movie). But when the child misbehaves (talks back or refuses to go to bed at night, for example), he or she would lose some points or tokens.

Behavior modification techniques such as these can be used alone or in combination with medication and other treatment methods to improve troublesome behavior related to ADHD. For further information about treatment, access to support groups, and some additional, helpful advice relating to this controversial but common disorder, visit the following Web sites:

- Children and Adults with Attention-Deficit/Hyperactivity Disorder (http://www.chadd.org/)
- National Attention Deficit Disorder Association (http://www.add.org/)
- U.S. Centers for Disease Control and Prevention (http://www.cdc.gov/ncbddd/adhd/)
- About.com (http://add.about.com/) SEE ALSO CONDUCT DISORDER; PERSONALITY DISORDER; RISK FACTORS FOR SUBSTANCE ABUSE; RITALIN.

Ayahuasca

Ayahuasca is a brew made by indigenous (native) peoples of South America. The brew is prepared from the roots of a vine, *Banisteriopsis caapi*, and sometimes other plant roots. It has been a part of ritual practices for hundreds of years in Colombia, Brazil, and Peru. People seeking alternatives to Western medicine have participated in rituals in which drinking ayahuasca tea is a central feature. These people report that the tea produces feelings of ecstasy and a sense of experiencing great insight. In southern Brazil, some psychotherapists bring patients to participate in such rituals. SEE ALSO DRUGS USED IN RITUALS; HALLUCINOGENS.

Babies, Addicted and Drug-Exposed

Addicted babies are infants who are born physically **dependent** on drugs because of drug use by the mother during her pregnancy. Doctors consider babies addicted if they have a high level of exposure to drugs before birth. Each year in the United States some 320,000 babies are born exposed to alcohol and illegally used drugs while in the

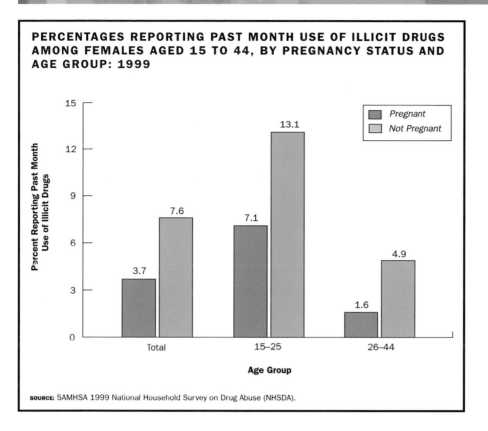

PERCENTAGES REPORTING PAST MONTH USE OF ILLICIT DRUGS AMONG FEMALES AGED 15 TO 44, BY PREGNANCY STATUS AND AGE GROUP: 1999

SOURCE: SAMHSA 1999 National Household Survey on Drug Abuse (NHSDA).

A much higher percentage of pregnant women between the ages of 15 and 25 report having used illicit drugs than pregnant women over the age of 26.

uterus, or in utero. A far larger number have been exposed in utero to **sedatives** and nicotine. Since the 1970s, an increasing number of women have begun to use both legal and illegal drugs. As a result, society is more aware of the problem of drug-exposed babies.

Drug-addicted women often use more than one substance at a time. Use of multiple drugs includes **depressants** (alcohol, marijuana, opioids such as heroin and methadone, and tranquilizers) and **stimulants** (cocaine and nicotine). The drugs are carried in the mother's blood across the **placenta** to the fetus. The baby's condition at birth depends on the substance the mother used, how much she used and how often, and the time between last use and delivery. The most severe withdrawal occurs in infants whose mothers have taken large amounts of drugs for a long time.

The Effects of Depressants

Infants exposed to heroin and other opioids suffer from the following problems:

- **withdrawal** in 55 to 94 percent of cases
- slowed growth rate in the uterus
- low birth weight
- premature birth

dependent someone who has a psychological compulsion to use a substance for emotional and/or physical reasons

sedative medication that reduces excitement; often called a "tranquilizer"

depressant chemical that slows down or decreases functioning

stimulant drug that increases activity temporarily

placenta in most mammals, the organ responsible for passing nutrients and oxygen from the mother to the developing fetus

withdrawal group of physical and psychological symptoms that may occur when a person suddenly stops the use of a substance or reduces the dose of an addictive substance

While this graph indicates the percentage use of illicit drugs by type among pregnant females over the past month in 1999, drug-addicted women often use more than one substance at a time.

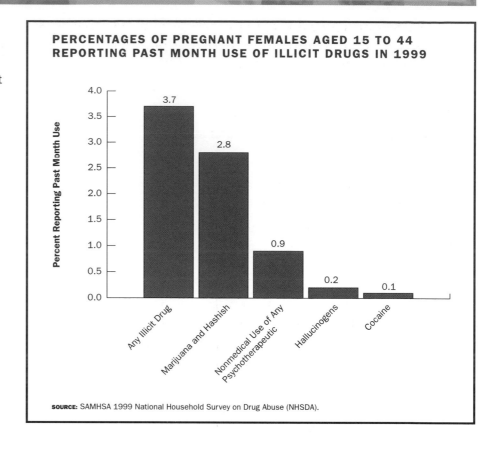

PERCENTAGES OF PREGNANT FEMALES AGED 15 TO 44 REPORTING PAST MONTH USE OF ILLICIT DRUGS IN 1999

SOURCE: SAMHSA 1999 National Household Survey on Drug Abuse (NHSDA).

resuscitation revival from unconsciousness; restoring energy, vitality

Premature birth or low birth weight can lead to such complications as immature lungs, difficulties in breathing at birth, bleeding in the brain, low sugar and calcium levels, infections, and jaundice. Low-birth-weight infants account for a large number of infants who test as mentally retarded (I.Q. of 70 or below), as well as children who have great difficulty in school because they are poor learners. In addition, low-birth-weight infants have an increased incidence of cerebral palsy and malformations that lead to death.

If the mother has used a large dose of a depressant drug (e.g., alcohol, any number of sedative-hypnotics, or heroin) immediately before delivery, the newborn, or neonate, may have difficulty breathing and may require **resuscitation**. If the mother has used one of these drugs regularly during pregnancy, the baby may have the following problems:

- neonatal withdrawal syndrome, with symptoms of irritability, tremors (shaking), and increased muscle tone
- nervous system irritability, which might include inconsolable fussiness and crying, involuntary twitching, excitability, and severe startling to sounds and movement
- gastrointestinal disorders that lead to poor feeding, vomiting, and diarrhea

- extreme difficulty with feedings because of a poor sucking reflex, leading to **malnutrition**, **dehydration**, weight loss, and, if symptoms go untreated, shock, coma, and death

- high-pitched crying

- difficulty in sleeping

- sneezing, sweating, yawning, nasal stuffiness, rapid breathing, and seizures

With heroin, the baby's withdrawal generally occurs within forty-eight hours of birth. With methadone, a longer-acting drug, the withdrawal can happen a bit later. In the withdrawal of alcohol-exposed infants, seizures are more likely to occur.

Sudden Infant Death Syndrome (SIDS). Sudden infant death syndrome is defined as the sudden and unexpected death of an infant between one week and one year of age. The infant's death remains unexplained after an **autopsy**, a full history of the child and family, and an investigation of the death site. Infants exposed to drugs appear to have an increased risk of SIDS, because drug-using groups share many other high-risk factors for SIDS. These include poverty, low birth weight, young age of the mother at the time of giving birth, black racial category, and maternal smoking. So the cause of higher rates of SIDS might not be the drug use itself but instead other

malnutrition unhealthy condition of the body caused by not getting enough food or enough of the right foods or by an inability of the body to appropriately break down the food or utilize the nutrients

dehydration state in which there is an abnormally low amount of fluid in the body

autopsy examination of a body after a person has died, to determine the cause of death or to explore the results of a disease

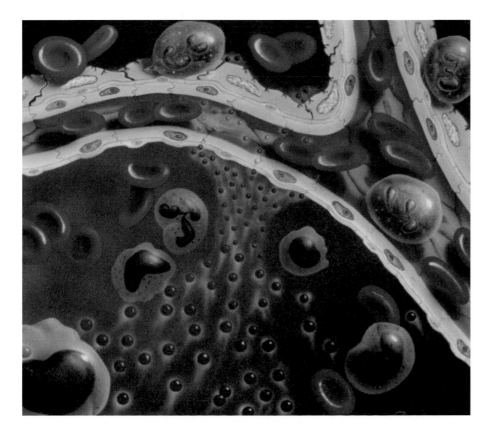

Alcohol—the small bubbles in this picture—is shown entering fetal membranes, demonstrating that the placenta can absorb harmful substances along with beneficial nutrients.

factors, such as poverty or the young age of the mother, that typically go along with drug use. In an extensive study of New York City SIDS rates, mothers who used opioids such as heroin had a three to four times greater risk of losing an infant to SIDS than did the general population.

The Effects of Stimulants

Expectant mothers who use stimulants such as cocaine and nicotine also put their newborns at risk.

Cocaine. Cocaine exposure in utero produces a chain of responses:

- constriction of blood vessels that deliver oxygen to the fetus
- decrease of oxygen delivery to the fetus
- neonatal stroke as a result of oxygen deprivation

Cocaine-exposed babies may suffer from growth problems and abnormal organ development and have an increased risk of brain hemorrhage and SIDS. Infants who were exposed to cocaine shortly before birth often appear less alert and less responsive to external stimuli, such as faces, voices, bells, lights, and rattles, than normal newborns. Babies exposed to cocaine in utero have an increased chance of language problems as they mature, and they may also show unusual behaviors, such as an inability to play, unresponsive moods, and difficulty paying attention.

Nicotine. Prenatal exposure to smoking is harmful in several ways. Carbon monoxide and high doses of nicotine obtained by inhaling tobacco smoke can reduce the oxygen supply to the fetus. This loss of oxygen may interfere with the development of the central nervous system. A child who was exposed to nicotine in utero may then have problems with:

- memory
- learning
- understanding

Other problems include:
- damaged respiratory system of the fetus
- respiratory illness in the infant
- low birth weight

Even passive smoking—that is, from the father or another person in the vicinity of the mother—seems to affect an infant's weight. The weight of newborns whose mothers smoked is on average 200 grams less than those with nonsmoking mothers. Heavy smokers are at the greatest risk for low-birth-weight babies. Women who stop smoking in pregnancy prevent the full effects of low birth weight, and studies have shown that the earlier a woman stops smoking during pregnancy, the lower the risk of a low-birth-weight baby.

One of the most dangerous risks of prenatal smoking is SIDS. A higher mortality rate exists for infants whose mothers have smoked compared to those who have not. The risk of SIDS is also greater among infants exposed to both prenatal and postnatal smoking compared to those only exposed to postnatal smoking. The greater the exposure to smoke both before and after birth, the higher the risk of SIDS.

Managing the Problem

Pregnant women with a drug addiction often stay away from medical facilities for fear of getting in trouble with authorities. Often they do not get badly needed prenatal care. Solving this major health problem requires that drug-treatment programs be designed to meet the specific needs of women.

Once a drug-addicted expectant mother seeks medical care, medical personnel should obtain a thorough alcohol and drug history from her. They should also test the urine of both mother and newborn for alcohol and other drugs. Newborns should be closely monitored for signs of withdrawal for a minimum of forty-eight to seventy-two hours, and longer when the mother has been on **methadone**-maintenance treatment. Because symptoms of withdrawal can be confused with a variety of infections or other medical problems, doctors and nurses should look for other simultaneous illnesses to explain any symptoms.

methadone potent synthetic narcotic, used in heroin recovery programs as a non-intoxicating opiate that blunts symptoms of withdrawal

Most hospital nurseries use a standard scoring system to determine whether a baby is in withdrawal. After the infant is born the hospital monitors the baby's sleep habits, temperature, and weight. If the newborn exhibits withdrawal symptoms, the infant is treated with intravenous fluids, swaddling, holding, rocking, a low-stimulation environment, and small feedings of a special formula with a high calorie count to help the baby gain weight. If symptoms continue or increase, the baby may need medication to calm and sedate its irritable nervous system until the effects of withdrawal pass. Common medications include paregoric, phenobarbital, and diazepam.

Medical personnel must also question the mother of an infant with withdrawal symptoms to get a sense of the home environment.

Addicted babies are often at high risk for either abuse or neglect or both. Normal bonding between mother and infant is difficult when the baby is irritable and unresponsive because of exposure to drugs. Irritability, poor feeding, inability to sleep regularly, and sweating may persist for three to four months. The mother may be feeling guilty and critical of herself, making bonding even more difficult. She may be poor and have inadequate housing as well as an abusive or absent partner or parent. In such cases health-care workers must contact child protection services, asking them to intervene to take steps to make sure the newborn is safe.

Some medical professionals and others involved in the care of addicted babies feel that separating them from their addicted mothers is the best course of action. But this solution may not be practical in cities where social services and courts are already understaffed and overworked. Decent foster care is expensive and hard to find. In general, pediatricians feel that mothers and infants should not be separated except in extreme situations. In addition to drug rehabilitation and medical treatment, these women need education, job training, outpatient care, and counseling to become productive citizens and loving mothers.

Outcome

Given the medical complications, the lack of prenatal care, and the prematurity of the infants at delivery, it is not surprising that the death rate for addicted babies is higher than for infants born to nonaddicts. The outcome for addicted babies depends on any permanent medical conditions resulting from addiction. It also depends on the quality of care the baby receives after leaving the hospital. After babies born with an addiction have been sent home, long-term follow-up on their care and development is very difficult. In some cases the effects of drug exposure on a child may not become apparent for many months or years.

The drug-addicted mother's lifestyle is often characterized by poverty, poor nutrition, violence, and prostitution, any or all of which may result in a high risk for medical problems. Needle use may cause the mother to become infected with hepatitis B and HIV. These conditions create a chaotic and potentially dangerous environment for babies and children. The mother will have great difficulty caring for an infant when she herself is in great need of care.

Methadone-maintenance programs for heroin-addicted mothers generally offer medical and social services to help new mothers cope with the effects of addiction. Although the mother continues to be addicted, these programs contribute to the improved outcome seen in their babies.

Babies born with drug exposure and addiction require ongoing special attention from doctors, schools, community organizations, and government agencies to ensure that they reach their highest potential. SEE ALSO COCAINE; FETAL ALCOHOL SYNDROME (FAS); GENDER AND SUBSTANCE ABUSE; HEROIN; NICOTINE.

Barbiturates

Barbiturates are a group of drugs that act as **depressants** on the central nervous system (the brain and spinal cord). They are derived from barbituric acid, a chemical discovered in 1863. Scientists looking for a drug to treat anxiety and nervousness that would not produce **dependence** (as do codeine and morphine) changed the structure of barbituric acid and **synthesized** barbital. Barbital, a depressant, was introduced as a medicine in 1903, followed by phenobarbital in 1913.

Since that time, more than 2,000 similar chemicals have been synthesized, but only about 50 of these have been sold as medicines. As more people took the drugs, the side effects of barbiturates became apparent. An overdose can result in respiratory depression (slowing or stopping normal breathing processes), which can be fatal. Doctors also realized that the barbiturates can be abused. People can become dependent on them, and a serious **withdrawal** syndrome can occur when a person abruptly stops taking the drugs. In the 1960s, the

depressant chemical that slows down or decreases functioning; often used to describe agents that slow the functioning of the central nervous system; such agents are sometimes used to relieve insomnia, anxiety, irritability, and tension

dependence psychological compulsion to use a substance for emotional and/or physical reasons

synthesize to produce artificially or chemically

withdrawal group of physical and psychological symptoms that may occur when a person suddenly stops the use of a substance or reduces the dose of an addictive substance

Barbiturates, which are highly addictive sedative drugs, are created in several steps.

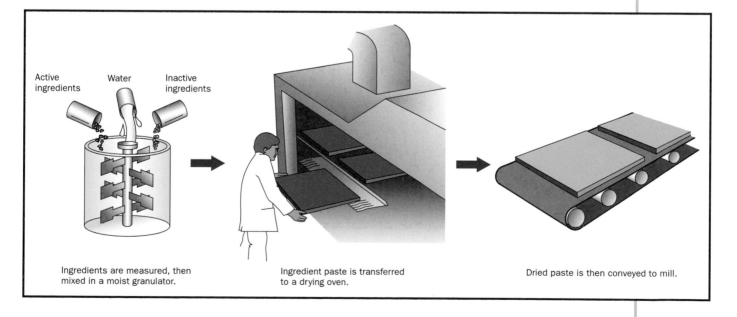

Ingredients are measured, then mixed in a moist granulator.

Ingredient paste is transferred to a drying oven.

Dried paste is then conveyed to mill.

CLASSIFICATION OF BARBITURATES

Drug Class and Generic Names	Trade Names
Ultrashort-Acting:	
methohexital sodium	Brevital
thiamylal sodium	Surital
thiopental sodium	Pentothal
Short-Acting:	
butalbital	
hexobarbital	Sombulex
pentobarbital	Nembutal
secobarbital	Seconal
Intermediate-Acting:	
amobarbital	Amytal
aprobarbital	Alurate
butabarbital	Butisol
talbutal	Lotusate
Long-Acting:	
phenobarbital	Luminal
mephorbarbital	Mebaral

SOURCE: Rall, 1990; Csáky, 1979.

Barbiturates are often called by slang names such as "blue birds" and "pink ladies," but their generic names and brand names are a little harder to pronounce.

euphoria state of intense, giddy happiness and well-being, sometimes occurring baselessly and out of sync with an individual's life situation

introduction of the benzodiazepines, a safer class of hypnotic drugs (drugs that bring on sleep), replaced barbiturates for certain prescribed uses.

Barbiturates are taken by mouth. Injecting the drug is a rare practice among barbiturate abusers. Barbiturates come in brightly colored capsules, with street names such as blue birds, blue clouds, yellow jackets, red devils, sleepers, pink ladies, and Christmas trees. The term "goofball" refers to barbiturates in general. The accompanying table lists the common barbiturates and their trade names.

The Effects of Barbiturates on the Body

Barbiturates work by affecting a neurotransmitter (brain chemical) that normally acts as a brake on the electrical activity of the brain. Barbiturates enhance, or increase, the braking effects of this chemical, causing sedation. The area in the brain called the reticular activating system is responsible for keeping people awake. It is the first area to be affected by the barbiturates. This is why an individual becomes tired and falls asleep after taking a barbiturate.

The various barbiturates differ mainly in how quickly they take effect and how long they keep acting. They can range from ultra-short-acting (taking effect within seconds and lasting a few minutes) to long-acting (taking effect in an hour and lasting six to twelve hours).

The effects of barbiturates range from mild sedation (decreased responsiveness), to hypnosis (sleep), to anesthesia (loss of sensation). A small dose will produce sedation and relieve anxiety and tension; a somewhat larger dose taken in a quiet setting will usually produce sleep; and an even larger dose will produce unconsciousness. How barbiturates affect an individual depends on the user's previous drug experience and the circumstances in which the drug is taken. For example, a dose taken at bedtime may produce sleep, whereas the same dose taken during the daytime may produce a feeling of **euphoria** and interfere with normal motor skills. This is similar in many ways to the effects of alcohol.

Barbiturate-induced sleep resembles normal sleep in many ways, but there are a few important differences. Barbiturates reduce the amount of time spent in rapid eye movement or REM sleep—a very important phase of sleep. Prolonged use of barbiturates causes restlessness during the late stages of sleep. Since the barbiturates remain in the body for some time after a person awakens, a feeling of drowsiness can interfere with judgment and moods for some time after the sedative effects have disappeared.

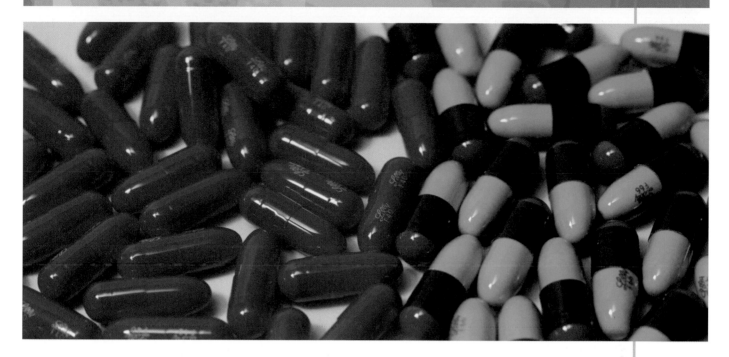

Medical Uses of Barbiturates

Doctors sometimes prescribe barbiturates to promote sleep in patients with insomnia. The general use of barbiturates as sleeping pills has decreased significantly, however, since they have been replaced by the safer benzodiazepines. Phenobarbital and butabarbital are still available as prescription medications used to treat inflammatory disorders. The ultrashort-acting barbiturates (such as thiopental) are given intravenously to induce anesthesia because of how easily and quickly they take effect.

Some barbiturates reduce seizures and so have been used to treat some forms of epilepsy. Phenobarbital is often used in hospital emergency rooms to treat convulsions such as those that develop during tetanus, cerebral hemorrhage (bleeding in the brain), and poisoning by convulsant drugs. The benzodiazepines are, however, gradually replacing the barbiturates in this setting as well.

Tolerance and Dependence

A person who takes barbiturates repeatedly develops tolerance to the drug's effects. This means that more and more drug is needed to achieve the effect the person got from the initial dose. However, tolerance does not develop equally in all of barbiturates' effects. For example, users do not develop tolerance to respiratory depression. Barbiturates reduce the drive to breathe and the processes necessary for maintaining a normal breathing rhythm. A person who takes a barbiturate for its sedative effect develops tolerance to that effect. But the dose now required to achieve that sedative effect has a **toxic**

Barbiturates are usually taken in pill form. They are highly addictive and are characterized with withdrawal symptoms that are worse than those for heroin.

toxic something that is poisonous or dangerous to people

101

effect on the respiratory system. Thus the higher dose can cause death by completely stopping breathing.

If tolerance develops and the amount of drug taken continues to increase, then physical dependence can develop. If the drug is suddenly stopped, withdrawal signs appear. In the case of barbiturates, mild signs of withdrawal include:

- fear
- insomnia
- excitability
- mild tremors (shaking)
- loss of appetite

If the dose was very high, more severe signs of withdrawal can occur, including:

- weakness
- vomiting
- decrease in blood pressure regulatory mechanisms (so that a person might pass out when rising from a lying position)
- increased pulse and respiratory rates
- epileptic seizures or convulsions
- delirium with fever, disorientation, and hallucinations

Unlike withdrawal from the opioids (such as morphine and heroin), withdrawal from central nervous system depressants such as barbiturates can be life threatening. The proper treatment of a barbiturate-dependent individual always includes a slow reduction in the dose to avoid the dangers of rapid **detoxification**.

detoxification
process of removing a poisonous, intoxicating, or addictive substance from the body

Abuse of Barbiturates

Many people who take barbiturates with a doctor's prescription to treat insomnia become dependent to some degree. Some of these individuals abuse the drug by taking increasingly larger doses to get the euphoric effect rather than to get the intended effect of sleepiness. In need of ever more drug, the person may obtain prescriptions from a number of doctors and take them to a number of pharmacists, or may buy the drug from illegal dealers. The person may abuse the drug daily or during binges that last from a day to many weeks at a time. This pattern of using barbiturates for the euphoric effect is more common among people who begin by buying barbiturates from illicit sources than among those who begin by seeking help for insomnia.

People who are dependent on a particular drug often take barbiturates to boost the first drug's effects. Alcohol and heroin are also commonly taken together in this way. Since barbiturates are "downers," people also take them to counteract the unwanted overstimulation that stimulant drugs produce. Abusers of stimulants such as cocaine or amphetamines ("uppers") use barbiturates to come down from the continued high. Also, barbiturates are used to ward off the early signs of withdrawal from alcohol.

Treating Barbiturate Dependence

Doctors must carefully control treatment for barbiturate dependence because of the potential dangers, such as seizures. Withdrawal must be closely supervised. Doctors give the patient phenobarbital or the benzodiazepines—chlordiazepoxide and diazepam—in gradually decreasing doses to reduce the severity of withdrawal symptoms. SEE ALSO ADDICTION: CONCEPTS AND DEFINITIONS; BENZODIAZEPINES.

Beers and Brews

Beers and brews are beverages that are produced by a process called fermentation. In fermentation, yeast is used to change the sugars in a mixture into alcohol. Beer making begins by allowing grains (such as barley) to sprout. These sprouted grains are called malt. Malt is mixed with water and the dried flowers of a vine (hops). Yeast is added to this mixture of malted grains, hops, and water, producing alcohol and carbon dioxide gas (carbonation). Beers generally contain 2 to 9 percent ethyl alcohol, although some may contain as much as 15 percent. Various types and flavors are created by adding different combinations of malts and cereals and allowing the process to continue for varying lengths of time.

Beer was an important food to the people of the Near East probably as far back as 10,000 years ago. The making of beer and of bread developed at the same time. Ancient Egyptians and ancient Romans valued beer, but the ancient Greeks preferred wine. Once the art of brewing reached England, beers and ales became the preferred drink of rich and poor alike. Beer was carried on the Mayflower, and American colonists quickly learned to make their beer with Indian corn. Much U.S. beer is still made with corn, although rice and wheat are also used in the mix with barley malt.

World and U.S. Consumption of Beers and Brews

About 128.6 billion liters of beer were commercially produced in the world in 1997. The United States led the world in beer production, producing 23.6 billion liters of beer in 1997. China followed with 17.0 billion liters, and Germany rounded out the top three in beer production volume with 11.5 billion liters. For the same year, the Czech Republic drank the most beer, consuming 161.4 liters per person. Other countries leading in beer consumption were the Republic of Ireland (152.0 liters per person) and Germany (131.2 liters per person). A 1999 study reported that the United States led the world in beer consumption, consuming over 17 billion liters. The top three brewers for 1997 were Anheuser-Busch, Heineken, and Miller Brewing.

Beer is the preferred form of alcohol among young people in the United States. In a national survey of more than 75,000 students in grades 6–12, conducted in between 2000 and 2001, 24.5 percent of junior high school students and 54.4 percent of senior high school students reported drinking beer in the past year. Among 12th graders, 40 percent reported drinking beer in the past month, compared to 46.4 percent who reported drinking any kind of alcohol in the past month. A recent study of drinking patterns and behavior revealed some interesting insights into beer drinking. The study compared drinkers of beer, wine, and distilled spirits. According to the authors of this study, beer drinking accounts for most of the hazardous alcohol consumption (defined as occasions in which five or more drinks were consumed in a day) reported in the United States. Moreover, hazardous beer consumption is more likely to lead to alcohol-related problems than hazardous consumption of wine or spirits. SEE ALSO ALCOHOL: CHEMISTRY; ALCOHOL: HISTORY OF DRINKING.

Benzodiazepine Withdrawal

benzodiazepine drug developed in the 1960s as a safer alternative to barbiturates; most frequently used as a sleeping pill or an anti-anxiety medication

therapeutic healing or curing

dependent someone who has a psychological compulsion to use a substance for emotional and/or physical reasons

To abruptly stop using **benzodiazepines** may produce a withdrawal syndrome. These withdrawal symptoms include increased anxiety and insomnia (the inability to fall or stay asleep)—the same conditions for which benzodiazepines are generally prescribed. Because the term "withdrawal" is usually applied to drugs of abuse (as opposed to drugs being taken for **therapeutic** reasons), the symptoms that occur when a person stops taking benzodiazepines are sometimes called abstinence syndrome or discontinuance syndrome.

Not all patients who take benzodiazepines will experience withdrawal symptoms when the person stops using the drug. Several factors determine whether the withdrawal symptoms will occur:

1. The benzodiazepine must be taken long enough so that the person has become **dependent** on the drug, producing changes

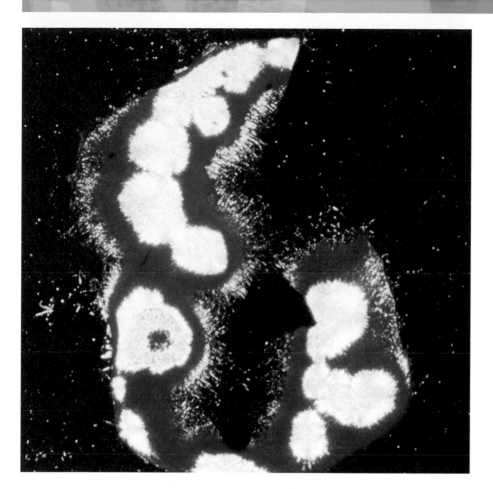

A micrograph of diazepam crystals, known more commonly by its trademarked name Valium. Diazepam is a benzodiazepine that is occasionally prescribed for anxiety disorders.

in the central nervous system that set the stage for withdrawal symptoms. The syndrome can occur after a person takes prescribed doses of benzodiazepines for several weeks to several months. Taking benzodiazepines once or twice during a crisis, or even for several weeks during a period of severe stress, ordinarily does not set the stage for withdrawal symptoms.

2. The dose of drug taken on a daily or nightly basis is also a critical factor. When a person takes more than the prescribed dose, then withdrawal symptoms may develop after a shorter period of use.

3. Stopping benzodiazepines abruptly can cause withdrawal symptoms to arise. Stopping abruptly causes blood levels of the drug to drop rapidly. This, in turn, causes levels of the drug in the central nervous system to drop rapidly. Gradual tapering down of benzodiazepines usually prevents the appearance or reduces the intensity of withdrawal symptoms.

4. The type of benzodiazepine that a person takes is also a factor. Benzodiazepines can be short acting or long acting. Short-acting benzodiazepines are cleared from the body very quickly,

When people stop taking benzodiazepines, they often experience a difficult process with many different withdrawal symptoms. Here are some that commonly occur:

- anxiety
- dizziness, lightheadedness
- headache
- insomnia
- altered taste
- ringing in ears
- confusion
- loss of appetite
- weakness
- poor concentration, memory
- muscle ache, stiffness
- seizures
- irritability
- nausea
- depressed mood
- sensitivity to light
- diarrhea

usually within four to about sixteen hours. In contrast, long-acting benzodiazepines may take anywhere from twenty-four to one hundred or more hours to be cleared from the body. The appearance of withdrawal symptoms depends, in part, on the rapidly decreasing blood level of the drug. As a result, a person who stops taking the short-acting benzodiazepines is more likely to experience withdrawal symptoms.

Symptoms of Benzodiazepine Withdrawal

The major symptoms of withdrawal from benzodiazepines are anxiety, restlessness, and difficulty falling asleep. These symptoms may be mild, causing little more than an annoyance for a few days. Or they may be quite severe and even more intense than the symptoms of anxiety or insomnia for which the drugs were initially prescribed. When the initial symptom, such as anxiety or insomnia, returns in a more severe form, this is known as the rebound symptom. Rebound symptoms usually occur within hours to days of stopping the drug and then gradually fade. In some cases, however, the symptoms may be so intense that the patient takes the benzodiazepine again for relief. The patient may continue to take the drug as a way to treat or prevent withdrawal symptoms, rather than to treat an anxiety or sleep disorder that was the original problem.

People who take benzodiazepines for sleep problems may also develop withdrawal symptoms. Rebound insomnia, the most common symptom, typically occurs on the first night and sometimes the second night after a person stops taking short-acting benzodiazepines. Rebound insomnia may be so intense during these nights that the patient may be unwilling to risk another sleepless night and so returns to taking the benzodiazepine. Rebound insomnia is less common with long-acting benzodiazepines.

If untreated, rebound symptoms can last for many months. When this occurs, it is difficult to determine whether the symptoms are still signs of withdrawal, or are signs that the person's original problem (anxiety, insomnia) has returned.

Sometimes new symptoms that did not exist before the patients took benzodiazepines appear after they stop taking the drug. These are true withdrawal symptoms, and they indicate that the functioning of the person's central nervous system has changed. True withdrawal symptoms include headache, anxiety, insomnia, restlessness, depression, irritability, nausea, loss of appetite, indigestion, and unsteadiness. Patients may also become more sensitive to sounds and smells and have difficulty concentrating.

People who previously have been dependent on benzodiazepines, alcohol, or other **sedative-hypnotic** drugs, such as barbiturates, are more likely to experience withdrawal symptoms after stopping use of benzodiazepines. It is especially important that such patients never stop taking their benzodiazepines abruptly.

Treatment

The best approach to withdrawal symptoms is to prevent them from occurring. Patients should take the medicine only if it is medically necessary, and they should not take larger doses than prescribed. If a person has been taking a prescribed benzodiazepine, that person should very gradually reduce the dose. Patients should never discontinue these medications abruptly if they have been taking them for more than a few weeks on a regular basis.

Even with gradual decrease of the dose, however, some patients may continue to have troubling symptoms. These patients can be treated with anticonvulsants. Alternatively, the person can start benzodiazepine treatment again, taking a long-acting type of the drug and then very gradually reducing the dose.

In Summary

For the great majority of patients, benzodiazepine withdrawal is a mild and brief syndrome. Most doctors agree that the benefits of taking benzodiazepines far outweigh any problems with withdrawal when drug treatment is no longer necessary. SEE ALSO BENZODIAZEPINES; NONABUSED DRUGS WITHDRAWAL; PRESCRIPTION DRUG ABUSE; TOLERANCE AND PHYSICAL DEPENDENCE.

Benzodiazepines

Tranquilizers are drugs that reduce feelings of anxiety and tension. Since the 1960s, benzodiazepines have been popular as prescription medications for the treatment of anxiety. Benzodiazepines are also effective at treating insomnia, an inability to fall asleep or stay asleep, and other sleep disorders. In the 1990s some health-care professionals as well as the public became concerned about the overuse of these drugs and possible complications.

Benzodiazepines that lessen the symptoms of anxiety include chlordiazepoxide (Librium), diazepam (Valium), lorazepam (Ativan), oxazepam (Serenid; Serax), clonazepam (Klonopin), and alprazolam

sedative-hypnotic drug that has a calming and relaxing effect; "hypnotics" induce sleep

Benzodiazepines are better known by the names that drug companies have marketed and trademarked, such as Valium, Ativan, and Rohypnol.

sedative medication that reduces excitement; often called a "tranquilizer"

(Xanax). Benzodiazepines that cause a person to fall asleep and stay asleep include short-acting drugs such as triazolam (Halcion), medium-acting drugs such as temazepam (Restoril), and long-acting drugs such as flurazepam (Dalmane) and nitrazepam (Mogadon).

The Medical Uses of Benzodiazepines

Many medical professionals prescribe benzodiazepines for anxiety, or fear that occurs in a situation where no clear threat exists. Benzodiazepines successfully treat the disorder known as "generalized anxiety," which is often quite severe and comes on without any apparent reason. High-potency benzodiazepines such as Xanax or Klonopin can prevent panic attacks. Tranquilizers can also be used to treat "normal anxiety," the anxiety that people feel when under stress or when challenged by life's problems. In these instances, the reasons for feeling anxious are clear, and the degree of anxiety seems to match the level of the stress the person feels. Because some people need help coping with these symptoms, doctors may prescribe benzodiazepines. Unfortunately, the line between anxiety as a medical disorder and anxiety as a normal response to stress is not always clear. This makes the decision to prescribe benzodiazepines a complicated one. As a result, some doctors avoid prescribing benzodiazepines, while others, particularly psychiatrists, recommend them for many patients.

Similar caution applies to the use of benzodiazepines as sleeping pills. Doctors generally agree on the safety of short-term use of these drugs—for example, for sleep upset by jet lag, severe stress, or shift work. However, doctors do not encourage long-term use in someone who has sleeping problems for long periods.

Benzodiazepines can also be used as **sedatives** before surgical operations, as light anesthetics during operations, and to lessen back pain and muscle spasms, such as those caused by sports injuries. Some benzodiazepines can be used to treat certain forms of epilepsy, a condition in which a person has seizures.

Side Effects of Benzodiazepines

Benzodiazepines, like most drugs, can have unwanted side effects. The most common side effects are drowsiness and tiredness, especially within the first few hours after large doses. People taking these drugs also complain of dizziness, headache, blurred vision, and feelings of unsteadiness. The elderly are particularly sensitive to tranquilizers and may become unsteady on their feet or even mentally confused.

Of course, a person unable to sleep does want a sleeping pill to produce drowsiness. However, the longer-acting benzodiazepines,

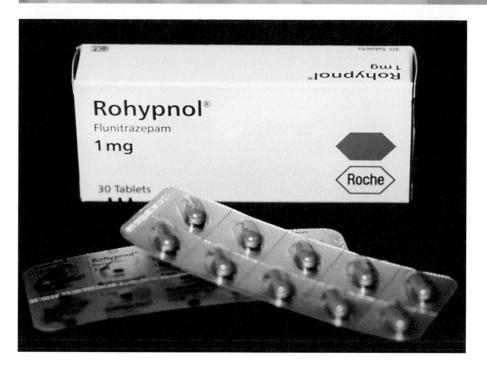

A blue dye has been added to the benzodiazepine Rohypnol (flunitrazepam) in order to make it more noticeable if it is added to a beverage, reducing the risk that an unwilling person will drink it.

and higher doses of medium-duration or short-acting drugs, can leave the person feeling drowsy the morning after taking the pill or even well into the afternoon. Again, the elderly are more likely to experience this continued sleepiness.

Benzodiazepines can interfere with alertness, coordination, performance at skilled work, mental activities, judgment, and memory. Patients should not make important decisions during their initial treatment. Nor should they drive or operate machinery, at least until a doctor assesses their reaction and adjusts the dose if necessary.

As with many drugs affecting the brain, benzodiazepines can interact with other drugs, especially alcohol. People taking tranquilizers or sleeping pills should not drink alcoholic beverages. Benzodiazepines can also enhance, or increase, the effects of antihistamines (such as for hay fever), painkillers, and antidepressants. Cigarette smoking may lessen the effect of some benzodiazepines.

Patients taking benzodiazepines may show responses that are paradoxical—the effects produced are the opposite of those intended. Their anxiety symptoms may worsen rather than lessen, and they have more trouble sleeping. A more disturbing side effect is a feeling of hostility or even aggression. A person's emotional responses might become extreme, such as uncontrollable weeping or giggling. Although these paradoxical effects may not last long, the best course of action is to stop taking the drug.

Benzodiazepines can affect breathing in individuals who already have breathing problems, such as those caused by chronic bronchitis or emphysema. Other occasional side effects include excessive weight gain, rash, problems with sexual functioning, and menstrual irregularities. Pregnant women should avoid benzodiazepines, as there may be a risk to the fetus. In nursing mothers, these drugs pass into breast milk and may sedate the baby. Finally, many people have taken an overdose of a tranquilizer in suicide attempts. Fortunately, these drugs are quite safe, and the person wakes up unharmed after a few hours' sleep.

Finally, benzodiazepines can have a different kind of side effect: They can turn a normal problem in someone's life into a medical problem. For example, taking the drug may lessen a symptom of nervousness, but it cannot solve the underlying problem—which might be an unhappy relationship or an unstable situation at work. In fact, by lessening the symptoms, the individual may feel less motivated to identify, confront, and tackle the basic problem. People can also develop personal problems after difficult events, such as the death of a loved one or a divorce. Events like these need to be worked through and mourned. Benzodiazepines can stop this normal process and actually prevent the individual from coming to terms with loss. For these reasons, benzodiazepines have become controversial as a treatment for certain conditions that are not necessarily medical problems.

Tolerance, Dependence, and Withdrawal

Tolerance to a drug develops when a person needs to increase the dose to achieve the effect of the original dose. When taking tranquilizers, people can become tolerant to the sedative effects. However, patients generally report that the drugs remain effective at controlling symptoms of anxiety. It is not yet clear whether benzodiazepines continue to be effective after long-term daily use. According to patients, side effects usually lessen over time. Problems with memory may continue, but most patients learn to cope with this by using written reminders.

psychosis mental disorder in which an individual loses contact with reality and may have delusions (i.e., unshakable false beliefs) or hallucinations (i.e., the experience of seeing, hearing, feeling, smelling, or tasting things that are not actually present)

Individuals who take benzodiazepines for long periods may become dependent on them, showing signs and symptoms of withdrawal when they stop taking the drugs. Minor symptoms of withdrawal include anxiety, insomnia, and nightmares. Less common and more serious symptoms include **psychosis**, seizures, and, very rarely, death. Serious withdrawal problems are more likely to occur in patients who have taken high doses for four or more months. Stopping the drug gradually can reduce the severity of withdrawal symptoms.

Some withdrawal symptoms that appear after the person stops taking a benzodiazepine may actually be a return of the symptoms for which the drug was originally prescribed. For example, a person who took Valium for anxiety might feel anxious again after he or she stops taking it. Because this is not true withdrawal, doctors sometimes use the term "abstinence syndrome," which is a set of symptoms that occur when a person stops taking a drug.

Although many patients may experience some symptoms of withdrawal, they are not addicted to benzodiazepines. This is because they have taken their medications for medical reasons, as directed by their doctors. It is also very unlikely that they will seek out benzodiazepines once their course of treatment has ended.

Abuse of Benzodiazepines

Patients who take a benzodiazepine drug with a doctor's prescription rarely abuse it by taking more than the recommended dose. However, if abusing the drug, the user may become **intoxicated**, with slurred speech and incoordination, or clumsiness. An estimated 2.7 million people aged 12 or older used tranquilizers such as benzodiazepines for nonmedical purposes in 2000, about the same number as in the previous few years. In 2001 about 6.5 percent of 12th grade students reported using tranquilizers such as benzodiazepines for nonmedical reasons within the past year, an increase from the previous year. Nonmedical use of these drugs increased in 2001 among 10th graders as well.

In general, benzodiazepines have a lower abuse liability—the likelihood that they will be abused—than **barbiturates**, **opiates**, or **stimulants**. However, benzodiazepines are frequently used by individuals who abuse other drugs. Some people with alcohol problems also abuse benzodiazepines. Alcoholics who have had no success in treatment programs for alcohol abuse have high rates of benzodiazepine abuse. People who use stimulant drugs such as cocaine and amphetamines may take benzodiazepines to relieve the nervous feelings that stimulants can produce.

Intravenous injection of benzodiazepines is an increasing problem. Some heroin addicts inject heroin along with benzodiazepines. Injection of benzodiazepines can result in clotting of the veins. It also carries the risk of getting infectious diseases from sharing dirty syringes, such as hepatitis and the AIDS virus. As a result of increased abuse by injection, the United States has established legal controls on the manufacture and prescription of benzodiazepines.

intoxicated state in which a person's physical or mental control has been diminished

barbiturate highly addictive sedative drugs that decrease the activity of the central nervous system

opiate derived directly from opium and used in its natural state, without chemical modification (e.g., morphine, codeine, and thebaine)

stimulant drug that increases activity temporarily; often used to describe drugs that excite the brain and central nervous system

Conclusion

Once hailed as wonder drugs, benzodiazepines were prescribed widely and for long periods of time. Health-care professionals now better understand the risks as well as the benefits of these medicines. For short-term treatment in the severely anxious and sleepless, they are still useful—although new and better drugs continue to be investigated and developed. SEE ALSO ADDICTION: CONCEPTS AND DEFINITIONS; ANXIETY; COMPLICATIONS FROM INJECTING DRUGS; SEDATIVE AND SEDATIVE-HYPNOTIC DRUGS; SLEEPING PILLS.

Betel Nut

stimulant drug that increases activity temporarily; often used to describe drugs that excite the brain and central nervous system

Betel nut, the seed of the betel palm, is prepared with other substances as a mixture for chewing. It is similar to chewing gum. More than 200 million people in areas of the western Pacific and parts of Africa and Asia chew or suck on betel nut for its mild **stimulant** effects. Its effects in some ways resemble those of nicotine. Others use it as a part of social customs, much as people in the West use alcohol. Regular use can damage the mouth, gums, and esophagus, stain the teeth red, and can cause **physical dependence**.

physical dependence condition that may occur after prolonged use of a particular drug or alcohol, in which the user's body cannot function normally without the presence of the substance; when the substance is not used or the dose is decreased, the user experiences uncomfortable physical symptoms

Betel nut is mentioned in ancient Greek, Sanskrit, and Chinese texts from more than a century B.C.E. Later it became an important aspect of the economy and social life in India, Malaysia, the Philippines, and New Guinea. Betel was probably brought to Europe by Marco Polo, around 1300, and became an important item in trade.

Bhang

Bhang, a word from Hindi, is a name given to the hemp plant (also the source of the active agent in marijuana) and its products. In India, people use bhang to make a beverage called *thandaii*. It is also used to make desserts and ice cream. Bhang is often served at weddings or religious festivals and is freely available from sidewalk stands in the major cities. Bhang can also be smoked. Bhang users report that it causes a high similar to that of marijuana, although much milder. SEE ALSO MARIJUANA.

Binge Drinking

A binge is a relatively short period of excessive behavior. For example, someone might go on an eating binge and consume an entire box of cookies and a whole bag of chips, or a shopping binge and buy many more items than the person can use or afford. Recently, binge drinking has become an increasing cause of concern. Dr. Henry Wechsler, the lead investigator of the Harvard School of Public Health College Alcohol Study, defined a binge episode as having five or more drinks on a single occasion for males, and four or more drinks on a single occasion for females. In this definition, a drink refers to the amount of alcohol found in a 12-ounce can or bottle of beer or wine cooler, a 4-ounce glass of wine, or a 1.25-ounce shot of liquor.

National surveys have used similar definitions to reveal patterns of drinking among adolescents and young adults in the 1990s. These surveys have revealed some troubling information about the extent of binge drinking and the negative consequences of drinking among young people. Although many people disagree with the use of the label of "binge drinking," occasional heavy drinking appears to be especially common during the period when adolescents enter adulthood.

The Patterns of Binge Drinking

Most middle and high school students and many college students drink little or no alcohol. However, some underage drinkers consume alcohol in large amounts. According to one study, the percentage of students who binge increases steadily from middle school to college. By 12th grade, nearly one-third of students report having consumed five or more drinks in a row in the last two weeks. Students who leave home to attend college drink more heavily than those who enter the workforce. Four out of ten college students (44 percent) have binged in the last two weeks. Half of this group (23 percent of the total) are frequent binge drinkers, binging three or more times in two weeks. These percentages tell only part of the story, for 19 percent of college students abstain from drinking, and another 36 percent drink lightly or moderately. Increasingly, however, students are drinking in more risky ways. Not only is the number of students who report frequent binge drinking growing, but the number who say that they drink in order to get drunk (48 percent) has also gone up in recent years.

Binge drinking is more common among certain groups of people. For example, male students are more likely to binge drink than female students, and white students binge more frequently than do African-American students. In addition, binge drinking is related to social and cultural groups. People who have a strong religious commitment have lower rates of drinking. In contrast, people who belong to fraternities or sororities (college social clubs) and are involved

PERCENTAGE OF PEOPLE REPORTING HEAVY ALCOHOL USE IN THE PAST MONTH BY AGE IN 1999 AND 2000

Age Category	"Binge" Alcohol Use 1999	2000
Total for all ages	20.2	20.6
12	1.1	1
13	2.5	3
14	6.4	6
15	11.7	12.6
16	17.3	17.9
17	21.5	22.9
18	29.9	30.9
19	36.3	34.8
20	38.4	38.5
21	44.9	45.2

NOTE: "Binge" alcohol use is defined as drinking five or more drinks on the same occasion on at least 1 day in the past 30 days.

SOURCE: SAMHSA, Office of Applied Studies, National Household Survey on Drug Abuse, 1999 and 2000. <http://www.samhsa.gov/oas/NHSDA/2kNHSDA/appendixf2.htm#f.42>.

Binge drinking is associated with a loss of control that can put drinkers at higher risk for unplanned sex, contracting sexually transmitted diseases, and physical injury.

The percentage of students who drink heavily enough to count as having "binged" increases dramatically between high school and college.

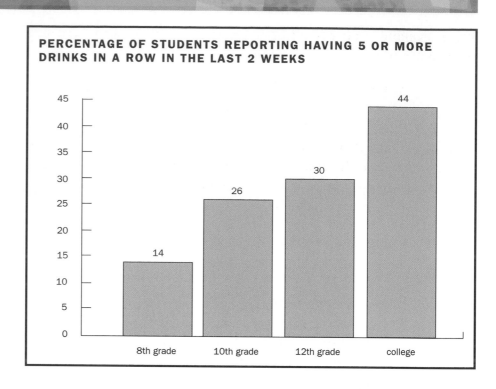

PERCENTAGE OF STUDENTS REPORTING HAVING 5 OR MORE DRINKS IN A ROW IN THE LAST 2 WEEKS

in athletics appear to drink more heavily. Academic performance tends to be associated with drinking patterns—heavier drinkers tend to get poorer grades in school.

The Reasons for Drinking

Drinking alcohol has long been considered a "rite of passage" or a normal step on the way to adulthood. Experimentation with drinking is one way to explore adult behaviors. The most common reasons for drinking given by high-school students suggest that they are simply curious. Over half say that the most important reasons for drinking are to have a good time with friends, and to experiment with the effects of alcohol. Nearly as many say they drink alcohol for other positive reasons: in order to feel good or high, because it tastes good, and because it relaxes them. However, a quarter of high-school seniors indicate that they drink alcohol because they are bored, they have nothing else to do, or they are trying to get away from problems. When drinking is being used to escape or avoid something, this can be a warning sign for future problems with alcohol.

Other reasons why young people may drink heavily have to do with general influences in the world around them. Many young people perceive that social **norms** support underage drinking. They base this perception on the information they have available to them. For example, if social events that involve drinking by peers are publicized and talked about more often than social events that do not in-

norm behavior, custom, or attitude that is considered normal, or expected, within a certain social group

volve drinking, students will perceive that the social norm supports drinking.

Also, research has shown that young people tend to overestimate how much and how often their peers drink. As a result, some students binge drink not because they like drinking alcohol that much, but because they feel that it is expected of them by their peer group. They also overestimate the approval they think they will gain from peers for drinking and drunken behavior. The mistaken belief that "everybody does it" may create an environment that encourages binge drinking.

The Negative Consequences of Binge Drinking

Binge drinking causes concern because it can have negative consequences. Drinking large quantities of alcohol places both the drinker and others around him or her in danger. Heavy drinking also affects the way people behave and think. In surveys of high-school seniors and college students, the most common negative consequence mentioned by both groups is doing something you later regret (52 percent for high school, 35 percent for college). In addition, many students who drink report that drinking has interfered with their ability to think clearly and keep up with their school work, and that drinking has hurt relationships with friends and family. Over 1 in 10 college drinkers report being hurt or injured as a result of their drinking since the beginning of the school year. Drinking in binges increases the chances of an alcohol-related injury: only 4 percent of non-binge drinkers but 26 percent of frequent binge drinkers report getting hurt or injured.

Binge drinkers, and especially frequent binge drinkers, are significantly more likely to experience negative effects of drinking alcohol. Despite the fact that the majority of college students are under the legal age to drink (21 in the United States), a surprising number of students report multiple (more than one) alcohol-related problems. Although only 3.5 percent of non-binge drinkers have experienced five or more problems since the beginning of the school year, almost 17 percent of occasional binge drinkers and nearly half (48 percent) of frequent binge drinkers reported five or more problems affecting their social relationships, personal well-being, or physical health. Examples of such problems include drinking and driving, engaging in activities that resulted in damaged property, injuries, decreased attendance at classes, and falling behind in class work.

Binge drinkers are more likely than non-binge drinkers to engage in behaviors that involve **risk**, including the risk of death. As a result,

risk increased probability of something negative happening

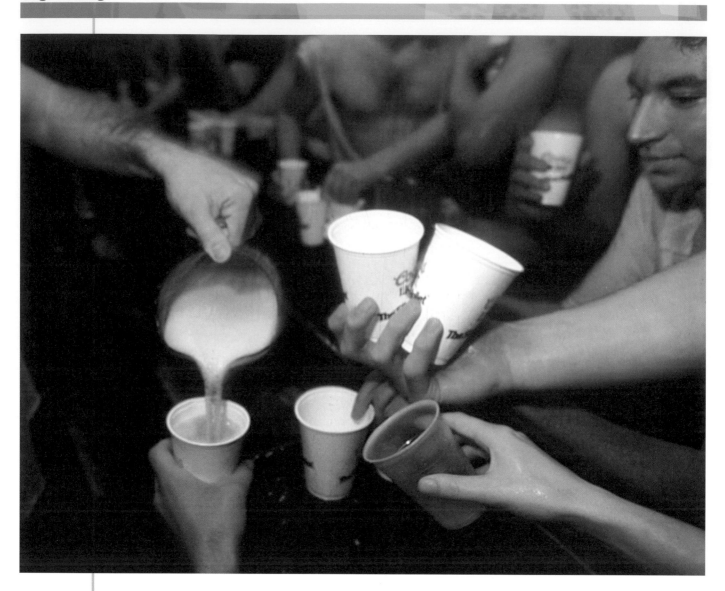

A student pours beer into cups at a "Kegs and Eggs" party. Studies show that students overestimate the amount of respect that they will get for drinking heavily, which becomes a factor in drinking games and other social occasions.

the people around them are more likely to experience the negative consequences of those behaviors. Many high-school seniors and college students report driving after drinking (19 percent for high school, 29 percent for college), a dangerous behavior for drivers, passengers, and others sharing the road with them. Binge drinkers are more likely than non-binge drinkers to report having unplanned sex and not using protection when they had sex. These behaviors carry risks of unintended pregnancy as well as sexually transmitted diseases such as HIV. In addition, drinking games continue to be popular among heavier drinkers. Because drinking games do not allow participants to control how much they drink, these games increase all of the risks of being drunk.

Even for students who do not binge drink, the presence of binge drinking around them can have unpleasant effects. Over half (60 percent) of college students who do not drink or who drink lightly have had their studies interrupted or lost sleep because of the drinking of other students. Nearly half (48 percent) have had to take care of a drunken student, and many (29 percent) have reported being insulted or humiliated by another student who was drunk. Considering the cases of vandalism and property damage to dormitories and physical assaults attributed to drunkenness, it is clear that binge drinking can affect the living and working environment of all students.

A Controversial Idea

The term "binge drinking" and its definition have caused a great deal of disagreement and controversy. Critics raise four major issues:

1. The term "binge drinking" has been used to describe at least two separate drinking styles. People who have worked in treatment facilities for addictions use the term "binge" to mean an extended period of excessive, alcoholic-style drinking. Many in the general population understand a binge to mean several days of out-of-control drinking, during which a person neglects responsibilities. As a result, using the same term to refer to consuming five drinks in one evening is confusing to people. In addition, some students reject being called binge drinkers because they do not feel that they drink alcohol irresponsibly.

2. Some people assume that binge drinking means drinking to the point of drunkenness, but this is incorrect. Drunkenness, or intoxication, is usually measured in terms of **blood alcohol concentration (BAC)**. Many factors affect BAC: how many drinks a person consumes, weight, gender, and the time taken to consume the drinks. Critics point out that it is possible for a 180-pound man to consume five drinks over several hours and never become intoxicated. In fact, studies have shown that many people who would be considered binge drinkers based on their last drinking event would not reach a BAC that indicated intoxication. Therefore, the number of drinks a person has consumed is not enough information to determine whether or not a person is intoxicated.

3. Some critics argue that binge drinking does not always have negative consequences. For example, a heavy drinker may still be on the honor roll. Although frequent binge drinkers are more likely, on the whole, to have alcohol-related problems, some individuals never do. Critics conclude that the effects of drinking for any given person must be evaluated on an individual basis.

4. Finally, defining binge drinking as five drinks in a row (four for women) has been criticized because it defines such a common

blood alcohol concentration (BAC) amount of alcohol in the bloodstream, expressed as the grams of alcohol per deciliter of blood; as BAC goes up, the drinker experiences more psychological and physical effects

behavior. If 44 percent of college students binged in the last two weeks, does that mean that nearly half of college undergraduates are problem drinkers? If binge drinking is almost normal for college students, then should it be a concern? There are two responses to these questions. First, students who binge drink do report significantly more negative experiences related to their drinking. Although not all of these problems are severe, they accumulate to reduce life satisfaction for many students. Second, heavier drinkers run risks related to higher BACs that lighter drinkers do not. While it is possible to run risks and never experience the negative outcome, it is hard to predict when a risk might turn into a real problem. Many people take risks, and only a few experience car crashes, or accidental injuries, or alcohol poisoning. However, binge drinkers do put themselves at greater risk for these outcomes.

The Dangers

Clearly, some adolescents and young adults are taking experimentation with alcohol to extremes. Almost half of drinkers in college report drinking for the purpose of getting drunk. Being drunk implies a lack of control over one's ability to make sound judgments, manage one's emotions, and maintain physical coordination. In addition, more than a quarter of college students have experienced an alcohol-induced blackout—forgetting where they were or what they did. Thus, binge drinking can result in BACs high enough to hurt the brain's ability to function. Regular drinking to intoxication increases the risks of harm to the drinker and those around him or her. Thus, binge drinking is cause for concern when it results in high BACs and intoxication. The frequency of binge drinking may be creating a climate in which heavy drinking and drunkenness are tolerated and considered acceptable.

tolerance condition in which higher and higher doses of a drug or alcohol are needed to produce the effect or "high" experienced from the original dose

physical dependence condition that may occur after prolonged use of a particular drug or alcohol, in which the user's body cannot function normally without the presence of the substance; when the substance is not used or the dose is decreased, the user experiences uncomfortable physical symptoms

Another danger of binge drinking is the development of **tolerance**. A drinker who is tolerant to alcohol must consume more drinks to achieve the positive, social, relaxing effects of alcohol. Tolerance to the many behavioral effects of alcohol develops at different rates, so that feeling unaffected by a given number of drinks does not always mean, for example, that one's reaction times or coordination are intact. Regardless of the perceived effects of alcohol, drinking higher quantities results in higher BACs, and more risk of being impaired in undesirable ways. Developing a tolerance to greater amounts of alcohol is a process that can result in **physical dependence** on alcohol. Once a person is dependent on alcohol, it is extremely difficult to stop drinking, even though a person may wish to quit.

In Summary

Although binge drinking does not always mean that a person is dangerously drunk or has an alcohol-abuse problem, consuming large quantities of alcoholic beverages in short periods of time is a risky behavior. In the short term, people who binge drink may feel tired and sick the next day, have conflicts with family and friends, suffer from injuries, or even die as a result of excessive drinking. In the long-term, heavy drinking may lead a person to rely on alcohol to have a good time and to develop tolerance to and physical dependence on alcohol. Despite a minimum legal drinking age of 21 in the United States, adolescents and young adults experiment with alcohol, drink enough to cause intoxication, and experience problems linked to their alcohol use. Prevention programs are needed to promote less risky drinking behavior. SEE ALSO ACCIDENTS AND INJURIES FROM ALCOHOL; ALCOHOL: CHEMISTRY; ALCOHOL: POISONING; BLOOD ALCOHOL CONCENTRATION; DIAGNOSIS OF DRUG AND ALCOHOL ABUSE: AN OVERVIEW.

Blood Alcohol Concentration

When a person drinks alcohol, the alcohol is absorbed from the stomach and small intestine into the bloodstream. The amount of alcohol in the blood is called blood alcohol concentration (BAC). As blood travels to the brain, the alcohol in the blood produces the signs and symptoms of inebriation, or drunkenness. BAC is expressed as the weight of alcohol in a fixed volume of blood, for example, grams per liter.

In addition to how much a person drinks, several factors affect the amount of alcohol in the blood. Eating along with drinking alcohol decreases the amount of alcohol that can be quickly absorbed into the blood. Having more than one drink in an hour causes the BAC to increase rapidly. The percentage of body fat in a person's total weight also affects BAC. More fat means less body water into which the alcohol can distribute, thus increasing BAC. This is why women

CONCENTRATIONS OF ALCOHOL (ETHANOL) IN BLOOD FOR LEGAL PURPOSES

Concentration Unit	Country	Legal Limit
Percent weight/volume (% w/v)	United States	0.10 g/100 ml
Milligrams per 100 milliliter (mg/dl)	Britain	80 mg/100 ml
Milligrams per milliliter (mg/ml)	Netherlands	0.50 mg/ml
Milligrams per gram (mg/g)	Sweden	0.20 mg/g
Milligrams per gram (mg/g)	Norway	0.50 mg/g

The legally acceptable amount of alcohol in the blood varies among countries.

As blood alcohol concentration increases, people's abilities decrease.

THE EFFECTS OF BLOOD ALCOHOL LEVELS ON PEOPLE

BAL	(BAC)	Effects
50	(0.05%)	There may be no observable effects on behavior, but thought, judgment, and restraint may be more lax and vision is affected. More errors in tasks that require divided attention such as more steering errors, and increased likelihood of causing an accident.
80	(0.08%)	Reaction time for deciding and acting increases. Motor skills are impaired. The likelihood of a crash increases to three to four times the likelihood when sober.
100	(0.10%)	Six times as likely to be involved in a crash. Reaction time to sights and sounds increases. Physical and mental coordination are impaired; movement becomes noticeably clumsy.
150	(0.15%)	Twenty-five times as likely to be involved in a crash. Reaction time increases significantly, especially in tasks that require divided attention. Difficulty performing simple motor skills. Physical difficulty in driving.
200	(0.20%)	One hundred times as likely to be involved in a crash. Motor area of brain significantly depressed, and all perception and judgment distorted. Difficulty standing, walking, and talking. Driving erratic.
300	(0.30%)	Confusion and stupor; inability to track a moving object with the eyes. Passing out is likely.
400	(0.40%)	Coma is likely.
450–500	(0.45–0.50%)	Death is likely.

SOURCE: Mothers Against Drunk Driving (MADD) and the National Safety Council.

---

generally have a higher BAC than men after having the same number of drinks.

Laws in the United States establish limits on how high a person's BAC can be while driving. The legal limit in the United States is 0.10 grams per 100 milliliters of blood, or a BAC of 0.10 percent. Some state laws set an even lower BAC. Law enforcement officers use Breathalyzer machines to measure BAC. The measurement of alcohol concentration in the breath is converted into a measurement of alcohol concentration in the blood. SEE ALSO ALCOHOL: CHEMISTRY; BREATHALYZER; DRIVING, ALCOHOL, AND DRUGS; DRUG TESTING METHODS AND ANALYSIS.

Boot Camps and Shock Incarceration

Boot camps, also known as shock incarceration programs, are short-term prison programs run like military basic training for young criminal offenders. Most programs target young offenders convicted of nonviolent crimes such as drug possession or sale, burglary, or theft. Participation is limited to those who do not have an extensive past history of criminal activity. Most programs require participants to sign an agreement saying they have volunteered. They are given information about the program and the difference between a boot-camp prison and a traditional prison. The major incentive for entering the

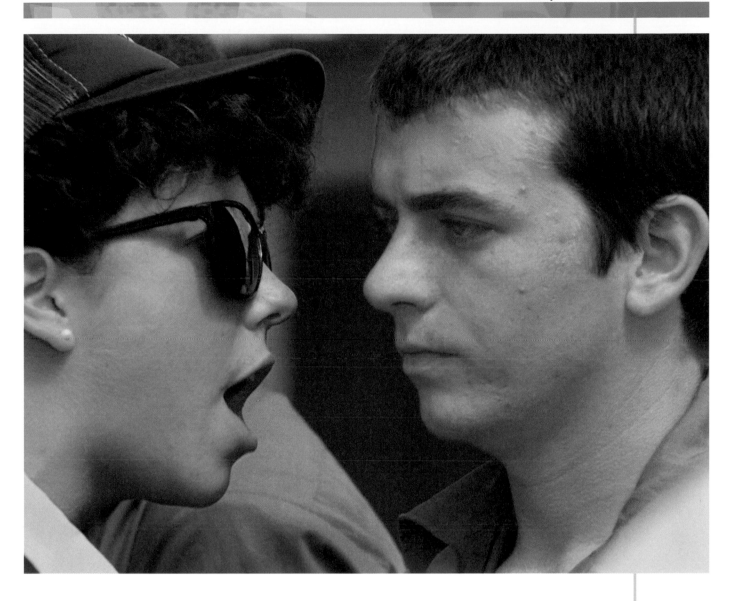

boot camp is that the boot camp requires a shorter term in prison than a traditional prison sentence.

Boot-camp prisons were first established in Georgia and Oklahoma in 1983, and since then all states and many counties have adopted this type of program. In the 1980s the number of convicted criminals rose sharply, and prisons became severely overcrowded. In addition, there were not enough probation officers to supervise the large numbers of offenders who were sentenced to probation in the community rather than jail time. Young offenders on probation were in special need of better supervision. Boot-camp prisons were developed in response to these problems. By 1999, more than 50 boot camps housed about 4,500 juveniles. Some boot camps house adult felons. The majority of boot camps have male participants, but some programs do admit women along with men. Other states have developed separate boot-camp prisons for women.

Authority is re-established and exercised upon entrance to boot camp.

Aspects of the Program

The first day of the boot camp involves a difficult in-take process, when the drill instructors confront the inmates. Inmates are given rapid orders about the rules of the camp, when they can speak, how they are to address the drill instructors, and how to stand at attention. The men have their heads shaved; the women are given short haircuts. This early period of time in the boot camp is physically and mentally stressful for most inmates.

Inmates of most boot camps are required to wake before dawn each day, clean their living quarters, and march to an exercise area to participate in rigorous physical training. During the day they practice military drill and ceremony, and perform six to eight hours of hard labor such as cleaning parks or public roads. They march to every meal and stand at parade rest while waiting to be served. After dinner, they attend rehabilitation programs until 9 P.M., when they return to their dormitories. Inmates are allowed few personal possessions, no televisions, and infrequent visits from relatives on the outside.

rehabilitation
process of restoring a person to a condition of health or useful activity

In other types of boot camps, offenders spend less time on work and military drill and a great deal of time in **rehabilitation** programs. Some camps emphasize academic education, while others focus on group counseling or treatment for substance abuse.

The correctional officers in the programs are referred to as drill instructors and are responsible for ensuring that inmates obey the rules and participate in all activities. When speaking to staff, inmates must refer to themselves as "this inmate." They must precede and follow each sentence with sir or madam, as in "Sir, yes, sir." Inmates who are disobedient are punished immediately, often in the form of additional physical activity, such as push-ups or sit-ups. Inmates who commit more serious rule violations may be dismissed from the program.

The programs last from 90 to 180 days. Those dismissed prior to graduation are considered program failures. They are either sent immediately to a traditional prison to serve a longer term of incarceration or they are returned to court for resentencing.

Offenders who successfully complete the boot camp participate in an elaborate graduation ceremony, in which inmates demonstrate the military drills they have practiced. Many programs encourage family members to attend the graduation ceremony. After graduating, offenders are supervised in the community for the rest of their sentence. Some programs closely supervise all offenders who successfully complete the boot camp; others offer a looser form of supervision similar to that of traditional probation sentences.

Program officials worry that graduates may have a difficult time making the transition from the rigid structure of the boot camps to the community environment. For this reason, some boot camps developed aftercare programs to help graduates make the change. These aftercare programs provide drug treatment, job counseling, academic education, and/or short-term housing.

Drug Treatment in Boot Camps

The earliest boot camps focused on discipline and hard work. More recently, they have begun to emphasize treatment and education. Corrections officials realized that many of the entrants were using drugs or involved in the drug trade. They realized that the punishment alone would not reduce drug use among these offenders. As a result, they introduced drug treatment or education into the daily schedule of boot-camp activities.

The type of treatment and the amount of time devoted to substance-abuse treatment varies greatly among programs. The ninety-day Florida program includes only fifteen days of treatment and education. In contrast, in the New York program, all offenders receive 180 days of treatment. In the New York program, each platoon in the boot camp forms a small community. They meet daily to solve problems and to discuss their progress in the shock program. They spend over 200 hours during the six-month program in substance-abuse treatment activity. The treatment is based on the Alcoholics Anonymous ☎ and Narcotics Anonymous ☎ strategies for recovery from addiction. All boot-camp inmates participate in the substance-abuse treatment regardless of their history of use and abuse.

Like New York's program, the Illinois boot camp also targets substance abusers. However, in Illinois different levels of treatment are provided to inmates depending on their needs. Inmates with no history of substance abuse receive only two weeks of education. Inmates who are identified as probable substance abusers receive four weeks of treatment in addition to drug education. Inmates considered to have serious drug addictions receive ten weeks of education and treatment. In addition to drug education and group therapy, they receive group sessions on substance-abuse **relapse**, **codependence**, family addiction, and roles within the family.

Pros and Cons

One problem with boot camps is that many participants are dismissed from the program. Depending upon the program, rates of dismissal vary from 8 percent to as much as 80 percent. In terms of their

☎ See *Organizations of Interest* at the back of Volume 1 for address, telephone, and URL.

relapse term used in substance abuse treatment and recovery that refers to an addict's return to substance use and abuse following a period of abstinence or sobriety

codependence situation in which someone, often a family member, has an unhealthy dependence on an individual with an addiction (e.g., to alcohol or gambling); the relationship is often characterized as "enabling" the addict to continue his or her addiction

Crossing a snowy river on a rope bridge in Glacier National Park, Montana, this drug rehabilitation program student learns about survival in nature as well as in addiction.

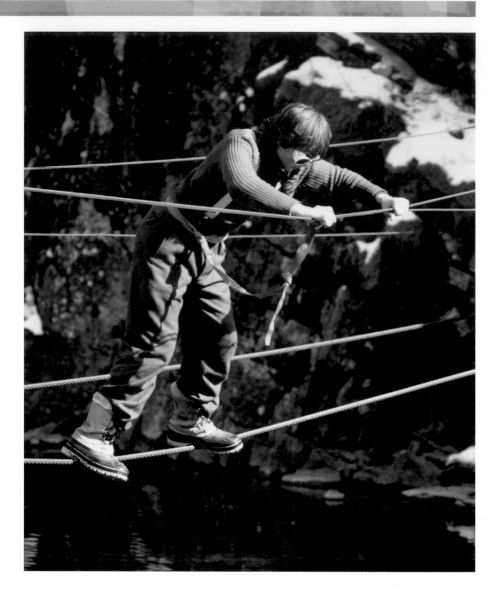

return to criminal activity, graduates of boot-camp prisons do not appear to perform better than offenders who served longer terms in prison or were sentenced to probation. Some programs have more success than others, but overall the results have been disappointing. The boot camps' military atmosphere alone does not appear to reduce repeat criminal activity. For drug-involved offenders, the drug-treatment therapy provided during the program and the aftercare treatment provided during community supervision do appear to be effective.

Studies conducted for the U.S. Justice Department found that the rate of repeat criminal activity for boot-camp graduates ranged from 64 to 75 percent. For those who served their time in traditional prisons, the rate ranged from 63 to 71 percent. Though juveniles often responded well while in the camps, they returned to the same neighborhoods where they first got into trouble. Colorado, North Dakota, and Arizona ended their programs, and Georgia, where boot-camp prisons started, is phasing out its camps.

Boot-camp prisons have sparked controversy. Critics point to evidence that this type of regimen does not reduce the likelihood that young offenders will commit more criminal acts after their release. Critics have also argued that participants may leave the boot-camp prison angry and damaged by punishments and verbal abuse, and that the military atmosphere designed to make a cohesive fighting unit may not be appropriate for these young offenders. In the late 1990s, state and federal prosecutors investigated allegations of abuse and misconduct by prison camp staff. By 2000 several states had either ended their programs or drastically reduced the size of their programs.

Advocates of the boot camp say that the program teaches discipline and responsibility. They argue that the strong relationship between the offenders and the drill instructors may be helpful to the inmates. Also, some aspects of the boot camps may be particularly helpful for drug-involved offenders. Although controversy exists about the boot-camp prisons, correctional officials still consider this type of "tough love" approach a good alternative to traditional prison terms. SEE ALSO LAW AND POLICY: COURT-ORDERED TREATMENT; LAW AND POLICY: HISTORY OF, IN THE UNITED STATES; TREATMENT TYPES: AN OVERVIEW.

Brain Chemistry

The brain is a chemical powerhouse, with each of its several billion cells churning out messages in the form of molecules, stored and ready to go. Precisely released in exquisitely tiny amounts, these molecular messages control the workings of the entire body. And it is the chemical nature of brain activity that reacts and adjusts to a person's use of an addicting drug.

The basic building block of the body's nervous system is the neuron, a cell with long fibers that make contact with other neurons. In spite of the fact that most of the signaling activity of a neuron is electrical, neurons use chemical messengers to communicate with each other. This is because neurons do not actually touch each other. Instead, they use different molecules to send messages that end up causing other neurons to either stay quiet, or activate an electric current. In turn, the current in the second neuron will cause more chemical messages to flow.

The body of the neuron is pretty ordinary in size as far as cells go, but the thin fibers reaching out from each neuron make this type of cell remarkable. Most cells in the body are of such small dimensions that they show up only under a microscope. But some neurons, while still not visible to the unaided eye, have to extend several feet, in order to let the brain know, for instance, what the big toe is doing.

Chemistry Carries the Message

Each neuron, when activated, will release molecules from the business end of its output fiber, the axon, to continue a message. The molecules must cross the microscopic gap that separates the end of the axon from the next nerve cell, a space called the synapse.

Many of the molecules that are released in synapses, the so-called neurotransmitters, have already been studied in detail. While more than 20 different molecules are known to serve as neurotransmitters, scientists believe that even more await discovery. Still, it is a single molecule, dopamine, that has been identified as the neurotransmitter responsible for addictive behavior.

When the nerve ending of one neuron meets the end of another neuron, the junction is called a synapse. Special chemicals, called neurotransmitters, are released, which meet and activate receptors.

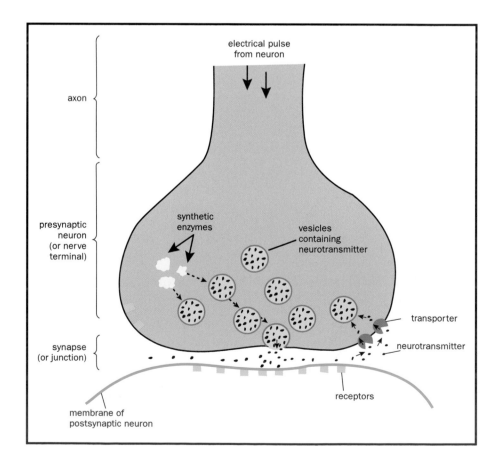

Dopamine. Neuroscientists have found that dopamine plays a key role in registering pleasure (allowing the person to feel pleasurable sensations), and that all drugs with addictive properties appear to affect dopamine transmission in the nervous system. The reason for all addictions, they say, lies in the particular way that dopamine is placed within, and controlled within, the brain. Dopamine serves as a key transmitter in those regions of the brain that scientists find are associated with creating pleasurable sensations. These regions include cell clusters within the middle of the brain, involved in emotions.

In these regions, dopamine is released when the neurons that make it are activated. Dopamine is immediately swept up from the narrow synaptic spaces between nerve cells after it spills from the sending neurons. The clean-up mechanism is perfectly tuned to react if more than the usual amount of dopamine is present, gearing up instantly

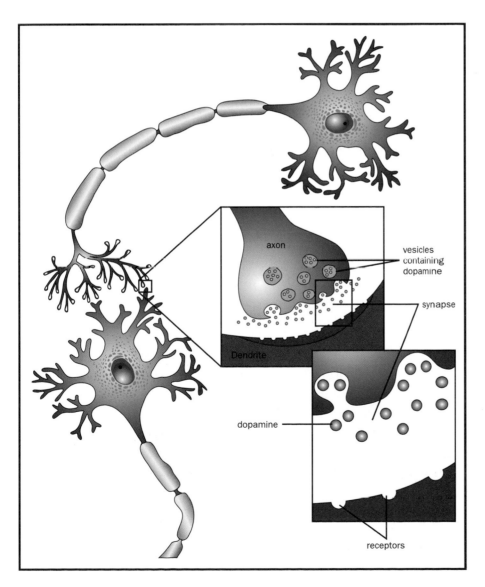

Dopamine is a neurotransmitter that many scientists believe is key to understanding addictions, because it allows people to feel pleasure.

to remove even more of it. This so-called reuptake mechanism also downshifts to low gear if less than the usual amount of dopamine is present.

In addition, receptors on the receiving neuron respond to maintain dopamine transmission. The receptor molecules for each neurotransmitter will respond to the message, with a change of shape. Triggered by the binding of the incoming transmitter molecule, the receptor rearranges itself to fit tightly to the messenger. By altering itself, the receptor sends its own signal. In turn, the messenger adjusts a set of reactions going on inside the receiving cell. In this way, the receptor carries the message along. Perhaps the next cell, as a result, will fire off its own message more readily, or more slowly.

If a receptor for a particular transmitter is present on the next cell across a synapse, that transmitter's message will be passed along. Dopamine receptors are able to respond instantly to how much dopamine is actually in use. They will be pulled from service if a lot of dopamine is let loose. On the other hand, more receptors will be sent to the synaptic front if a dopamine shortage is sensed.

Thus the chemical balance within the nervous system is kept in tight control. The brain and nerves try to stay in a stable state so that the body runs smoothly and reacts just so to what it needs to sense. Addiction is a disturbance of the nervous system's chemistry, and actually is the result of the body's attempts to bring itself back into chemical balance.

Opiates as an Addicting Example

Morphine, heroin, and codeine are examples of addicting substances. They are known as opiates, because they are made from the opium poppy. In a person who takes one of these drugs, the brain's response to the first dose changes with repeated doses.

A dose of morphine will enter the brain through the bloodstream. There, at synapses, a receptor sees and recognizes the morphine molecule, which looks a lot like certain molecules normally present in the brain. Morphine binds to these opiate receptors, studding the surface of dopamine-making neurons. Contact with the morphine molecules in turn prods these neurons to release dopamine. Because the brain likes to stay in chemical balance, it responds to a flooding of outside substances by cutting back on certain aspects of its own chemistry. Responses to the excess dopamine must be scaled back.

Here then is the essence of addiction. Addicting drugs resemble, at the molecular level, neurotransmitters that are made by the body itself. In turn, most if not all of these substances eventually alter dopamine. But the brain and nervous system throughout the body fight to maintain the usual level of chemical activity, and the balance of dopamine.

When morphine is added, and dopamine floods receptors, the reuptake mechanism goes into overdrive. Then, when the morphine is finally broken down by the body's metabolism, revved-up reuptake leaves the fewer receptors empty. This translates into the feelings that make the user crave more drug. The more morphine taken, the more reuptake, the fewer receptors, and the greater the interruption of dopamine transmission when the morphine is stopped.

An opiate abuser who abruptly stops taking the drug goes through a **withdrawal** syndrome. The symptoms of opiate withdrawal include anxiety, restlessness, yawning, flu-like symptoms including muscle and bone pain, diarrhea, wakefulness, vomiting, chills and goose bumps, and involuntary movement of the legs. All aspects of withdrawal are the **physiological** opposite of the initial effects of the drug: at first morphine causes sleepiness, relaxation, constipation, lessened sensation of pain, and, because of the dopamine release, euphoria (a feeling of intense well-being). It takes days to weeks to get the synapse back into **metabolic** balance after opiate abuse ends, depending on the dose that the user had built up to and how long the abuse had continued.

A person who steadily uses morphine develops tolerance to the drug. This means that more and more drug is needed to produce the same effect of the original dose. A tolerant morphine user can take massive doses that would kill a first-time user. The usual dose of morphine prescribed for medical purposes is 5 to 20 milligrams. However, cancer patients as well as street addicts may take several hundred milligrams a day. In extreme cases, thousands of grams a day of morphine may be taken.

Another Example: Cocaine

Cocaine, a drug that is rapidly addicting, also causes a person to feel pleasure because of its action on dopamine. In the case of cocaine, the reuptake mechanism itself is directly affected. Cocaine molecules bind especially well to the uptake molecules that normally sweep released dopamine back into the neuron that let it out. Cocaine essentially blocks the reuptake process by occupying the reuptake sites. As a result, dopamine stays in the synapses. Increased impulses spread out from the reward circuit when cocaine is present. But the reaction of the reuptake mechanism to too much dopamine is to boost the

withdrawal group of physical and psychological symptoms that may occur when a person suddenly stops the use of a substance or reduces the dose of an addictive substance

physiological the functions and activities of life on a biological level

metabolic describing or related to the chemical processes through which the cells of the body break down substances to produce energy

number of reuptake molecules. Once the cocaine is gone, the synapses are so empty of dopamine that the user feels an immediate and intense craving for more drug.

Morphine and its drug relatives act to increase the release of dopamine. Cocaine makes more dopamine stay in the synapse. The end result on the reward system from both these drugs is the same, an increase in dopamine. Other addicting substances, such as alcohol and nicotine, also act to increase dopamine transmission through the reward circuitry, although in a less direct way.

Addiction and Other Brain Chemicals

Despite the current emphasis on dopamine, neuroscientists realize that it is not just dopamine that is involved in addiction. Some drugs that end up as addicting have actions that are clearly caused by changes in another major transmitter system, the adrenergic system. This set of nerve cells use the transmitters adrenaline and noradrenaline (also called epinephrine and norepinephrine).

The adrenergic system is the same system that you feel going into action when you are under stress. A person who faces immediate danger experiences the so-called fight-or-flight response: racing heart, butterflies in the stomach, and trembling muscles readied for action. These responses occur because adrenaline is released from the adrenal gland sitting on top of the kidneys. Adrenaline is also squirted out by nerves.

Opiates dampen the signals coming from a tiny group of adrenergic cells in the upper brain stem. When an opiate abuser stops taking the drug after constant use, he or she feels anxiety. This anxiety may be triggered by the adrenergic system. A new approach to treating addicts in withdrawal involves adding a drug called clonidine, which calms the anxiety produced by the adrenergic system in an addict trying to quit.

Progress in Addiction Research

People have known for centuries that opium and more refined chemicals made from the sap of the unripe poppy seed pod can soothe pain and induce sleep. But only in the 1970s did scientists stumble on the fact that opium, morphine, codeine, heroin, and all manmade opiate drugs closely mimic the molecular structure of a set of natural neurotransmitters. These neuroscientists had identified the brain's own morphine, calling it endorphin.

Even caffeine, the active ingredient in coffee, cola drinks, and chocolate, mimics a natural neurotransmitter within the brain called

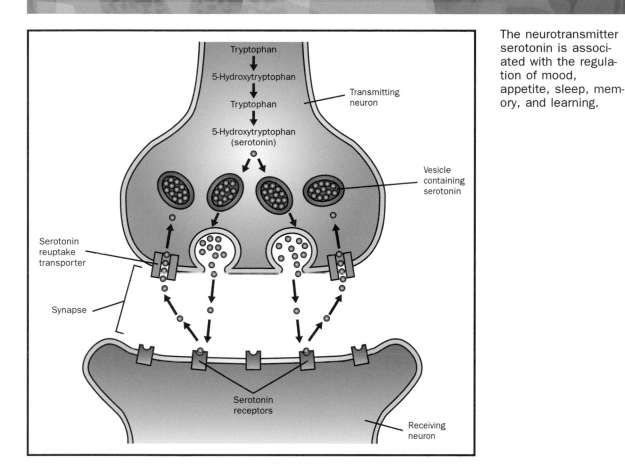

Tryptophan

5-Hydroxytryptophan

Tryptophan

5-Hydroxytryptophan
(serotonin)

Transmitting neuron

Vesicle containing serotonin

Serotonin reuptake transporter

Synapse

Serotonin receptors

Receiving neuron

The neurotransmitter serotonin is associated with the regulation of mood, appetite, sleep, memory, and learning.

adenosine. Caffeine's ability to boost alertness and change the rates of contraction of some smooth muscles comes from its actions at adenosine receptors.

Scientists have identified the purpose of the brain's own opioids. Say an animal has been injured. Because of the actions of brain opiates, the animal does not yet notice the sensation of pain. This allows the injured animal to escape the source of the injury. Once the animal is away from danger, the injury itself then needs to be noted so that the animal can hide and heal—in other words, it is then necessary for the animal to feel its pain. So the body's own opiates are crafted by evolution to work in an emergency, but to then fade away and allow pain to assert itself. The poppy makes its own molecules, morphine and codeine, most likely to counter insects. These substances just happen to fit in the receptors that have evolved in animals for their own needs.

Similarly, caffeine, and its chemical relatives in tea (theophylline) and chocolate (theobromine), were probably meant to affect insects chewing on the plants, but also turn out to affect people who eat or drink the foods and beverages brewed from the seeds and leaves. When people chew the leaves of the coca plant, from which cocaine is made, the cocaine serves up its effect to the dopamine reuptake system, though the plant is merely equipped to defend against chewing bugs with far simpler nervous systems.

Beyond the Surface Receptors

Many brain researchers now study second messengers, which guide the reactions that take place within neurons after transmitters bind to the surface receptors. When morphine binds to its opiate receptors, these altered receptors in turn activate an enzyme inside the nerve cell that governs the firing of the cell. Repeated activation of this enzyme, adenylate cyclase, eventually leads to a weakened response that will require more drug, simply to maintain the enzyme's normal function.

Just as response to transmitter is adjusted in addiction, so too are the activities of the second messengers. New drugs may soon be invented to treat addiction inside the neuron by targeting the second messenger systems within it.

The Future of Research

Drug addiction is the brain's response to the interruption of its normal chemical balance. By coincidence, drugs that people have taken from plants and purified and copied through chemistry are able to mimic the basic means by which one nerve cell communicates with another. By understanding the intricate workings of the brain's chemistry, scientists hope to find ways to interrupt an addict's self-destructive impulses, which in fact arise from the impulses within the brain. SEE ALSO BRAIN STRUCTURES; COCAINE; HEROIN; IMAGING TECHNIQUES: VISUALIZING THE LIVING BRAIN; RESEARCH; TOLERANCE AND PHYSICAL DEPENDENCE.

Brain Structures

Consider the human brain: Somehow, its several billion invisible cells serve to produce emotions, thoughts, and dreams. The deeply wrinkled surface of the brain's identical halves contains the substance that makes a mind, able to soar on the notes of a bird or the colors of a sunrise, suffer the deepest anguish from pain or loss, or simply be bored. Millions of tiny changes in molecular currents within the brain, each instant, create all of these emotions, and can lead a person to seek the source of all things in the universe.

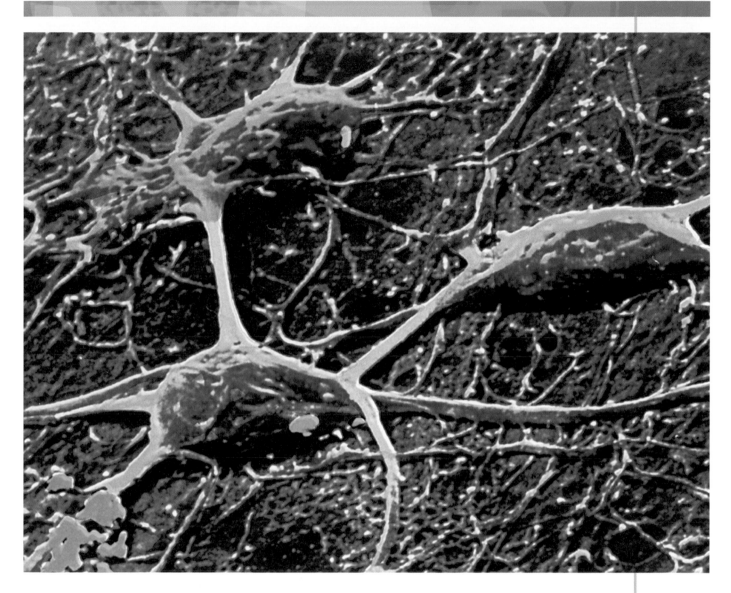

While humans, the great apes, and perhaps the whales, dolphins, and elephants, have the most complicated brains, all mammalian brains share similar structures. As animals evolved more complex behaviors, their brains tended to add outer layers to primitive core structures. Thus, a rat has a basic mammalian brain structure that monkeys and humans share, but monkeys and humans have more complicated coverings, containing added circuitry.

Nerve cells in the cerebral cortex have many nerve fibers branching from them. These fibers provide thousands of possibilities for different connections to be made in the brain, and facilitate rational thought, planning, and problem solving.

The Ancient Brain: The Limbic System

If you split open the two halves of the human brain, as you would split the halves of a walnut, the inner face would show a small part of what neuroscientists call the limbic system. Most of this limbic system lies hidden deep within each half, buried below the covering folds of the cortex, the outermost layer of the brain. The outer, cortex

The brain consists of several major sections or lobes, such as the frontal lobe. Within these lobes are interior sections of the brain (right), which control specific processes such as emotions, reasoning, and breathing.

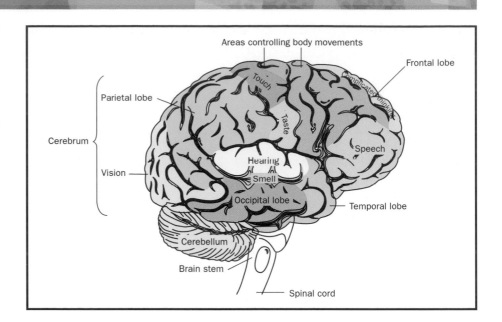

covering of the brain is the source of reasoning, neuroscientists have found, while the inner, limbic system is the source of reacting.

Reptiles have the beginnings of a limbic system, and all animals further along on the evolutionary tree share this reptilian heritage, but have built on it. Parts of the limbic system seem to respond in emotionally charged situations. Memories of an emotional nature are stored here as well.

Most knowledge of the limbic system was gained through experiments on animals. For example, in cats, scientists placed wires finer than a hair into the limbic structure called the *amygdala* (named for the Latin word for almond, because of its shape). By passing a small electric current through that wire, the very picture of rage could be created: a cat's fur would instantly rise up, its back would arch, and it would hiss and show its claws. Other cats, with the amygdala removed surgically, would stay placid no matter what.

Such experiments on animals gave hints on how the human brain works. Careful studies of people who had disease or accidents that affected specific parts of their brains confirmed what scientists had found in animals. For instance, people with epilepsy, a disorder involving uncontrolled electrical activity within the brain, had unusual rage reactions if the electrical storm took place within the temporal lobe. The temporal lobe is the part of the brain beneath the skull's temples that surrounds the amygdala.

One man who had epilepsy of the temporal lobe would pick up a kitchen knife and for no reason threaten his wife during one of his epileptic attacks. He had surgery to remove part of the temporal lobe, which successfully interrupted the abnormal brain activity. The man then no longer fell into these uncontrolled rages.

Many structures besides the amygdala make up the limbic system. These different regions of the limbic system are all clusters of the cell bodies of many millions of nerve cells. These nerve cells are also called neurons. Fibers leading from one set of clustered neurons make connections to other sets of neurons in the limbic system, and also to other parts of the brain. The covering of the human brain, known as the cerebral cortex, is complexly wrinkled and convoluted (having many folded, crumpled curves). This allows more surface area to pack in more cortical neurons. The neurons of the cortex carry out the rational thoughts that, in people, are able to govern emotions. Planning and thoughts based on situations recalled from the past can help suppress, or prevent, immediate emotional reactions generated in the limbic system.

A Basic Blueprint of the Brain

The two halves of the brain each contain regions that control the movement of the limbs and receive sensations from the skin, with each half of the brain responsible for the opposite side of the body. The brain also makes sense of reports from the sense organs in the head. Even special sensors in joints tell the brain how the body is arranged in space—that is, they register the body's posture. Unconsciously, the brain monitors the degree of tension in each muscle, and adjusts to allow coordinated movement. (A good deal of coordination is carried out by the cerebellum, the structure underneath the main part of the mammalian brain.)

The somatosensory area, which receives sensations, and the motor cortex, which sends out commands for moving the body's parts, spread down the middle sides of the cortex, midway between the front and back of the brain. In the back of the brain is an area called the optic cortex, which records and analyzes sights from the eyes. In between the optic cortex, and the somatosensory and motor cortex, are areas that govern hearing. Language comprehension is generated by a region near the hearing center. Producing speech is enabled by a place in the cortex near the motor area for the face.

More complex processes are carried out in other cortical regions, primarily in the temporal lobe (mentioned earlier) and in the frontal lobes of the cerebral cortex. These regions at the front end of the brain are involved in planning and judgment.

All of these areas in the cortex interact with the limbic system below the brain's surface. Deeper still in the core of the brain, joining the halves, are clusters of neurons providing the controls over breathing, heart rate, and other basic bodily functions. The structure called the thalamus, which is located between the brain's core and the limbic system, registers pain and relays painful messages to the limbic system and cortex.

The Electrical Nature of the Brain

The brain's cells, the neurons, work by tiny electric currents that in turn release molecules to relay a message to the next neuron. An example of these connections and relays is what would take place if you stub your toe. The pressure and resulting damage to the toe stimulates pain fibers, which are the endings of nerve cells. These fibers are a thousand times finer than a human hair. The pain fibers are entwined within the cells just below the surface of the skin. An electrical impulse is generated in these microscopic fibers, and travels to the main body of the pain-sensing neurons, which lie within the spinal cord.

The pain message then proceeds up along the even longer fiber coming out of these spinal, pain neurons, traveling toward the brain. The pain neurons thus have one fiber reaching to the skin that receives the pain impulse, called the dendrite, and another that runs through the spinal cord and delivers pain to the brain, the axon.

At the thalamus, the pain impulse reaches the pain fiber's axon terminal, and here, the electrical message becomes chemical. At this

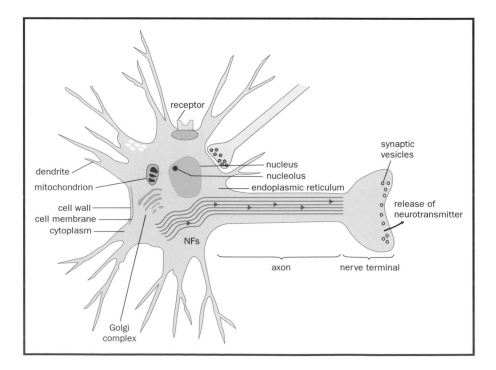

A neuron cross-section. Neurons are brain cells that communicate with each other through electric currents, which in turn signal the release of molecules to relay information.

special ending of the neuron, the current causes tiny amounts of chemicals called neurotransmitters to be released. Neurotransmitters continue the message to the next neurons. In this manner, pain from the big toe is relayed all the way to the cortex.

Different Brain Areas, Different Neurons

The pain neuron is simple, with its two main fibers. Other neurons in the brain have elaborately branching dendrites, resembling the bare branches of a tree. (*Dendrite* is a Latin word meaning "branches.") These two types of neurons are shown in the accompanying figure. Each of these many dendrites are covered all over with thousands of spines—and each spine is clasped by the ending of the axon of another neuron. This complicated, branching structure of the brain explains its amazing ability to carry out complex mental processes. Try to calculate how many connections are possible among a few billion neurons, each equipped with several thousand spines studding its hundreds of dendrites.

Brain Structures in Addiction

The brain must have ways to regulate the vast array of impulses and the flow of chemicals that create its activity. In fact, scientists have only begun to explain how the brain is controlled. Drug addiction is

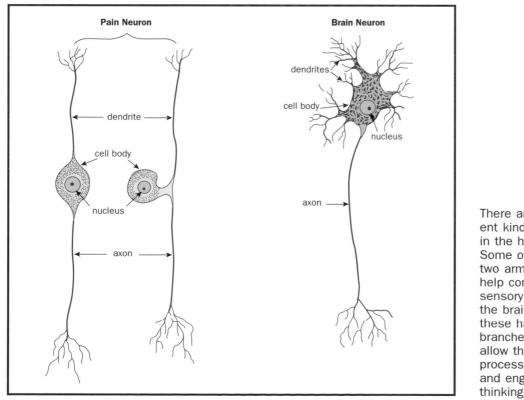

There are many different kinds of neurons in the human body. Some of these have two arms (left), and help communicate sensory messages to the brain. Some of these have many branches (right), and allow the brain to process information and engage rational thinking.

a response to an introduced substance that at first disrupts the precisely controlled actions of the brain. In response, the brain attempts to bring itself back into balance despite the drug.

Reward System. Animals learn to find food, comfortable places to sleep and hide, and mates based on feelings of pleasure that are generated within the structures of the limbic system. Even animals with more complex behaviors, such as people, still depend on the primitive reward system for meeting basic needs as well as the ability to enjoy the more complex rewards of human culture. Scientists have traced a limbic circuit governing pleasure, and it is this system that is responsible for the addictive nature of abused drugs.

A key limbic structure involved in generating rewarding feelings is termed the nucleus accumbens. It receives messages by means of a messenger molecule called dopamine, and so does part of the brain's cortex, called the prefrontal cortex (toward the front end of the brain). The prefrontal cortex is a region that recruits memories and higher thought processes needed for rational planning. The prefrontal cortex appears in humans but is primitive or absent in most other species.

Studies of addiction in rats can be used to study the basic chemistry behind human addiction. These studies might also help scientists to develop ways to make quitting easier. With rats that are made addicted to drugs, researchers can try out existing **therapeutic** drugs or discover new ones. Then, clinical trials are carried out in people.

Researching the Brain

By the close of the 1990s, brain researchers had new tools to look inside the living brain and watch it work. Neuroscience has also uncovered a range of growth factors that are critical in building and maintaining a brain. These new tools and discoveries have been employed in the field of addiction research.

Data from research on animals provide evidence that **opiate** abuse causes toxic (poisonous) actions on a number of brain cells in a key limbic region responsible for memory. In adult rats, the number of newly formed cells in this region, called the hippocampus, was cut back by long-term exposure to morphine. For existing brain cells in animals, morphine was found to decrease the length and number of the spines on neurons that receive incoming transmitter messages.

Drug abuse can also literally shrivel neurons. Repeated injections of morphine directly into a brain region known to be part of the limbic pleasure circuit in rats made certain neurons in this region 25 percent smaller. The injections cause the neurons to make lots of their

therapeutic healing or curing

opiate drug derived directly from opium and used in its natural state, without chemical modification (e.g., morphine, codeine, and thebaine)

WANT TO BE A BRAIN SURGEON?

A really fun way to learn how the brain is organized is to be a "virtual" neurosurgeon on the Internet. Check out this URL: <http://www.pbs.org/wgbh/aso/tryit/brain/> to try your hand at playing doctor.

messenger molecule, dopamine, and they apparently adapt by shrinking to shut down production.

In Summary

Addictive drugs are chemicals that are able to hijack the brain's own chemistry. By mimicking molecules that the brain uses to send messages, the drugs activate regions of the brain that guide the body's movements and emotions. Research is showing that long-term use of these drugs not only changes brain chemistry, but that abusing drugs may also permanently change the structures of the brain on which they act. SEE ALSO BRAIN CHEMISTRY; IMAGING TECHNIQUES: VISUALIZING THE LIVING BRAIN; RESEARCH; TOLERANCE AND PHYSICAL DEPENDENCE.

Breathalyzer

Breath-analysis machines detect and measure the alcohol present in air that is breathed out. When an individual drinks alcohol, the alcohol crosses from the intestine into the bloodstream. When the blood circulating around the body gets to the lungs, some of the alcohol in the blood crosses into the air contained in the tiny sacs of the lungs. The air that is breathed out of the lung will contain alcohol that can be measured by breath-analysis machines.

Researchers have determined the ratio of breath alcohol to blood alcohol. The Breathalyzer result allows the tester to estimate the concentration of alcohol in the blood. Blood alcohol concentration (BAC) is approximately 2,300 times greater than breath alcohol concentration, with some variation among individuals. Breath-alcohol analysis is quick and **noninvasive**. This makes the Breathalyzer breath-test machine a useful tool for law enforcement agencies to monitor drinking and driving.

noninvasive not involving penetration of the skin

If a person's BAC measures 0.10, it means that there are 0.10 grams of alcohol per 100 milliliters of blood. According to the American Medical Association, a person can become impaired when the BAC hits 0.05. The legal standard for drunkenness in the United States varies slightly according to state. Many states have now adopted a legal limit of 0.08, replacing the legal limit of 0.10 that was used across the United States in the past. The federal government has encouraged states to lower the legal limit by making more federal funding available to states that lower the limit from 0.10 to 0.08.

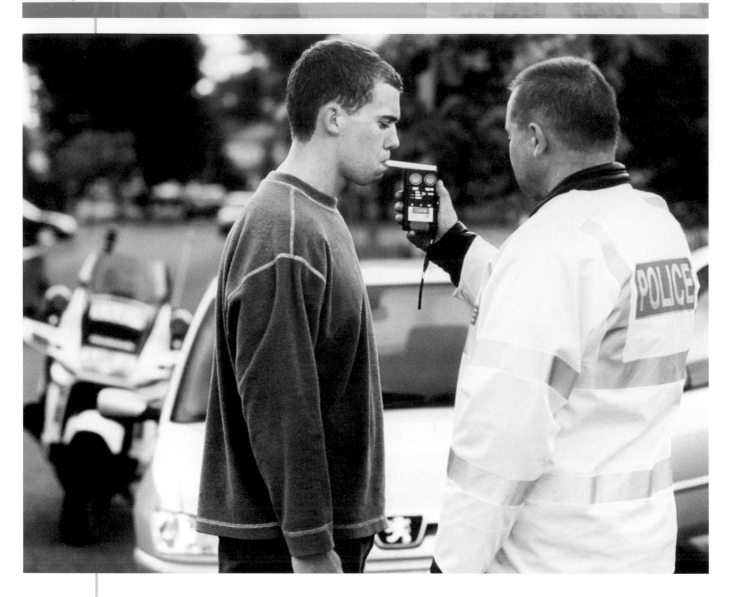

Because Breathalyzer tests are relatively easy to administer—compared, for example, to blood tests—they have become widely used.

intoxicated state in which a person's physical or mental control has been diminished

corroborate to independently find proof or support

Officers routinely conduct field sobriety tests on motorists they suspect of driving while **intoxicated**. An officer first requests that the motorist perform certain physical tests, such as walking a straight line, putting a finger to the nose, or balancing on one foot, in order to **corroborate** the officer's suspicion. If the officer concludes that the motorist has failed one or more of these tests, the officer requests that the motorist submit to a Breathalyzer test. The results of the test can be used to support and corroborate the police officer's opinion in testimony at trial. In those states that set blood-alcohol intoxication levels, the results can demonstrate that the motorist's blood-alcohol level exceeded the permissible level.

A motorist can refuse to take a Breathalyzer test. However, under some state laws, the motorist's driver's license will then be automatically suspended for a set period of time. In the late 1990s some states, including New York and California, approved laws that made it a crime to refuse a Breathalyzer test. Legislators concluded that the penalty of a license suspension was not severe enough for drunk drivers.

Because Breathalyzer test results serve as powerful evidence, defendants and their lawyers often obtain experts who question the way the test was administered and the reliability of the Breathalyzer machine itself. If the Breathalyzer machine has not received proper and timely maintenance, this information can be used to cause a jury to have a reasonable doubt about the accuracy of the results. This failure has led to an acquittal (failure to convict) in a number of trials.

In recent years, schools have begun to use the Breathalyzer breath-test machine as well. Some schools now use Breathalyzers at school functions such as proms to bar entrance to students whose test results show that they have blood alcohol levels above the legal limit. Such use of the Breathalyzer is controversial. Some students and others see this use as an infringement on students' rights; others see it as a way to save lives and to discourage the use of alcohol among minors. SEE ALSO BLOOD ALCOHOL CONCENTRATION; DRIVING, ALCOHOL, AND DRUGS; DRUG TESTING METHODS AND ANALYSIS.

Bulimia *See Eating Disorders*

Caffeine

Caffeine is a chemical found in the beans, seeds, leaves, or bark of many plants. Caffeine is considered a chemical stimulant of the nervous system. A chemical stimulant speeds things up both mentally and physically, increasing alertness, interfering with sleep, and raising heart rate and blood pressure.

Foods and beverages made from caffeine-containing substances are widely available in and accepted by most contemporary societies. In North America, the most common food sources of caffeine include coffee, tea, and chocolate. More than 80 percent of adults in North America consume caffeine regularly. Average per capita (per person) caffeine intake in the United States has been estimated at 211 milligrams per day, in Canada at 238 milligrams, in Sweden at 425 milligrams, and in the United Kingdom at 444 milligrams per day. The world's per capita caffeine consumption is about 70 milligrams per day.

A model of caffeine as produced by a computer. Drinking caffeinated beverages, such as coffee and soda pop, is popular in North America.

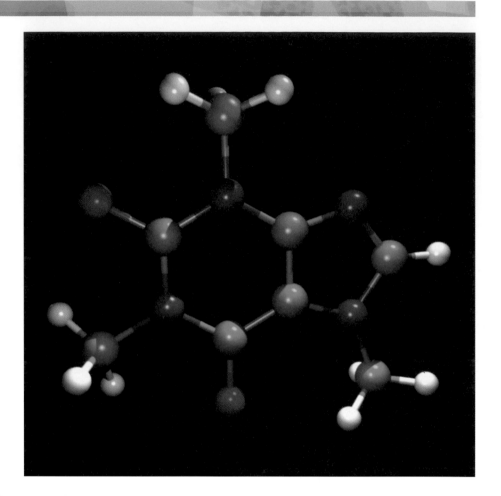

physical dependence condition that may occur after prolonged use of a particular drug or alcohol, in which the user's body cannot function normally without the presence of the substance; when the substance is not used or the dose is decreased, the user experiences uncomfortable physical symptoms

tolerance condition in which higher and higher doses of a drug or alcohol are needed to produce the effect or "high" experienced from the original dose

withdrawal group of physical and psychological symptoms that may occur when a person suddenly stops the use of a substance or reduces the dose of an addictive substance

Even though caffeine-containing foods and beverages are perfectly legal and very commonly used, caffeine can affect behavior in ways that are similar to the effects of drugs of abuse. People who regularly use caffeine can experience both **physical dependence** and **tolerance**.

Caffeine has known effects on the brain. As little as 32 milligrams of caffeine, less than the amount of caffeine in most 12-ounce cola soft drinks, can improve alertness, performance, and reaction time. Doses as low as 10 milligrams, less than the amount of caffeine in some chocolate bars, can alter mood. Regular use of only 100 milligrams of caffeine per day—in other words, drinking one cup of coffee every day—can cause severe **withdrawal** symptoms if the daily caffeine is stopped abruptly.

Sources of Caffeine

Coffee and tea are the world's primary dietary sources of caffeine. Consumption of tea was first documented in China in 350 C.E., although there is some evidence that the Chinese first consumed tea as early as the third century B.C.E. Coffee cultivation began around 600

C.E., probably in what is now Ethiopia. Other commonly used items containing caffeine include soft drinks, cocoa products, and medications.

Caffeine is found in more than sixty species of plants. Coffee is derived from the beans (seeds) of several species of *Coffea* plants, and the leaves of *Camellia sinensis* plants are used in caffeine-containing teas. Chocolate comes from the seeds or beans of the caffeine-containing cocoa pods of *Theobroma cacao* trees. In developed countries, soft drinks, particularly colas, provide another common source of dietary caffeine. Only a portion of the caffeine in soft drinks comes from the kola nut (*Cola nitida*); most of the caffeine is added during manufacturing. Since the 1960s, a marked decrease in coffee consumption in the United States has been accompanied by a substantial increase in the consumption of soft drinks. Matt leaves (*Ilex paraguayensis*), guarana seeds, and yoco bark are other sources of caffeine for a variety of cultures. The accompanying table shows the amounts of caffeine found in common dietary and medicinal sources. As can be seen in the range of values for each source in this table, the caffeine content can vary widely depending on the method of preparation or commercial brand.

Effects on Mood and Performance

It has long been believed that caffeine stimulates mood and behavior, decreases fatigue, and increases energy, alertness, and activity. Although caffeine's effects in experimental studies have sometimes been subtle (difficult to detect) and variable, dietary doses of caffeine have a variety of effects on mood and performance. Doses below 200 milligrams have been shown to improve vigilance (alert watchfulness) and reaction time and postpone sleep. In addition, the subjects of these studies report increased alertness, energy, motivation to work, desire to talk to people, self-confidence, and well-being. Higher doses can both improve or disrupt performance of complex tasks and can cause nervousness, jitteriness, restlessness, and anxiousness.

Medical Uses of Caffeine

Caffeine is an ingredient in a variety of over-the-counter medications such as analgesics or painkillers (particularly to treat headaches), stimulants, and decongestants. It is also used in treatments for menstrual pain and appetite suppressants. Although caffeine is a common ingredient in headache preparations (including some prescription drugs to treat migraine headaches), evidence for caffeine's effectiveness for relieving headaches is limited, as is the evidence for its appetite-suppressant effects. Caffeine has also been used to treat:

CAFFEINE CONTENT OF COMMON FOODS AND DRINKS

Source	Standard Value (in milligrams)
Coffee (6 oz./180 ml)	
ground roasted	102
instant	72
decaffeinated	4
Tea (6 oz./180 ml)	
leaf or bag	48
instant	36
Cola Soft Drink (12 oz./360 ml)	43
Chocolate Milk (6 oz./180 ml)	4
Chocolate Bar (1.45–1.75 oz./40–50 g)	7
Milk Chocolate (1.5 oz)	10
Dark Chocolate (1.5 oz)	31
Caffeine-containing over-the-counter medications	
analgesics and cold preparations	32
appetite suppressants and stimulants	100

Caffeine can be found in a wide range of common foods and beverages, including chocolate bars and tea, as well as in over-the-counter medications.

- chronic obstructive pulmonary disease
- asthma
- breathing problems in newborns
- overdoses with opioid drugs

The Medical Risks of Caffeine

Although more research is needed, some researchers are concerned that there may be an association between caffeine intake and such diseases as benign fibrocystic breast disease and cancer of the pancreas, kidney, lower urinary tract, and breast. In a recent survey of physician specialists, more than 65 percent recommended reductions in caffeine in patients with cardiac arrhythmia (irregular heartbeat), palpitations, tachycardia (rapid heartbeat), esophagitis/hiatal hernia, fibrocystic disease, or ulcers, as well as in patients who are pregnant.

Caffeine Abuse

Case reports have described individuals who consume large amounts of caffeine—more than one gram (1,000 milligrams) per day. This excessive intake is called caffeinism, and occurs most often in psychiatric patients, drug and alcohol abusers, and anorectic patients. Caffeinism can produce a range of symptoms—muscle twitching, anxiety, restlessness, nervousness, insomnia (inability to fall asleep or stay asleep), rambling speech, tachycardia, cardiac arrhythmia, and sensory disturbances including ringing in the ears and flashes of light. Some research has also linked caffeinism with **psychoses** and **anxiety disorders**. Extremely high doses of caffeine—between 5,000 and 10,000 milligrams—can produce convulsions and death and have been shown to produce birth defects in mammals.

The American Psychiatric Association recognizes a condition known as caffeine intoxication, in which high doses of caffeine produce adverse effects. Substantial amounts of caffeine are also used by a small percentage of competitive athletes, who believe that caffeine will enhance their athletic performance, despite rules against such use.

Tolerance and Physical Dependence

Regular caffeine use can decrease a person's responsiveness to its effects. This result is known as tolerance. At first, daily doses of 250 milligrams of caffeine can cause blood pressure to go up and increase the production of urine and saliva. After several days of caffeine use, however, tolerance develops. With tolerance to caffeine, blood pressure and urine and saliva production return toward normal. Caffeine tolerance has not been well researched, although there is some sug-

psychosis mental disorder in which an individual loses contact with reality and may have delusions (i.e., unshakable false beliefs) or hallucinations (i.e., the experience of seeing, hearing, feeling, smelling, or tasting things that are not actually present)

anxiety disorder condition in which a person feels uncontrollable angst and worry, often without any specific cause

gestion that sleep-disturbing effects and jitteriness noticed when caffeine is first used both lessen after regularly using caffeine.

Uncomfortable symptoms occur when caffeine use is suddenly stopped. Caffeine withdrawal is typically characterized by reports of headache, fatigue, drowsiness, and decreased alertness. Severe withdrawal can interfere with normal functioning and include flu-like symptoms, fatigue, severe headache, nausea, and vomiting. In general, caffeine withdrawal begins twelve to twenty-four hours after stopping caffeine use and lasts from two to seven days. Caffeine withdrawal can occur following termination of caffeine doses as low as 100 milligrams per day, an amount equal to one strong cup of coffee, two strong cups of tea, or three soft drinks. These data indicate that the large majority of the adult population of the United States is at risk for significant disruption of mood and behavior when there are interruptions of daily caffeine consumption. SEE ALSO ADDICTION: CONCEPTS AND DEFINITIONS; CHOCOLATE; COFFEE; COLA DRINKS; TEA.

Cancer, Drugs, and Alcohol

Medical researchers are constantly trying to determine which substances cause cancer. Among the substances they study are alcohol and drugs—both legal, prescription medications and illegal drugs of abuse. Another area of concern is the treatment of cancer patients who are or have been substance abusers.

Identifying Carcinogens, or Cancer-Causing Agents

There are several ways to study whether a substance is a "carcinogen," or a substance that causes cancer.

1. Cancer cells have certain abnormalities in their cell structures. Cells can be grown in a test tube to see if these cell-structure abnormalities develop.

2. The substance can be given to animals to see if cancers result.

3. Doctors and medical researchers can analyze the course of a disease in a human patient.

4. Researchers can compare the outcomes in a group of people who use a certain substance to outcomes in those who do not.

Identifying carcinogens is complex and difficult, partly because of the long time delay between the use of a carcinogen and the appearance of cancer symptoms. It can take as long as thirty years for those symptoms to appear. This is why early studies of new medications are rarely successful at identifying carcinogens. Also, cancers can have many causes other than carcinogenic drugs, such as environmental, nutritional, and genetic factors. It is often difficult to separate one cause from another.

Drugs of Abuse and Cancer

Alcohol. Research conducted on animals does not show that alcohol alone causes cancer. However, the body **metabolizes** alcohol to produce acetaldehyde, an enzyme that has been shown to be carcinogenic. Animals who were exposed to alcohol in combination with known carcinogens had higher rates of several kinds of cancerous tumors than did animals only exposed to the known carcinogen.

Studies show that alcoholics are more likely to have cancers of the digestive tract than nonalcoholics. The risk for cancer increases with the amount of alcohol consumed. Overall, it has been estimated that as many as 10 percent of all cancer deaths are due to alcohol.

Illicit Drugs. The role of illicit drugs as a cause of cancer is still unclear. Research reports show that heavy marijuana users sometimes get cancers in the respiratory tract, primarily the lungs. Cocaine users, who usually take the drug by inhaling it, can get cancers of the nasal passages. Opium smokers have increased rates of cancer of the esophagus.

Substance Abuse and Cancer Treatment

Cancer patients have used marijuana to reduce the nausea that chemotherapy treatment sometimes produces. Marijuana may also be used to provide pain relief. However, opinion varies sharply about whether a drug that is an illegal source of abuse should be used for these medical purposes. Doctors often give cancer patients morphine or other **opioids**, drugs known to have the potential for addiction, to control pain. Patients with no history of substance abuse very rarely become addicted to these drugs. In contrast, treatment is complicated for patients who have abused opioid drugs in the past. A history of substance abuse may shorten a cancer patient's life expectancy, and drugs used to manage pain may not be as effective. SEE ALSO COCAINE; LAW AND POLICY: DRUG LEGALIZATION DEBATE; OPIATE AND OPIOID DRUG ABUSE; TOBACCO: MEDICAL COMPLICATIONS.

metabolize the breakdown of various substances in the cells of the body to produce energy and allow the body to function

opioid substance that acts similarly to opiate narcotic drugs, but is not actually produced from the opium poppy

Cannabis Sativa

Cannabis sativa is the botanical name for the hemp plant, which originated in Asia. It is the source of tetrahydrocannabinol (THC), which is the active agent in the drugs marijuana, hashish, ganja, and bhang.

An herb of the mulberry family, *Cannabis sativa* grows in tropical, subtropical, and temperate regions. Due to genetic differences, some plants produce strong fibers but little THC, and others produce a substantial quantity of THC but weak fibers. The fiber-producing plant is grown commercially for cloth, rope, roofing materials, and floor coverings. The drug-producing variety is widely cultivated in societies that approve of its use. Illegal crops are also planted, some in the United States. When harvested, the leaves often resemble lawn cuttings, which accounts for the slang term "grass." SEE ALSO ADOLESCENTS, DRUG AND ALCOHOL USE; BHANG; MARIJUANA; MARIJUANA TREATMENT.

Causes for Substance Abuse *See Risk Factors for Substance Abuse*

Child Abuse and Drugs

In the United States, on average, about twelve out of every 1,000 children are abused or neglected each year. A precise number may be impossible, as many cases are never reported, but the U.S. Department of Health and Human Services estimated that 826,000 children were abused or neglected in 1999 in the United States. This abuse can take the form of physical abuse, neglect, sexual abuse, and emotional maltreatment. In addition, each year a higher percentage of American children are being raised in poverty, often by overstressed and drug-abusing parents.

Child-welfare authorities consider parental substance abuse to be a major risk factor for child abuse. In other words, when parents abuse drugs, they are more likely to engage in child abuse as well. Under the influence of alcohol and other drugs, adults are less inhibited—they feel free to act on their desires and wishes. They lose a sense of good judgment and emotional control. For these reasons, some adults who abuse alcohol or drugs are more likely to hurt their children or behave in harmful ways.

Researchers have noted that families in which child abuse occurs and families in which substance abuse occurs have certain features in common:

In the United States, 85 percent of state caseworkers listed substance abuse as one of two top contributors to child abuse.

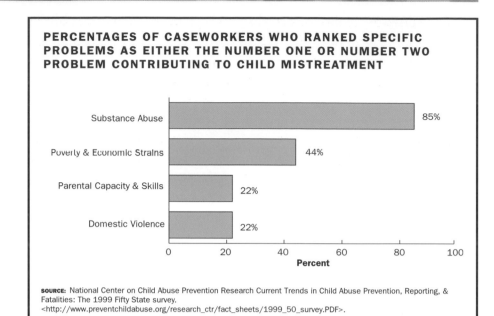

PERCENTAGES OF CASEWORKERS WHO RANKED SPECIFIC PROBLEMS AS EITHER THE NUMBER ONE OR NUMBER TWO PROBLEM CONTRIBUTING TO CHILD MISTREATMENT

SOURCE: National Center on Child Abuse Prevention Research Current Trends in Child Abuse Prevention, Reporting, & Fatalities: The 1999 Fifty State survey. <http://www.preventchildabuse.org/research_ctr/fact_sheets/1999_50_survey.PDF>.

depression state in which an individual feels intensely sad and hopeless; may have trouble eating, sleeping, and concentrating, and is no longer able to feel pleasure from previously enjoyable activities; in extreme cases, may lead an individual to think about or attempt suicide

psychosis mental disorder in which an individual loses contact with reality and may have delusions (i.e., unshakable false beliefs) or hallucinations (i.e., the experience of seeing, hearing, feeling, smelling, or tasting things that are not actually present)

antisocial personality disorder condition in which people disregard the rights of others and violate these rights by acting in immoral, unethical, aggressive, or even criminal ways

- parents often have poor parenting skills—parents spend little time with children, speak harshly and critically to them, discipline them in extreme ways or not at all
- family disorganization—the family members do not communicate with each other, the children's needs are not met, and there is frequent conflict and possibly violence
- parents are more likely to resort to criminal activity, often to obtain illegal drugs
- high rates of mental illness, such as **depression**, **psychosis**, and **antisocial personality disorder**
- high rates of physical illness due to chaotic lifestyle, lack of health care, and the risks of intravenous drug use

How Children Are Abused

Child abuse takes different forms: prenatal exposure to drugs, postnatal exposure to drugs, physical abuse, and sexual abuse.

Prenatal Drug Exposure. The laws of several states define exposure of a fetus to alcohol and other drugs as child abuse. In some states the law requires that a child be removed from the mother when drug tests show that she has abused drugs during pregnancy. Laws also require medical or social services personnel to report such cases to state agencies. Unfortunately, because of this rule, pregnant, drug-abusing women may avoid getting prenatal care for fear that they will be punished or lose their children. For this reason, a number of states have placed a priority on making drug treatment more readily available to pregnant women.

The abuse of alcohol or drugs by a pregnant woman can result in abnormalities in the fetus. In addition, substance-abusing women are likely to have poor nutrition, to have more illness and stress, and to fail to get medical prenatal care, all of which can harm their babies. Babies born to alcoholic mothers can suffer from fetal alcohol syndrome (FAS), which causes facial deformities, retarded growth, and abnormalities of the heart, kidneys, ears, and skeletal system. The long-term effects of FAS appear to include reduced intelligence, attention deficits, learning disorders, hyperactivity, and more antisocial behaviors than the norm.

When the pregnant mother has abused drugs such as cocaine, heroin, and phencyclidine (PCP), babies can suffer from **withdrawal** symptoms in infancy. Their development is often delayed, and some have long-term damage to the **central nervous system**. The major effects at birth of most drugs, including alcohol and tobacco, are premature birth, low birth weight, and a slowed rate of growth that may affect both brain and physical development. Sudden infant death syndrome is also two to twenty times higher in infants exposed to cocaine and **opiates**.

If babies exposed to drugs come home to a nurturing environment, where a caregiver responds to their needs and provides stimulation and early childhood education, these babies can overcome the problems of drug exposure. But if the baby is in the care of a mother who returns to taking drugs, the baby's needs are unlikely to be met.

Postnatal Exposure to Drugs. Children can be hurt by inhaling cigarettes or cigarette smoke, by accidentally swallowing drugs, by being given drugs by a minor, and by deliberate poisoning. In addition, alcohol, nicotine, and other drugs are all present in the breast milk of women who use these substances, so nursing infants may be exposed to these drugs. Some parents who abuse drugs allow their children to drink alcohol or use the drugs they find lying around the house. In a disturbing form of child abuse, some parents deliberately give their children alcohol or other drugs (such as tincture of opium) to make them stop crying, to **sedate** them, or to make the children **intoxicated** to amuse the parents.

Physical Abuse. Physical abuse can involve any of a variety of violent acts against a child, including beatings, burns, strangulation, and biting. Children who are physically abused have unfulfilled needs and low self-esteem. They distrust others and have problems with aggression and anxiety. Research on the physical abuse of children shows a strong overlap between physical abuse and parental alcoholism.

withdrawal group of physical and psychological symptoms that may occur when a person suddenly stops the use of a substance or reduces the dose of an addictive substance

central nervous system the brain and spinal cord

opiate derived directly from opium and used in its natural state, without chemical modification (e.g., morphine, codeine, and thebaine)

sedation process of calming someone by administering a medication that reduces excitement; often called a tranquilizer

intoxicated a state in which a person's physical or mental control has been diminished

149

In a survey of child welfare professionals, crack cocaine dominated as the most commonly used illicit drug among parents who mistreat their children.

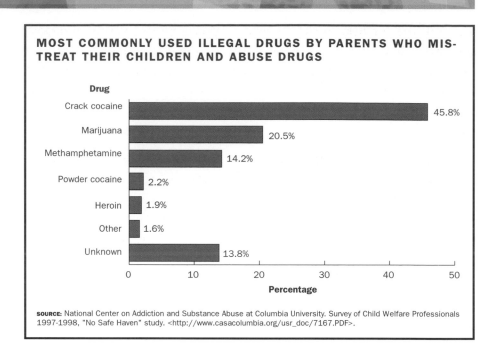

MOST COMMONLY USED ILLEGAL DRUGS BY PARENTS WHO MISTREAT THEIR CHILDREN AND ABUSE DRUGS

Drug

Drug	Percentage
Crack cocaine	45.8%
Marijuana	20.5%
Methamphetamine	14.2%
Powder cocaine	2.2%
Heroin	1.9%
Other	1.6%
Unknown	13.8%

Percentage

SOURCE: National Center on Addiction and Substance Abuse at Columbia University. Survey of Child Welfare Professionals 1997-1998, "No Safe Haven" study. <http://www.casacolumbia.org/usr_doc/7167.PDF>.

Unfortunately, less research has been conducted on the role of other kinds of drug abuse in child abuse cases. However, according to the Child Welfare League of America, substance abuse exists in 40 to 80 percent of families in which the children are victims of abuse. Furthermore, children whose parents abuse alcohol and other drugs are three times more likely to be abused and more than four times more likely to be neglected than children from non-abusing families. Drug abusers often belong to social groups in which violence is common. Children raised in violent homes are more likely to become abusers as adults, thus continuing the cycle of violence.

Child Sexual Abuse. Child molesters are often intoxicated when they commit the acts of abuse. Research shows that in about 30 to 40 percent of child sexual-abuse cases, particularly when girls are abused, the abuser had been drinking. A study of incest victims and perpetrators showed that 48 percent of fathers who had committed incest were alcoholic, and that 63 percent of this group were drinking at the time of the abuse.

A very high percentage of drug abusers in treatment programs report being sexually abused as children. In fact, childhood sexual abuse is often a hidden factor contributing to drug abuse and **relapse** into drug abuse after treatment. Sexually abused children find it difficult to maintain a sense of themselves that is separate from other people. As a result, survivors of childhood sexual abuse often do not see themselves as individuals separate from the desires or demands of others. They may not know how to refuse another person access to their bod-

relapse term used in substance abuse treatment and recovery that refers to an addict's return to substance use and abuse following a period of abstinence or sobriety

ies, and in later life, to their privacy, time, physical space, and possessions. They are especially vulnerable to the coercion of others, and may begin to use drugs or keep using them because they are unable to say no to the urgings of another person.

What Can Be Done?

Because of the high overlap between child abuse and drug abuse, drug treatment agencies should routinely ask their clients if they have been or are being physically or sexually abused. Similarly, child welfare agencies should routinely investigate whether substance abuse by a parent or caregiver is contributing to the maltreatment of children.

Because it is not possible to remove all children from risky family environments, both government-funded and private agencies must find other ways to protect children. Caregivers and professionals can help maltreated children learn how to avoid abuse. Social welfare agencies need to teach parenting skills to addicted mothers and fathers, who must be made to understand that their chaotic street lives damage their children. Positive steps include parent-and-family-skills training programs, locating good early-childhood education for the child and outside child care, and considering foster care or adoption. SEE ALSO BABIES, ADDICTED AND DRUG-EXPOSED; CHILDHOOD BEHAVIOR AND LATER DRUG USE; FAMILIES AND DRUG USE; FETAL ALCOHOL SYNDROME (FAS); POVERTY AND DRUG USE.

Childhood Behavior and Later Drug Use

Certain inappropriate behaviors, tendencies, and conditions during childhood may predict whether a child will use drugs or engage in deviant (unacceptable and unlawful) behavior later on. The factors that may indicate risk include the child's personality traits, family experiences, and general environment.

Personality Traits. A child who is irritable and easily distracted, who throws temper tantrums, fights often with siblings, and behaves in unacceptable ways is more likely than other children to use drugs in adolescence. An aggressive child has an especially high risk of adolescent drug use and deviance.

Often, adolescents who use marijuana could not control their impulses and had difficult temperaments as children. They may have been unable to control strong emotions, such as anger. They also may have had trouble with "delayed gratification," the ability to wait beyond the immediate moment to have a personal desire fulfilled. Those qualities often carry over into adolescence. The use of illicit drugs and the effects of those drugs may then worsen the adolescent's feelings of irritability and aggressiveness. Temper tantrums, acts of aggression, and delinquent behavior may continue to cause problems. Adolescents who do not learn how to cope with typical feelings of frustration until a difficulty can be resolved may be more likely to turn to drugs to ease feelings of discomfort and anxiety.

Family Experiences. Family experiences can also predict whether a young person will take drugs. In a long-term study investigating the early childhoods of adolescent drug users, researchers found that greater involvement by the mother with the child protected against later drug use. Children who become frequent drug users as adolescents often have mothers who were cold and who gave them little encouragement.

Environment. The environment a child is raised in can also play a role in later drug use. Studies show, for example, that a child growing up in a neighborhood with a high crime rate and readily available drugs is more likely to experiment with drug use as an adolescent. The risk for drug abuse increases in low-income households where money is not available to pay for positive experiences such as camps or extracurricular activities that provide a supportive drug-free environment.

It is important to understand that a person's childhood experiences do not directly determine whether he or she will use drugs in adolescence. Adolescence has its own types of experiences, which shape the influences absorbed from childhood. Together, experiences from both periods of a person's life become risk factors for drug use.

Risk Factors

During adolescence, there are three major risk factors for drug use:

- the adolescent acts in unconventional ways, usually some form of rebelliousness
- the parent-child relationship is difficult and involves a great deal of conflict, with the parent showing little affection for and attachment to the child
- the adolescent spends a great deal of time with peers whose behavior is deviant

Changes in any one of these factors can reduce the chances that the adolescent will use drugs.

Prevention and Treatment

Because childhood risk factors often contribute to adolescent risk factors for drug use, the best chance for prevention is early intervention. Through early intervention, therapists or social workers try to identify personality traits (such as inability to tolerate frustration, thrill-seeking, antisocial personality traits, poor judgment) and difficult childhood experiences that might lead to later drug use. Early intervention can spur the development of drug-resistant personality traits, foster a positive parent-child bond, and encourage friendships with appropriate peers. SEE ALSO CHILD ABUSE AND DRUGS; CONDUCT DISORDER; FAMILIES AND DRUG USE; POVERTY AND DRUG USE; RISK FACTORS FOR SUBSTANCE ABUSE.

Chocolate

Chocolate is an ingredient of many popular treats, such as candies, baked goods, hot drinks, and ice cream. It is prepared, often as a paste, from the roasted crushed seeds (called cocoa beans) of the South American cacao tree (*Theobroma cacao*). Chocolate contains theobromine and caffeine, both of which produce a mild stimulating effect. The word "chocoholic" was coined to describe people especially attracted to chocolate flavor. SEE ALSO CAFFEINE.

Club Drugs

Clubs and rave scenes have been a popular part of American and European youth culture since the 1990s. The drugs people take as part of the club experience are known as club drugs. These drugs vary in terms of their effects and their **toxicity**. An important element of club drugs is novelty, so no list of club drugs can pretend to be complete at any time. Commonly used club drugs include MDMA, GHB, ketamine, Rohypnol, methamphetamine, and LSD. Users see most of these drugs as relatively **benign** compared to "older" drugs such as cocaine. This perception is often mistaken.

toxicity condition of being poisonous or dangerous to people

benign harmless; also, noncancerous

The history of much drug use in the United States is cyclical. For example, the cocaine epidemic of the 1980s was in fact the second cocaine epidemic in this century, the previous one having ended in the 1930s. In the 1980s, just as in the 1930s, users believed that cocaine was a safe drug. The later generation had no idea of the harsh lessons the earlier generation had learned about its effects. In

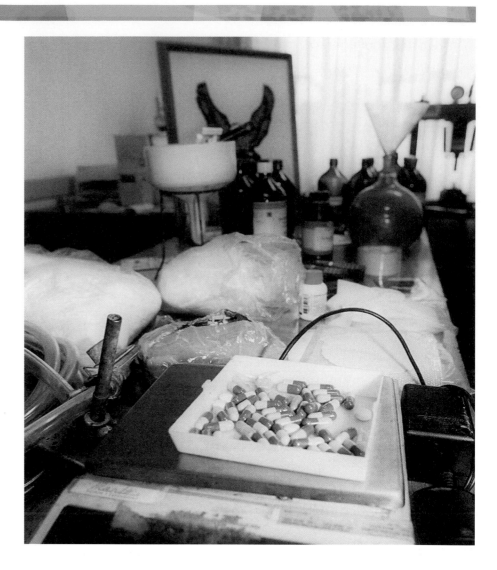

An illegal laboratory designed for making the stimulant-hallucinogenic drug ecstasy after being raided on August 18, 2000, by São Paulo police in Brazil. That same year, the U.S. Customs Service seized 9.3 million smuggled tablets of ecstasy.

recreational drug use casual and infrequent use of a substance, often in social situations, for its pleasurable effects

psychoactive term applied to drugs that affect the mind or mental processes by altering consciousness, perception, or mood

hallucinogen a drug, such as LSD, that causes hallucinations, or seeing, hearing, or feeling things that are not there

comparison, club drugs are relatively new, so few have had direct experience with their negative consequences. **Recreational use** of MDMA, for instance, began only in the 1980s. But being new does not mean being safe. History suggests that such confidence in a drug's safety is unwarranted.

The **psychoactive** drug MDMA is a **hallucinogen** derived from amphetamine. Popularly called "ecstasy," it gives the user enhanced or increased feelings of emotional and physical closeness to others. Though it has a reputation as a benign "love drug," ecstasy has contributed to hundreds of deaths in its short time as an abused drug. It has also been linked to seizures as well as kidney and cardiovascular failure. Ecstasy has produced long-term damage to the nervous system in animals, and long-term use has resulted in damage to mental and emotional functioning in a number of humans.

Two popular club drugs, Rohypnol and GHB, have been used for more than mere recreational purposes. In a number of criminal cases, men convicted of rape were found to have given Rohypnol or GHB to their victims without their knowledge. Rohypnol, known as the "date rape drug," can be slipped undetected into an unsuspecting victim's drink. Rohypnol and GHB can impair a person's memory and cause unconsciousness, which makes the intended female target an easy victim for a prospective rapist.

Again, these drugs are fairly new to the world of recreational drug use, although Rohypnol belongs to the same class of drugs, the benzodiazepines, as Valium, a drug with a well-known history of abuse. This group of drugs is especially dangerous when used with alcohol, which enhances their effects as **depressants**. A person who takes these drugs and then drinks alcohol can end up in a **stupor**, with dangerously slowed breathing. The combination can in some cases cause coma and death. Like alcohol, GHB and Rohypnol seem to cause an increase in violent behavior in some users. These drugs have been linked to so many negative consequences that many countries have increased restrictions on their use. Both GHB and Rohypnol are illegal in the United States.

Unlike other club drugs, methamphetamine, a **psychostimulant**, is not new. In fact, "speed" has a long and well-documented history of abuse and toxic effects. Its appearance on the club scene seems to be linked to its low cost and the negative image of cocaine as an alternative stimulant. Ironically, methamphetamine is substantially more toxic to the brain and liver than cocaine, while sharing some of cocaine's potentially deadly effects on the cardiovascular system. Amphetamine use has also been linked to toxic psychosis, a condition in which an individual loses touch with reality due to the effects of a substance and may suffer from hallucinations and delusions.

Ketamine, another club drug often called "special K," is an anesthetic formerly used in humans but now largely restricted to veterinary use. Ketamine, like phencyclidine (PCP), can produce many of the symptoms of **psychosis** in humans, including hallucinations and indifference to pain or death. Previous generations often referred to PCP as "angel dust." Chronic PCP use has been associated with the development of long-term psychosis, and it is likely that ketamine will cause the same risk.

LSD (lysergic acid diethylamide, often referred to as "acid") is another drug with a well-known history of misuse and abuse. Its major dangers lie in its hallucinogenic properties, which may cause users to do physical harm themselves or others. LSD also seems to worsen depression and psychosis. Outside of its intense and dangerous psychological effects, LSD has few side effects on the body.

depressant chemical that slows down or decreases functioning; often used to describe agents that slow the functioning of the central nervous system; such agents are sometimes used to relieve insomnia, anxiety, irritability, and tension

stupor state of greatly dulled interest in the surrounding environment; may include relative unconsciousness

psychostimulant medication that is prescribed to control hyperative and impulsive behaviors

psychosis mental disorder in which an individual loses contact with reality and may have delusions (i.e., unshakable false beliefs) or hallucinations (i.e., the experience of seeing, hearing, feeling, smelling, or tasting things that are not actually present)

Club drugs are not risk free, and the public is likely to face more examples of their dangers. The most dangerous aspect of the club drug phenomenon is that most club drug users mix several of these drugs, and may also use tobacco and/or alcohol. With such a variety of drugs being abused by individual users, toxic results are far more likely to occur. The long-term consequences of such multiple use are yet to be discovered. SEE ALSO ECSTASY; LYSERGIC ACID DIETHYLAMIDE (LSD) AND PSYCHEDELICS; RAVE; ROHYPNOL; SPEED.

Coca Plant

The coca plant is a shrub found in the highlands of the Andes Mountains and the northwestern areas of the Amazon River in South America. The plant is also grown in Asia and other parts of the world. Coca plants have long histories of use as medicines and **stimulants**. The stimulant effects are due to the cocaine the plant contains. However, only two varieties of the more than 200 species of the coca plant contain significant amounts of cocaine.

stimulant drug that increases activity temporarily; often used to describe drugs that excite the brain and central nervous system

Legends of native South Americans describe the coca plant's origin and supernatural powers. The Inca called the coca plant a "gift of the Sun God," and believed that it had many magical functions. The Inca and the other civilizations of the Andes chewed coca leaves during social ceremonies and religious rites, as well as for medicine. Because coca leaves also increase energy levels, soldiers used them during the military campaigns of these civilizations, as did messengers who traveled long distances in the mountains.

In the 1500s, under the Spanish conquest of South America, coca plants were systematically cultivated. Chewing coca leaves or drinking coca tea became part of daily life for Indians in South America. Today, Indians living in the Andean highlands continue to use coca leaves as a medicine, as well as for its **psychoactive** effects. Their society sets standards for acceptable use of coca leaves, and individuals rarely go against those standards.

psychoactive term applied to drugs that affect the mind or mental processes by altering consciousness, perception, or mood

Chewing coca leaves along with an alkaline substance produces numbing in the mouth and a generally stimulating effect. This effect lasts for about an hour. The cocaine from the plant is absorbed from the inner wall of the cheek as well as from the gastrointestinal tract after saliva containing coca juice is swallowed. SEE ALSO COCAINE; DRUG PRODUCERS; PSYCHOACTIVE DRUGS.

Cocaine

The abuse of cocaine is a major public-health problem in the United States. In the 1970s, people began taking cocaine as a **recreational drug**. Experts believed that cocaine was harmless. Many movies and books from this decade show cocaine use as a popular, sophisticated social activity. By the mid-1980s, when many people were using cocaine in large quantities, experts and the public began to recognize the drug's dangers. Cocaine use can cause severe medical and psychological problems.

Cocaine (also known as "coke," "snow," "lady," "crack," and "ready rock"), is an alkaloid that can act both as a local anesthetic and as a stimulant. Users generally take cocaine in binges: They take the drug repeatedly for several days, and then use no cocaine for several days or weeks. Many users resist getting treatment. Users caught possessing or selling cocaine face stiff criminal penalties, but these punishments have not been effective at reducing the rate of heavy cocaine use. In fact, the number of people who used cocaine rarely or occasionally declined during the 1990s. However, the number of frequent or heavy users only decreased slightly.

Medical Uses of Cocaine

The major medical use of cocaine is as a local anesthetic, particularly for procedures that involve the nose, throat, or mouth. It is the only local anesthetic that causes vasoconstriction, or narrowing of the blood vessels. For this reason, cocaine is useful in surgeries that require a minimum of bleeding. In addition, cocaine shrinks membranes, giving the surgeon a better view. When used in appropriate doses for necessary surgeries, and with appropriate medical caution, cocaine appears to be both useful and safe as a local anesthetic.

Methods of Abuse

As an illegal drug, cocaine can be taken in a number of ways. These "routes of administration" include oral (by mouth), intranasal (through the nose), intravenous (by injection into the veins), and smoking. The effects of cocaine are similar no matter what the route. However, the way in which a person takes cocaine influences the likelihood that he or she will abuse it. This is because some methods of taking the drug act more quickly to increase levels of cocaine in the brain. The amount of cocaine in the brain determines the sensations that the user will feel. A person who gets the largest and quickest changes in cocaine brain levels is more likely to take the drug again.

recreational drug substance used casually and infrequently, often in social situations, for its pleasurable effects

DID YOU KNOW?

Cocaine was first synthesized in 1855. It was not until 1880, however, that the medical world studied its effects. In 1886 John Pemberton included cocaine as the main ingredient in his new soft drink, Coca-Cola, contributing to public acceptance of cocaine. It was cocaine's energizing effect on the consumer that was initially responsible for Coca-Cola's popularity.

Public disapproval over the use of that substance forced Pemberton to remove cocaine from Coca-Cola in 1903. Eventually people became so concerned about the dangers of cocaine that it was outlawed in 1920. Today cocaine—in any form—is illegal.

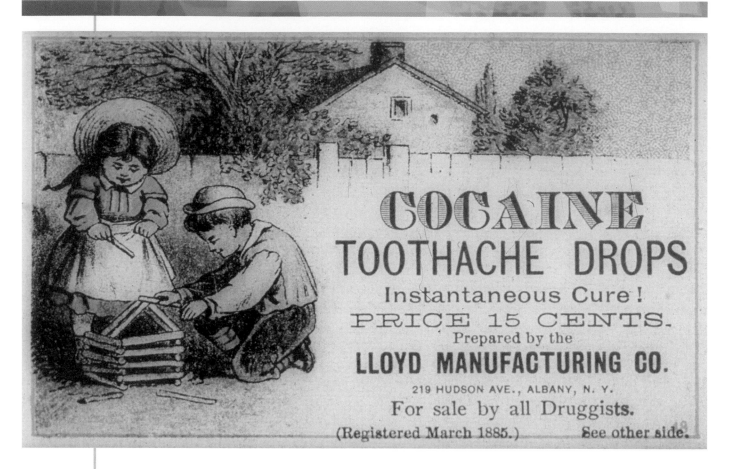

Cocaine has been used in the past as an anesthetic.

Cocaine abusers do not take cocaine orally, because cocaine taken by mouth is absorbed into the brain slowly. By this method, it takes more than an hour to reach peak brain levels of cocaine. Abusers are more likely to inhale cocaine into the nose as a powder. By this method, the drug is quickly absorbed from the mucous membranes in the nose. Because of its local anesthetic actions, cocaine numbs or "freezes" the mucous membranes. A person buying cocaine on the street will test its purity by inhaling a small amount to see if this numbing occurs. When cocaine is inhaled, or "snorted," cocaine blood levels peak about twenty to thirty minutes later. Users who inhale cocaine report that they are ready to take a second dose of the drug within thirty to forty minutes after the first dose. Snorting was the most common way for people to use cocaine in the mid-1980s. Later, users discovered that smoking or injecting cocaine gets the drug to the brain faster. These became the preferred methods for taking the drug.

When taken by intravenous injection, cocaine reaches peak blood levels immediately, and users experience a "rush." Brain levels of cocaine increase quickly, so the user feels the drug's effects just as quickly. As blood levels of cocaine decrease, so do the effects, and users are ready for another intravenous dose within thirty to forty minutes. Users who inject cocaine are more likely to combine their

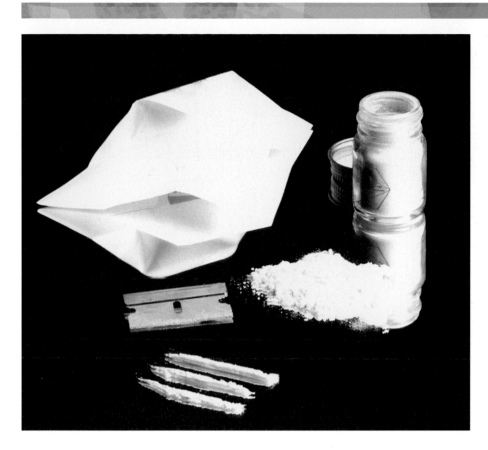

Powder cocaine is often sold with a cutting agent such as mannitol or baking powder. A cutting agent is a white powder used to dilute pure cocaine.

cocaine with heroin (a combination known as a "speedball") than are users who take it in other ways.

The smokable form of cocaine came into widespread use in the mid-1980s. Freebase, or crack, is a form of cocaine that is not destroyed when heated. As with injected cocaine, blood levels peak almost immediately and the user feels a strong rush. Users can prepare their own freebase from the powdered form they buy on the street, or they can buy it in the form of crack.

Freebase and crack offer an instant high. They are easier to use than other forms of the drug and also less expensive. As a result, users tend to take the drug repeatedly. Repeated high doses of cocaine are very toxic, or poisonous, causing serious damage to the user's health.

Cocaine is frequently taken in combination with other drugs such as alcohol, marijuana, and heroin. In fact, almost 75 percent of cocaine deaths reported in 1989 involved the use of other drugs. Relatively low doses of cocaine can be highly toxic when taken together with alcohol.

Medical Complications from Cocaine Use

Cocaine use leads to a broad range of medical complications affecting nearly every one of the body's organ systems. At low doses,

This map shows the source countries for cocaine, indicating where coca plants are grown and how cocaine travels to the United States.

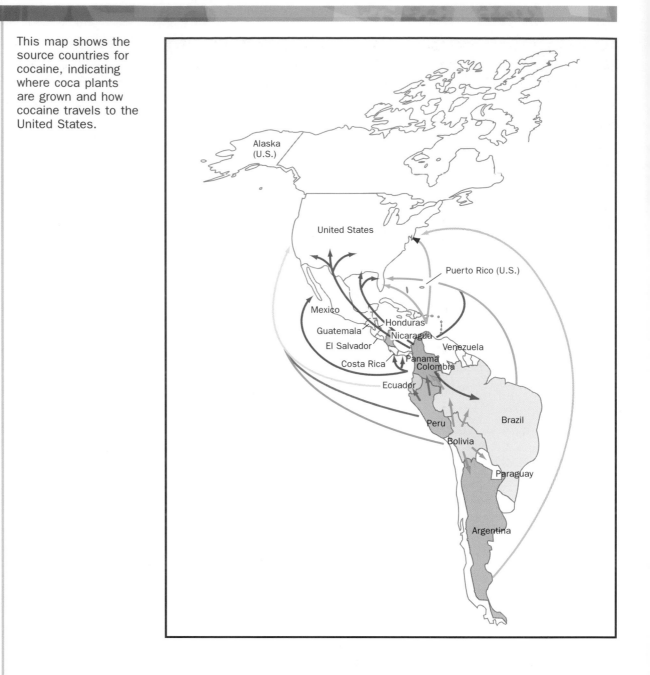

paranoid someone who is excessively or irrationally suspicious

psychosis mental disorder in which an individual loses contact with reality and may have delusions (i.e., unshakable false beliefs) or hallucinations (i.e., the experience of seeing, hearing, feeling, smelling, or tasting things that are not actually present)

cocaine causes increases in heart rate, blood pressure, respiration (breathing), and body temperature. A person intoxicated by cocaine can suffer from heart attacks, stroke, contractions of blood vessels (which interferes with blood flow), and cardiac arrhythmia (irregular heartbeat).

When taken repeatedly over long periods, cocaine can cause changes in behavior, including irritability, hypervigilance (being overly watchful or alert), **paranoid** thinking, excessive activity, and eating and sleep disturbances. Repeated cocaine use can also cause severe mental disturbances. The user may develop a **psychosis** in which he or she feels paranoid and anxious and has hallucinations. Some users display unpredictable, odd behavior that may become violent.

Stopping cocaine use after a binge often causes a crash, in which the user becomes **depressed**, feels tired, and has eating and sleep disturbances. At first during the crash, the person does not crave more cocaine. But as time goes on, the user may think of little else other than finding the next dose.

How Cocaine Affects Behavior

A major effect of cocaine on human behavior is its ability to change a person's moods. The user's desire to feel this effect again is what makes cocaine a drug of abuse. Research shows that cocaine produces a feeling of euphoria, or intense well-being. People feel more energetic and friendly when on cocaine. These effects occur whether a person injects or smokes cocaine.

A person who takes cocaine repeatedly will develop tolerance to many of its behavioral effects. When the original dose no longer has much of an effect, the user must take increasingly larger amounts of cocaine to achieve the high. These larger doses present greater risks to the user's heart and blood vessels.

Users of cocaine and other stimulant drugs claim that the drug improves their performance of many activities. No evidence exists to support this claim. In general, cocaine has little effect on performance except when a person is unable to perform up to usual standards because of fatigue. In this situation, cocaine can enable the person to perform as if he or she were not tired. But this effect lasts for only a short time. SEE ALSO COCA PLANT; COCAINE: WITHDRAWAL; COCAINE TREATMENT: BEHAVIORAL APPROACHES; COCAINE TREATMENT: MEDICATIONS; COMPLICATIONS FROM INJECTING DRUGS; CRACK; USERS.

Cocaine: Withdrawal

The signs and symptoms of withdrawal from **depressant** drugs, such as alcohol or heroin, are much easier to recognize than the symptoms of withdrawal from the **stimulant** drug cocaine, because a cocaine abuser who stops taking the drug has no immediate physical symptoms. Instead, the person feels a severe change in mood. Because of the lack of physical withdrawal symptoms, both medical professionals and the public long believed that cocaine was not an addicting drug. The cocaine epidemic of the 1980s led to greater concern about how cocaine affects users. Researchers studied the drug to determine whether cocaine use leads to **dependence** and withdrawal.

depressed someone who has begun to suffer from depression and who feels intensely sad and hopeless

depressant chemical that slows down or decreases functioning; often used to describe agents that slow the functioning of the central nervous system; such agents are sometimes used to relieve insomnia, anxiety, irritability, and tension

stimulant drug that increases activity temporarily; often used to describe drugs that excite the brain and central nervous system

dependence psychological compulsion to use a substance for emotional and/or physical reasons

Signs and Symptoms

By conducting interviews with outpatients who had been cocaine users, researchers have identified three phases that occur after a person stops taking the drug:

1. The crash occurs when a person who has used cocaine for an extended period suddenly stops taking the drug. In this state, the person becomes extremely exhausted. The crash can last between nine hours and four days. At the beginning of the crash, the person feels a **craving** for cocaine, irritability, **dysphoria**, and agitation. In the middle of the crash, the individual yearns for sleep. In the late crash, the person sleeps excessively. Some individuals may suffer from extreme **depression** in the early stages of the crash (especially those who have suffered from depression in the past). They may think about or try to commit suicide. Even first-time users of cocaine can experience the crash, depending on how high the dose and how long the period of use.

2. As depression worsens and the desire for sleep increases, the person feels less craving. After waking from a long sleep, the individual enters a brief normal period with mild craving. This is followed by a long period of milder withdrawal, lasting from one to ten weeks. During this time the craving for cocaine returns, and the person enters a state known as anhedonia. With anhedonia, the person can no longer feel pleasure from activities or experiences he or she used to enjoy.

3. The final phase of cocaine withdrawal is called extinction. The extinction phase usually begins two weeks after a person stops using cocaine. The person returns to a normal mood but still feels an occasional craving for cocaine. Because of continued cravings, the chance for **relapse** is high.

Alcohol and Cocaine. When an individual has drunk alcohol in addition to taking cocaine, the depression of the crash phase can be even worse. Alcohol reduces a person's control over his or her impulses, such as the impulse to commit suicide. Therefore, alcohol use combined with the despair of the crash period can put a person at high risk for suicide. In addition, cocaine has important interactions with alcohol in the body. For example, cocaine plus alcohol in the body produces a compound called cocaethylene. This compound produces more intense and longer euphoria (a feeling of intense well-being), but it also increases the risk of death from cardiac arrhythmia (irregular heartbeat).

Recent studies of cocaine withdrawal suggest that not all users go through three separate phases. One four-week study examined twelve

craving powerful, often uncontrollable desire for drugs

dysphoria depressed and unhappy mood state

depression state in which an individual feels intensely sad and hopeless; may have trouble eating, sleeping, and concentrating, and is no longer able to feel pleasure from previously enjoyable activities; in extreme cases, may lead an individual to think about or attempt suicide

relapse term used in substance abuse treatment and recovery that refers to an addict's return to substance use and abuse following a period of abstinence or sobriety

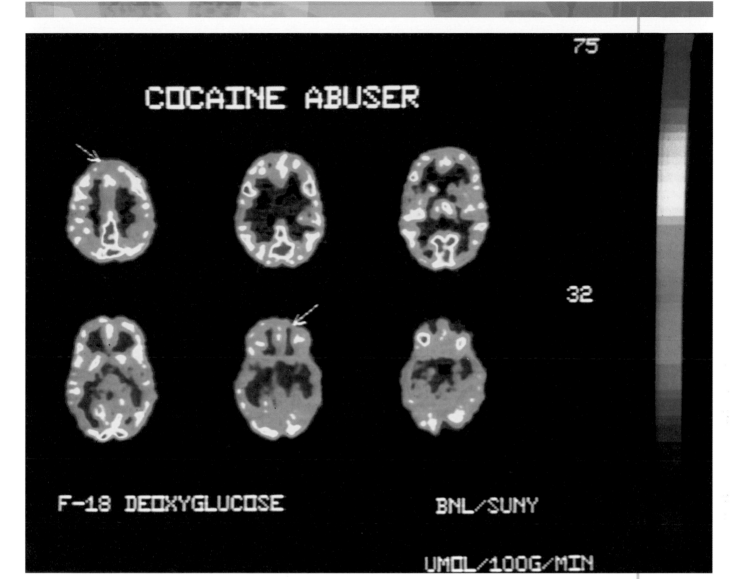

COCAINE ABUSER

75

32

F-18 DEOXYGLUCOSE

BNL/SUNY

UMOL/100G/MIN

inpatients who were dependent on cocaine. During withdrawal, the subjects suffered from depression, craving, and anxiety. These symptoms improved steadily during the four weeks. By the end of the fourth week, the cocaine users had come out of withdrawal. An important difference between this study and earlier studies is that the researchers worked with inpatients. Inpatients live in the protected setting of a hospital or treatment center. They are not constantly reminded of cocaine by certain people or places in their lives, as are cocaine users who go through outpatient treatment while living on their own. As a result, the phases of cocaine withdrawal may be less distinct for inpatients.

The red and yellow areas of the brain in this PET scan indicate high brain activity. Brain activity is reduced among cocaine users. Note the decreased activity in the frontal lobes of this cocaine abuser (arrows). The frontal lobes are where a person's thoughts and memories are formed.

Treating Cocaine Withdrawal

Treatment for cocaine withdrawal can include treatment as an inpatient or outpatient or a combination of both. Cocaine craving is the

detoxification
process of removing a poisonous, intoxicating, or addictive substance from the body

major cause of relapse in individuals trying to quit using cocaine. Reminders of drug use in the person's environment—areas where the person used to buy drugs, the people they used to get high with, and so on—can stimulate craving at any time. As a result, people with severe addiction trying to quit cocaine often do better in an inpatient treatment program. A heavy cocaine user with the support of family or friends and resources may benefit from an inpatient **detoxification** program that lasts a minimum of one week. This is the peak period for craving. The person may then need to continue as an outpatient for a minimum of one to two years.

Individuals who lack the support of family or friends and who do not have a stable living situation can often benefit from weeks to months as inpatients in a residential treatment center. The crash phase may be milder for inpatients, and addicts who experience less distress may be better able to concentrate on therapy and education. Inpatients may also feel a greater sense of control over themselves. Control is especially difficult to achieve when craving for cocaine is high. However, many patients can develop a false sense of control over their addiction because, as inpatients, they are protected from environmental cues that trigger craving. Inpatients need to be reintroduced gradually to life outside the treatment center.

The depression and despair that follow an end of long-term cocaine use may occur because of conditions in the user's life. When addicts stop using drugs, they must face the shambles of their lives—the destruction of their families, loss of jobs, financial ruin, poor health, injured relationships, and low self-esteem. Addicts may feel that they have entered a state of crisis. During withdrawal, the craving for cocaine may be caused by their desperate wish to feel better. As a result, cocaine users who receive treatment only as outpatients may suffer from more intense depression during withdrawal. Inpatients may feel more protected from the difficult conditions of their lives while living in a treatment center.

neurotransmitter
chemical messenger used by nerve cells to communicate with other nerve cells

opioid substance that acts similarly to opiate narcotic drugs, but is not actually produced from the opium poppy

Treatment for the crash phase of cocaine withdrawal can include prescription drugs. The two major drugs that have been useful during the crash phase are bromocriptine and amantadine. Both of these drugs enhance or increase the transmission of dopamine, a **neurotransmitter**. After a cocaine binge, a person generally has reduced levels of dopamine in the brain. Researchers believe that reduced dopamine levels cause the depression, irritability, agitation, and drug craving during the crash phase.

Treatment involving medicines is especially important for cocaine addicts who are also dependent on alcohol or **opioids** such as heroin.

It is very common for users to be dependent on more than one substance. A benzodiazepine drug is usually prescribed for alcohol withdrawal; for opiate withdrawal, the drug of choice may be methadone, clonidine, naltrexone, or combinations of these. SEE ALSO COCAINE; COCAINE TREATMENT: BEHAVIORAL APPROACHES; COCAINE TREATMENT: MEDICATIONS; TOLERANCE AND PHYSICAL DEPENDENCE.

Cocaine Treatment: Behavioral Approaches

In the medical community, there is no general agreement as to the best way to treat cocaine dependence. This is alarming given that in 2000, an estimated 1.2 million Americans were current cocaine users. One form of treatment takes a behavioral approach towards cocaine dependence. Behavioral therapy works to change how a person thinks, feels, and behaves. Behavioral therapy uses a number of different approaches to work on breaking an individual of his or her drug use. The behavioral approach uses various methods depending on the doctor's own preferences and the needs of the patient. Many consider it particularly useful because it can be combined with other treatments, such as medication. However, the effectiveness of behavioral treatment is in the early stages of being tested.

Outpatient versus Inpatient Treatment

People dependent on drugs can get treatment as an outpatient—meaning the person lives at home but visits a hospital or other treatment center regularly—or as an inpatient—meaning the person lives at the treatment center. Inpatient treatment is not usually recommended for people dependent on cocaine. This is because, in general, recovering from cocaine dependence requires that the patient learn to cope with circumstances in his or her environment that have led to cocaine abuse. The best chance for accomplishing this task lies outside the hospital. However, inpatient treatment is necessary if the patient (1) fails to make progress or worsens during outpatient treatment; (2) has severe medical or psychiatric problems; (3) is physically dependent on other drugs; or (4) has a history of criminal activity.

Inpatient treatment takes place in a therapeutic community. The patient lives in this community for a period of time determined in advance, from six to twelve months. One study has shown that patients who stayed for longer periods at treatment centers were less likely to relapse, or return to drug use, after treatment. Inpatient treatment focuses on helping the individual readjust to living and functioning in

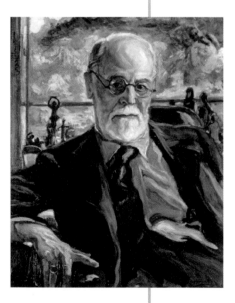

In the 1880s, Sigmund Freud (above) tried cocaine and recommended it to his associate, Dr. Ernst von Fleischl-Marxow, who became severely addicted. Freud quit his usage and backed away from his initial praise of the drug.

PERCENTAGE OF PATIENTS REPORTING WEEKLY OR MORE FREQUENT COCAINE USE BEFORE AND AFTER TREATMENT

	In the year before treatment	In the year after treatment	Percent difference
Outpatient Methadone Programs	41.9	21.7	20.2
Long-Term Residential Programs	66.4	22.1	44.3
Outpatient Drug-Free Programs	41.7	18.3	23.4
Short-Term Inpatient Programs	66.8	20.8	46

SOURCE: The Drug Abuse Treatment Outcome Study, 1991 and 1993, National Institute on Drug Abuse. <http://www.nida.nih.gov/NIDA_Notes/NNVol12N5/Study.html>.

According to the Drug Abuse Treatment Outcome Study, 1991 and 1993, the two most effective cocaine treatments (judging from the percentage drop in cocaine use after one year) are short-term inpatient programs and long-term residential programs. They share in common the practice of completely removing the abuser from the circumstances in which they used cocaine.

rehabilitation
process of restoring a person to a condition of health or useful activity

☎ See *Organizations of Interest* at the back of Volume 1 for address, telephone, and URL.

society without taking drugs. In addition to support services, the individual may receive **rehabilitation** through working at a particular trade.

Cocaine Anonymous

Cocaine Anonymous (CA) ☎ is a community-based organization that offers self-help to cocaine users. CA takes Alcoholics Anonymous (AA) ☎ as its model and applies the same basic principles. The goal for members is to stop using cocaine and remain drug-free by following the Twelve Steps of CA (which are based on the original Twelve Steps of AA).

CA is available to anyone who expresses a desire to stop using cocaine and other drugs. All that is necessary to become a group member is to attend meetings. Meetings vary from large, open sessions that anyone can attend to small, closed discussions reserved for specific groups. For example, young people, professionals, or women might organize their own groups to address their specific concerns. At most meetings, members share their experiences and offer advice and support to each other. In addition, CA offers sponsors, or members who have been in recovery for a substantial period of time, to provide support and guidance to a person attempting to recover. Many treatment professionals recommend CA for people with cocaine problems.

Group Therapy

Many professionals suggest that group therapy is an essential part of cocaine-abuse treatment. These groups are led by a therapist and include people of different backgrounds and at different stages of recovery from cocaine dependence. Group therapy aims (1) to help individuals overcome the feeling that they are suffering alone with their drug problem; (2) to provide positive role models for those in the early stage of treatment; and (3) to encourage hope for success. Doctors who recommend group therapy believe that peer pressure and support are necessary to persuade individuals that stopping cocaine use is the right thing to do.

People in group therapy may discuss their feelings of guilt, problems in their personal relationships, or how cocaine has changed their lives. The therapist points out the negative effects of cocaine. Group therapy occurs in outpatient or inpatient settings. It is sometimes used as the sole source of treatment or combined with individual counseling and other forms of treatment. Group therapy has some drawbacks, including the individual's loss of confidentiality and the possibility that some peers in the group may have a negative influence on the other participants. Research continues on the effectiveness of group therapy as compared to individual therapy alone or a combination of both approaches.

Psychotherapy

Inpatient and outpatient treatment for cocaine dependence usually includes individual therapy with a psychotherapist. Psychotherapy tries to discover the underlying personality disturbances that bring about cocaine abuse. These disturbances include painful emotional states, such as depression. Psychotherapists believe that the individual's emotional and psychological problems must be solved before he or she can become **abstinent** from cocaine.

Supportive Psychotherapy. Supportive or supportive-expressive psychotherapy is often used for cocaine dependence. In this type of therapy, the patient must acknowledge the negative consequences of cocaine use, accept the need to stop using the drug, and learn to control the impulses that lead to cocaine use. The therapist and the patient explore ways to stay away from other users and environments where drug use is common. The focus of treatment then shifts to exploration of the underlying reasons for the cocaine abuse. The patient tries to gain insight into his or her personality and understand why he or she has turned to cocaine. However, a study from the 1990s has led some researchers to conclude that psychotherapy of this type was ineffective with the majority of their subjects.

Interpersonal Psychotherapy. Interpersonal psychotherapy (IPT) is based on the idea that drug abuse is one way in which an individual attempts to cope with problems in interpersonal relationships. In this therapy, the therapist and patient discuss the negative effects cocaine has had on the patient's functioning. They then compare those effects with any supposed benefits the patient might have believed he

abstinent describing someone who completely avoids something, such as a drug or alcohol

or she was getting from cocaine use. After the patient stops using cocaine, the therapy then addresses difficulties in relationships, including the role of drug use in these relationships.

IPT patients must recognize that drug use cannot help them achieve the goal of satisfying relationships or a rewarding social life. For example, the cocaine abuser may be using the drug to meet new people or to feel relaxed in a social situation. IPT tries to offer patients different and better ways to achieve their social goals.

Behavioral Therapy

Like all drugs, cocaine produces particular effects on the brain. In the view of some drug-abuse therapists, dependence on cocaine is a behavior that begins and continues because of those biological effects. Cocaine produces a reaction in the brain that increases the likelihood that a person will take the drug again.

Environmental factors also determine whether a person will become dependent on cocaine. These factors include (1) the person's peers, (2) a desire for acceptance by others, and (3) the person's belief that drug use will have no negative consequences. In addition, research has clearly demonstrated that cocaine users try to obtain and use the drug at certain times of day, in response to certain events, and in response to certain of their own emotional states. The goal, then, of behavioral therapy is to change these "using" conditions and creating new conditions that encourage abstinence from cocaine.

Behavioral therapy for cocaine dependence is often conducted through group therapy. The idea behind the therapy is to make drug use less attractive and to create alternatives to drug use. Patients learn how to change their external environments and their own internal responses. They also learn to recognize situations in which they are most likely to use cocaine, to avoid these situations when they can, and to cope more effectively with problems and problematic behaviors associated with drug abuse. For example, individuals learn how to cope with boredom, anger, frustration, and depression, and how to handle social pressure to use drugs. Sometimes individuals act out social situations in therapy sessions so that they can better handle such situations in real life. Individuals are also urged to give up other drugs, especially alcohol, because drinking makes a person more likely to use cocaine and weakens his or her resolve to avoid cocaine.

Behavioral therapy acknowledges that people will sometimes have a lapse and use cocaine while under treatment. A typical group therapy session might address why temporary lapses occur and try to help

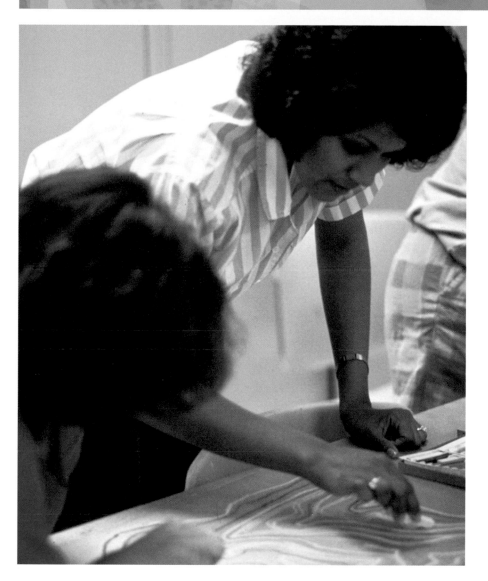

Some therapies, such as art and dance or movement therapy, help people understand themselves better, cope with trauma and illness, or manage stress through means that are not exclusively verbal.

individuals work to prevent total relapse. Family and friends are also encouraged to join therapy groups, as many researchers believe that such support is one of the most effective ways to encourage abstinence.

Reward System. Some behavioral therapy uses a system in which the patient receives a reward for staying in treatment and remaining cocaine-free (proven through drug-free urine tests). The patients earn points that can be exchanged for items that encourage healthy living, such as joining a gym or going to a movie and dinner. This reward system has shown positive results among many cocaine users.

Negative Incentive System. In another behavioral treatment method that sometimes works, the cocaine addict writes a letter admitting to cocaine use. The addict then agrees that the letter can be made public if a urine test turns out positive for cocaine. This system uses a negative incentive. The patient avoids the drug in order to avoid a negative consequence rather than to win a positive reward. Researchers believe that a negative incentive works for some cocaine users who have something to lose, such as a good job.

Environmental Factors. Another behavioral approach focuses on people, places, and things in a person's environment that produce a craving for cocaine. These might include drug-using friends, drug **paraphernalia**, white powder, and places where cocaine is used. In therapy, the person is exposed repeatedly to those aspects of his or her environment. The difference is that, in the controlled conditions of therapy, cocaine is not available. As a result, the events or places that used to produce a craving gradually lose their ability to do so. Once the person breaks the connection between cocaine and certain places or certain things, he or she is less likely to use cocaine when in those places or exposed to those things.

Relapse Prevention Treatment. Relapse prevention treatment (RPT) focuses on ensuring that brief lapses to cocaine use do not become full relapses. In this approach, the therapist communicates to the patient that a lapse is not uncommon in recovery and that it does not negate the progress the patient has made. The first test of RPT's effectiveness at treating cocaine dependence showed that relapse prevention helped individuals stay in treatment and did help them to become abstinent.

Motivational Therapy

Most studies of drug treatment show that a large number of patients drop out of their treatment programs. Studies also show that most individuals who do remain in treatment succeed in breaking the habit. As a result of these findings, researchers believe that a cocaine user's commitment to stop taking drugs is the most important factor affecting chances for success. Motivational therapy focuses on the person's motivation to change and aims to strengthen his or her desire to quit.

The Best Treatment Method

No single treatment for cocaine abuse has proven more effective than any other. The treatment of cocaine addiction is complex and must address a variety of problems. Like any good treatment plan, cocaine treatment strategies must match the needs of particular patients. Programs that combine several treatment methods may prove the most effective. In general, researchers believe that recovery from cocaine addiction will be difficult unless the individual has something to lose

---

paraphernalia equipment that enables drug users to take the drugs (e.g., syringes and needles)

THE BIOLOGICAL MYSTERY OF COCAINE ADDICTION

For a long time, the human brain has remained clouded in mystery—including the mystery of why some drugs, such as cocaine, lead to such intense cravings that users will destroy marriages, careers, and families in order to get their "fix." Recently scientists who study the human brain have begun testing more than 500 chemicals in order to locate an "anticocaine," or a medication that will eliminate these cravings without causing negative side effects.

While such a discovery will never substitute for an addict's desire for recovery, a chemical breakthrough could make relapses rarer and greatly help individuals who are struggling to quit their cocaine use.

and unless the individual believes that he or she has the power to change and make positive choices. SEE ALSO COCAINE TREATMENT: MEDICATIONS; RISK FACTORS FOR SUBSTANCE ABUSE.

Cocaine Treatment: Medications

When cocaine abusers seek treatment for their addiction, medications can help them to stop using cocaine. These medications can also reduce the chances of relapse, or an addict's return to using cocaine. A person who suddenly stops using cocaine generally goes through a withdrawal syndrome, with symptoms of depression, anxiety, and **craving** for cocaine. This craving often lasts for several weeks after a person stops using the drug. Places or things associated with cocaine use in the past, called cues, can continue to trigger cocaine craving for many months. Because of this ongoing craving, it is easy for the abuser to relapse at any time after he or she becomes **abstinent**. Preventing relapse is an important function of medication treatment.

Cocaine **dependence** causes changes in the brain, decreasing the ability of the brain chemical dopamine to function normally within the brain. This effect continues for at least two weeks after a patient stops using cocaine. Interference with dopamine within the brain may be involved in causing the cravings for cocaine that create the risk of relapse. Several medications work by reversing these changes in the brain.

Cocaine's effects on the brain may cause some of the symptoms of cocaine withdrawal. The early phase of this syndrome, called the "crash," involves depression, agitation, and increased risk of suicide. Medications that can treat these complications include **antipsychotic drugs**, such as chlorpromazine and haloperidol. The antipsychotic drug flupenthixol may help with other aspects of cocaine abuse and dependence. In several studies, this drug decreased the intense giddy happiness and/or **paranoid psychosis** that cocaine abusers experience after they use cocaine. Flupenthixol may be particularly useful as a treatment for cocaine abusers with **schizophrenia**.

In the crash phase of withdrawal, large doses of **benzodiazepine** can be used to calm highly agitated patients. Because the crash phase usually lasts for no more than several days, medication does not need to be taken for long periods.

Medications play a more important role during the later phase of withdrawal from cocaine, which may last for several weeks. During

craving powerful, often uncontrollable desire for drugs

abstinent describing someone who completely avoids something, such as a drug or alcohol

dependence psychological compulsion to use a substance for emotional and/or physical reasons

antipsychotic drugs drugs that reduce psychotic behavior; often have negative long-term side effects

paranoid psychosis symptom of mental illness characterized by changes in personality, a distorted sense of reality, and feelings of excessive and irrational suspicion; may include hallucinations

schizophrenia medical condition in which people lose the ability to function normally, experience severe personality changes, and suffer from a variety of symptoms, including confusion, disordered thinking, paranoia, hallucinations, emotional numbness, and speech problems

benzodiazepine drug developed in the 1960s as a safer alternative to barbiturates; most frequently used as a sleeping pill or an anti-anxiety medication

antidepressant medication used for the treatment and prevention of depression

binge relatively brief period of excessive behavior, such as eating an unusually large amount of food

attention-deficit/ hyperactivity disorder long-term condition characterized by excessive, ongoing hyperactivity (overactivity, restlessness, fidgeting), distractibility, and impulsivity

behavioral therapy form of therapy whose main focus is to change certain behaviors instead of uncovering unconscious conflicts or problems

☎ See *Organizations of Interest* at the back of Volume 1 for address, telephone, and URL.

this later phase, patients feel depressed and anxious, and crave cocaine. **Antidepressants** can be given to patients to reduce these symptoms. Studies show that the antidepressant drug desipramine can reduce cocaine craving. As a result, it can help a patient to remain abstinent from cocaine. In one study, cocaine use declined several weeks before cocaine craving was reduced. Another study suggested that the antidepressant drug venlafaxine may be an effective treatment for patients who suffer from both depression and cocaine dependence.

A wide range of medications other than antidepressants have also been tried as treatments for cocaine abuse and addiction. These medications affect the actions of dopamine, serotonin, and other neurotransmitters in the brain. Known as dopaminergic drugs, they appear to take effect within a day after a person begins treatment with them. Because of this quick action, they may reduce the severity of early withdrawal symptoms after cocaine **binges**. These drugs include amantadine, bromocriptine, and methylphenidate. Studies of amantadine show that it reduces cocaine craving and use for several days to a month. Methylphenidate was effective in reducing cocaine cravings in cocaine users with **attention-deficit/hyperactivity disorder** (ADHD). People with ADHD may use cocaine as a way to medicate themselves for their problem. They then can become addicted to the drug.

Studies have begun on the development of a cocaine vaccine. The vaccine would produce antibodies that bind to cocaine in the bloodstream and prevent it from traveling to the brain. This action would block the effects of cocaine. The vaccine may be helpful in combination with **behavioral therapy**.

Multiple-Drug Use

According to the National Institute on Drug Abuse, ☎ most cocaine-dependent people also abuse other substances. More than half are dependent on alcohol, and many are dependent on opioids (such as heroin) and benzodiazepines. The use of these drugs in combination has serious medical consequences—often more severe than the use of each drug alone.

People who are dependent on other substances in addition to cocaine may be treated with a combination of medications. Cocaine abusers who are also dependent on alcohol can take disulfiram (Antabuse), a drug used to treat alcohol abuse. Taking disulfiram before using cocaine may block the pleasurable effects of cocaine and cause such negative effects as anxiety and paranoia. These undesirable effects may discourage a person from cocaine use.

Cocaine abusers who are also dependent on heroin can take the drug naltrexone, which is used to treat opioid abuse. Heroin addicts sometimes take cocaine to increase the euphoria from heroin. As a result, control of heroin abuse in many patients may directly reduce cocaine abuse. Researchers are also studying the possibilities of giving patients who are dependent on both cocaine and opioids an opioid drug that is less addictive than morphine, such as buprenorphine. However, substituting one drug of abuse with another is a very risky treatment approach.

Patients who are dependent on opiates, alcohol, or benzodiazepines in addition to cocaine require **detoxification**. While cocaine withdrawal does not usually lead to major medical complications, withdrawal from these other drugs can have serious medical consequences. Medications are especially important in the treatment of multiple-drug abuse. SEE ALSO COCAINE; COCAINE: WITHDRAWAL; COCAINE TREATMENT: BEHAVIORAL APPROACHES; NALTREXONE.

detoxification process of removing a poisonous, intoxicating, or addictive substance from the body

Codeine

Codeine, a natural product of the opium poppy, is one of the most widely used analgesics (painkillers) for mild to moderate pain. Most codeine medications combine a dose of codeine with mild analgesics such as aspirin, acetaminophen (e.g., Tylenol), and ibuprofen (e.g., Advil). The presence of the mild analgesics permits far lower codeine doses. Using lower doses of codeine can reduce its side effects, such as constipation and nausea. SEE ALSO ANALGESIC; OPIATE AND OPIOID DRUG ABUSE.

Codependence

When someone is addicted to alcohol or drugs, that person's problems affect the entire family. The family members often share some of the addicted person's beliefs and behave in similar ways. The term "codependence" refers to these shared beliefs and behaviors. Codependence has become a popular topic of discussion, and bookstores are full of works on the subject. Many of these books deal with the emotional damage suffered during childhood and the need to heal the "inner child."

Although currently popular, the idea that alcohol and drug problems affect family members is not new. In a 1973 book called *I'll Quit*

Tomorrow, Vernon Johnson wrote that, "While there may be only one alcoholic in a family, the whole family suffers from the alcoholism. For every harmfully dependent person, most often there are two, three, or even more people immediately around him who are just as surely victims of the disease. They too need real help."

The people who live with an alcoholic or drug abuser have experiences that damage their sense of well-being. As the addicted person fails again and again to quit using alcohol or drugs, the family members also meet failure after failure. They may blame themselves for the other person's failure to quit. This failure may lead to feelings of fear, frustration, shame, inadequacy, guilt, resentment, self-pity, and anger. They may have a growing sense of worthlessness, and in response they may build emotional defenses against their feelings. Like the addicted person, they may begin to project some of the angry, negative feelings they have about themselves onto other family members, including children. They take the anger and disgust they feel about themselves and apply it to others, acting as if these other family members deserve the same feelings of anger and disgust. They do not see that this behavior makes them weaker rather than stronger, or that they have become out of touch with reality. Like the addicted person, they may deny that they need help.

Characteristics

The following six characteristics form the common thread weaving through the lives of many, if not most, family members of alcoholics, drug addicts, and people with other addictions such as gambling or eating disorders:

1. *Codependents change who they are, and what they are feeling, to please others.* Like the chameleon that changes its coloring to blend in safely with its current environment, codependents give up their own identity in an effort to get others to love them. They do this for two reasons. First, they fear being abandoned if people know how they really feel or who they really are. Second, they have so little sense of who they are that they need to be in relationships in order to feel complete. Unless they are in a relationship, they feel desperately lonely and worthless. As a result, codependents are split between the false version of themselves they show to other people, and the way they truly feel—chaotic, fearful, and empty.

2. *Codependents feel responsible for meeting other peoples' needs, even at the expense of their own needs.* Codependents are so afraid of rejection that they will do anything to keep other people happy, including sacrificing their own needs to keep people from leav-

ing them. They actually get more upset if others are disappointed or hurt than if their own problems go unsolved. This habit of focusing more on others often leads to the problem of enabling. Enabling means that the codependent person protects the addicted person from the negative consequences of his drinking or other addictive behavior. The enabler tries to keep the other person from having to feel any pain or embarrassment. For example, if an alcoholic's drinking prevents him from going to work, the enabler may phone the employer to say he is "sick." This kind of "protection" prevents the alcoholic from facing natural consequences for his behavior.

3. *Codependents have low self-esteem.* Most people who are dependent on drugs or alcohol feel ashamed of themselves. Other family members also begin to feel bad about themselves. For codependents, low self-esteem comes from having very little sense of self to begin with. By always pleasing others and taking their whole identity from others, codependents end up not knowing who they are apart from the relationships they are in. As a result, they do not respect themselves. Low self-esteem also comes from believing that they truly are responsible for someone's alcohol or drug use. Once they believe this, they will always feel inadequate when they fail to control the addict's behavior. This mistaken sense of what should be under their control is at the very core of both codependence and dependence.

4. *Codependents are driven by compulsions, or a sense of extreme responsibility and urgency that a particular action be taken.* The codependent believes that success or failure will depend on acting in a certain way or completing a particular task. Initially, the compulsion may appear to be a positive force for the codependent, such as making lists. However, the codependent cannot abandon the compulsion without feeling anxious or fearing failure. Codependents feel they do not have any real choices about what is happening to them. They feel compelled to do any number of things: keep the family together, stop the drinking or other drug use, save the family from shame, work, eat or diet, be religious, keep the house clean, and on and on. Compulsions create excitement and drama. As people battle their compulsions, simple decisions, such as what to eat or how much to work, are turned into life-or-death struggles. These dramas temporarily give the codependent a feeling of purpose and vitality. Compulsions also take up a lot of time and keep people from confronting their deeper feelings. Codependents often get locked into compulsive behaviors to avoid more painful feelings of fear, sadness, anger, and abandonment.

5. *Like the addicts in their families, codependents deny reality.* Alcoholics often deny that they are abusing alcohol and remain unaware of its impact on their lives and their relationships with family members, friends, and coworkers. Codependents show exactly the same denial. They often refuse to see that a family member is addicted, or they refuse to acknowledge that their children are being hurt. Shame and the compulsion to keep things under control cause codependents to deny the problem.

6. *Like addicts, codependents are unwilling to accept that human willpower has its limits.* Just as alcoholics believe they can control their own drinking problem, codependents think they can control their loved one's alcoholism if they just use enough willpower. They keep trying to control the situation through their own force of will, not admitting that they need help with their problem.

Codependents firmly believe that their failure to cope is caused by their personal inadequacy. When they cannot control the drinking, drug use, or other addiction of someone they love, they blame themselves for not trying hard enough—or for not trying the right way. When codependents take too much responsibility for another person's recovery, it keeps the alcoholic or addict from seeing that only he or she is responsible for his or her own recovery. In this way, codependence actually increases the likelihood that a drug or alcohol problem will continue.

Children and Codependence

Codependence can be a serious problem for children. In all families, children must balance two competing childhood needs: (1) Children need to be unconditionally loved by their parents and to feel that they are at the center of things and (2) children also have the opposite need to rely completely on powerful and good parents; or in other words, to have others be at the center of things. Parents who have problems with alcohol or drug addiction are often unable to put their children at the center of family attention. They cannot tolerate not being the center of relationships, even at the expense of their children's needs. Children then sacrifice their own need for attention, allowing the parent to remain at the center. In this way children can become codependent.

Professionals who work in the field of addiction agree that huge numbers of people have found help for their problems through the concept of codependence. By understanding the concept, they can learn how to cope with their own problems and stop blaming themselves for the problems and failures of a loved one.

Many support and self-help groups incorporate efforts to break people of their tendencies to be codependent. Some groups include Adult Children of Alcoholics, ☎ Al-Anon, ☎ Alateen, ☎ and Nar-Anon. ☎ SEE ALSO ADULT CHILDREN OF ALCOHOLICS (ACOA); AL-ANON; ALATEEN; FAMILIES AND DRUG USE.

☎ See *Organizations of Interest* at the back of Volume 1 for address, telephone, and URL.

Coffee

Coffee is the world's most common source of caffeine, a **stimulant**. In the United States, coffee is usually made by percolation or infusion from the roasted and ground or pounded seeds of the coffee tree (genus *Coffea*). This tree was native to Africa but now is grown widely in warm regions for commercial crops. More than half of adolescents and adults in the United States drink some type of coffee beverage. SEE ALSO CAFFEINE; COLA DRINKS; TEA.

stimulant drug that increases activity temporarily; often used to describe drugs that excite the brain and central nervous system

Cola Drinks

Cola drinks are carbonated soft drinks that contain extract of the kola nut. Kola nuts, the seeds of the African kola tree, contain the **stimulant** caffeine. Coca-Cola, one of the first sodas to contain kola extracts, originally also contained extracts of the coca plant (cocaine). In the early 1900s the cocaine was removed and replaced by additional caffeine.

Drinking cola is part of American and worldwide culture, with many brands competing for a huge and growing consumer market. Colas are now available with sugar or artificial sweeteners, with or without caffeine, and with or without caramel coloring. People seem to like them regardless of the specific ingredients. SEE ALSO CAFFEINE.

Complications from Injecting Drugs

Many injectable drugs are used for medical purposes. Some of these prescription drugs are used illegally, as are a variety of street drugs. Illegal and abused injectable drugs can include nearly any drug that can be produced in a liquid form. The user takes these drugs to experience a high by injecting them into veins or under the skin. Injecting drugs puts a user at risk for a variety of medical complications.

Injecting drugs into one's system can cause a wide range of health problems and even lead to death.

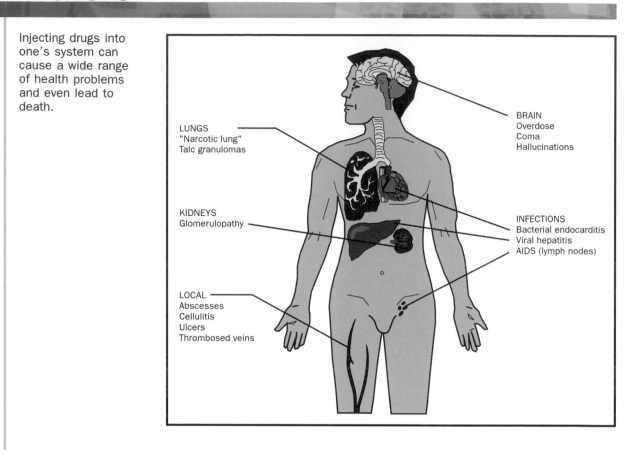

LUNGS
"Narcotic lung"
Talc granulomas

KIDNEYS
Glomerulopathy

LOCAL
Abscesses
Cellulitis
Ulcers
Thrombosed veins

BRAIN
Overdose
Coma
Hallucinations

INFECTIONS
Bacterial endocarditis
Viral hepatitis
AIDS (lymph nodes)

Transmitting Disease through Injection

Injections are the source of the greatest number and variety of medical complications from drug use. The most common complication, and the one with the most frequent fatal and disabling consequences, is transmitting disease through the use and sharing of dirty needles. Injecting drug users feel an intense desire to get high. They will inject drugs even if their needles and other injection equipment are not sterile. Injecting drug use can also affect a person's ability to exercise good judgment. Users are more likely to engage in risky behaviors, resulting in disease or even death.

Human Immunodeficiency Virus (HIV). The use of injected drugs is the second greatest risk factor for HIV (the first is sex between men). The majority of heterosexual HIV transmission occurs through injecting drug use. Injecting drug users transmit the virus directly through blood when they share used, unsterilized hypodermic needles and syringes, cotton, cookers (items such as a spoon or bottle top used to heat heroin prior to injection), rags, and water that has been contaminated with the infected blood of others. HIV may live in a needle contaminated with blood for up to four weeks. HIV is also transmitted when bodily fluids, including semen, saliva, and blood, are exchanged during sexual acts.

At least half of all new HIV infections in the United States are among people under age 25, with females making up 47 percent. According to one study, African Americans account for 56 percent of HIV cases reported among 13- to 24-year-olds. Because all needle-using drug abusers are considered at extremely high risk for HIV infection, HIV screening is performed routinely at most drug-treatment centers.

Hepatitis B and C. Hepatitis B and Hepatitis C, diseases of the liver, are the most common diseases caused by injecting drug use. Like HIV, hepatitis can also spread during sexual intercourse or other direct sharing of blood and bodily fluids. Hepatitis can cause hepatic fibrosis, the development of fibrous tissue in the liver, which can interfere with liver function. Hepatitis can also cause or worsen cirrhosis (scarring of the liver), although this is most often a result of chronic alcohol abuse. A vaccine is available to prevent hepatitis B. However, there is no vaccine for hepatitis C, and infection progresses more rapidly to liver damage in HIV-infected individuals. In fact, the majority of HIV-infected drug users also have hepatitis C.

Tetanus and Malaria. Between 70 and 90 percent of all cases of **tetanus** are among drug abusers. Tetanus most often occurs from injecting drugs under the skin, also known as "skin-popping." **Malaria** has been spreading in the United States among injecting drug users who have been to areas where malaria is common, such as Africa or Asia. The spread of both these diseases among needle-sharing drug abusers (particularly on the East Coast and in Chicago) is generally contained because of the quinine added to heroin. (Dealers add quinine to stretch the heroin's profitability.)

tetanus rare but often fatal disease that affects the brain and spinal column

malaria disease caused by a parasite in the red blood cells; passed to humans through the bite of mosquitoes

Complications to Heart and Blood Vessels. Endocarditis is an infection of tissues in the heart, usually a heart valve. This condition can prevent the free flow of blood through blood vessels, and can cause progressively worsening heart damage. Endocarditis can also cause severe heart-valve destruction that can be fatal if not treated. This disease can result from repeated injection of the infective agents into the blood system, usually from nonsterile needles.

Other Complications

There has been considerable concern over the hazards of cocaine, especially when it is self-administered into a vein. Chest pain is a very common effect of injecting cocaine. The physical conditions causing this pain place a cocaine user at significant risk for an acute coronary syndrome, a heart condition in which the heart muscle is deprived of oxygen, risking heart attack and damage.

People who inject amphetamines may experience inflamed and swollen arteries that can, in turn, lead to blood-vessel changes and tissue loss. This blockage of blood flow in the vessels of the brain may trigger a stroke. Intravenous users of amphetamines may also develop lung problems caused by materials that are included as cutting agents or as buffers and binding agents in drugs that come in pill form but are liquefied and injected. These substances do not dissolve, so particles may lodge in the lungs, causing damage. These same buffers and binding agents may also become lodged in various capillary systems, including the tiny blood vessels in the eye.

Bone infections (osteomyelitis) are a common complication of injecting drug use. Gangrene can develop from cutting off circulation to the limbs and may lead to amputation or death. Injecting drug use also contributes to reduced immune system functioning, making the user more susceptible to disease and related complications.

Occasionally drugs are accidentally injected into an artery (rather than into a vein or under the skin). This produces intense pain, swelling, cyanosis (blueness), and coldness of the part of the body injected. Injecting a drug into an artery creates a medical emergency and, if untreated, may produce gangrene of the fingers, hands, toes, or feet and result in loss of these parts.

Preventing Complications Among Injecting Drug Users

The best way to avoid complications from injecting drugs is to never start. Once a person becomes a user, the best course of action is to

Drugs users who take their drugs through injections are much more likely to be men and, in particular, to be white men.

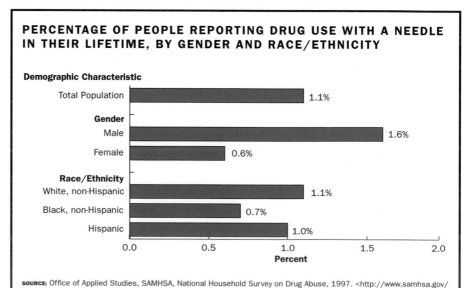

PERCENTAGE OF PEOPLE REPORTING DRUG USE WITH A NEEDLE IN THEIR LIFETIME, BY GENDER AND RACE/ETHNICITY

Demographic Characteristic

Total Population	1.1%
Gender	
Male	1.6%
Female	0.6%
Race/Ethnicity	
White, non-Hispanic	1.1%
Black, non-Hispanic	0.7%
Hispanic	1.0%

Percent (0.0 – 0.5 – 1.0 – 1.5 – 2.0)

SOURCE: Office of Applied Studies, SAMHSA, National Household Survey on Drug Abuse, 1997. <http://www.samhsa.gov/oas/NHSDA/1997Main/nhsda1997mfWeb-96.htm#Table 10.5>.

enroll in a drug treatment program. However, until a user stops, he or she should take certain precautions to keep personal risk at a minimum. For example, the user should use new, sterile syringes for each injection. Syringes, needles, water, or drug equipment should never be shared or reused. Needle exchange programs in some areas will exchange clean, sterile needles for used, dirty needles. The goal of these programs is to keep infection rates down by offering clean needles. When sterile syringes are not available, individuals should wash syringes and other equipment with bleach, even though this procedure is not as safe as using a new, sterile syringe. Toothbrushes, razors, and personal care items that might be contaminated with blood should not be shared. Injecting drug users and their partners should also practice safer sex such as using a **condom** or **dental dam** during every sex act. SEE ALSO ACCIDENTS AND INJURIES FROM DRUGS; COCAINE; HEROIN; NEEDLE EXCHANGE PROGRAMS; SUBSTANCE ABUSE AND AIDS.

condom covering worn over the penis; used as a barrier method of birth control and disease prevention

dental dam piece of latex used to protect the mouth; can be used in dentistry, or can be used to prevent the oral transmission of sexually transmitted diseases

Conduct Disorder

Conduct disorder refers to a behavioral disturbance in children. Children with the disorder behave repeatedly in ways that violate the basic rights of others and that society does not consider appropriate for their age. The behavior is different from general misbehavior, which occurs among nearly all children: usually it lasts longer, is more severe, and involves different kinds of actions. It also has more serious consequences than typical childhood mischief. Conduct disorder is the behavioral problem that child psychiatrists most often treat. Reports of the number of children who have conduct disorder range from less than 1 percent to more than 10 percent of all children. These children are often called antisocial, and one-quarter to one-half of such children will have **antisocial personality disorder** as adults.

antisocial personality disorder condition in which people disregard the rights of others and violate these rights by acting in immoral, unethical, aggressive, or even criminal ways

Characteristics

The behaviors that characterize conduct disorder include:

- theft
- vandalism
- physical fights—sometimes with weapons
- fire setting
- running away from home
- truancy

- repetitive lying
- forcing sexual activity on others
- physical cruelty to animals and to people
- substance abuse

Law enforcement may become involved when children commit these acts.

Conduct disorder appears to be more common in boys than in girls and more common in urban areas than in rural areas. Girls with a conduct disorder are likely to run away from home and/or become involved in prostitution. Children with this disorder rarely perform at an academic level in keeping with their intelligence or age, and they often have poor relationships with peers. They are more likely than other children to suffer from depression, to have suicidal thoughts, to make suicidal attempts, and to commit suicide.

Factors That Contribute to the Disorder

Some of the factors that contribute to conduct disorder have to do with biology, while others have to do with the family and social life of the child. Social factors include:

- a family history of antisocial personality disorder or alcohol dependence (or both)
- parents who have poor parenting skills
- early rejection by the mother
- early institutionalization (placement at a young age in a group home or institutions)
- large family size and crowding in the home
- a chaotic home environment
- lower economic status

Biological factors that contribute to conduct disorder include:

- mild abnormalities of the central nervous system (the brain and spinal cord)
- neurological damage during the birth process
- insensitivity to physical pain

Often, children with conduct disorder are also diagnosed with attention deficit disorder or attention-deficit/hyperactivity disorder and some developmental disorders.

As adults, these children frequently have psychiatric problems. They are less likely to do well in higher education and hold on to jobs, and more likely to commit crimes, to smoke, to abuse alcohol, and to use illegal drugs. Many will have problems with **dependence** and will seek treatment many times in their lives for drug abuse.

Conduct Disorder and Drug Use

In individuals with both conduct disorder and substance abuse, a common combination, the conduct disorder usually appears before the drug abuse. Many individuals have a genetic **predisposition** to both substance abuse and conduct disorder. This means that they have inherited a trait that makes it likely they will both use drugs and behave in antisocial and violent ways.

Drug use during adolescence almost always involves illegal behavior plus a deviant peer group. As a result, drug use increases the risk for violent assault as well as getting arrested and convicted for drug possession or selling. The use of drugs in early to mid-adolescence sets up a pattern of antisocial behaviors that may last into adulthood.

Treating Conduct Disorder

Conduct disorder in children and adolescents can be treated through family therapy, individual therapy, and residential treatment programs. The most promising treatment, however, appears to be a training program for parents in which they learn skills for managing their children and encouraging them to behave in positive ways. The children also receive training in the use of problem-solving strategies.

Four drugs have been tested as treatments for conduct disorder in children. One test showed that lithium and methylphenidate (Ritalin) can reduce aggressiveness in children. Tests of the other two drugs, carbamazepine (Tegretol) and clonidine (Catapres), showed they were also effective in reducing aggressiveness but had many side effects.

Conduct disorder is a very difficult condition that presents risks to individuals, families, and society. More research into conduct disorder may eventually reveal ways to prevent it or to treat it effectively once it is diagnosed. SEE ALSO ANTISOCIAL PERSONALITY; ATTENTION-DEFICIT/HYPERACTIVITY DISORDER; CRIME AND DRUGS; FAMILIES AND DRUG USE; RISK FACTORS FOR SUBSTANCE ABUSE; RITALIN.

dependence psychological compulsion to use a substance for emotional and/or physical reasons

predisposition condition in which one is vulnerable or prone to something

Costs of Substance Abuse and Dependence, Economic

Substance abuse and dependence on substances continue to be major health problems in the United States. The abuse of alcohol and drugs

☎ See *Organizations of Interest* at the back of Volume 1 for address, telephone, and URL.

costs the nation billions of dollars in health-care costs and reduced or lost productivity each year. Since the mid-1980s, researchers have made estimates of these rising economic costs of substance abuse and dependence in the United States. In 1998, the National Institute on Drug Abuse ☎ and the National Institute on Alcohol Abuse and Alcoholism ☎, which are parts of the National Institutes of Health, released a study on these costs based on 1992 survey data. This article is based on the 1998 report.

The Extent of the Problem

The economic cost to society from alcohol and drug abuse was $246 billion in 1992. Alcohol abuse and alcoholism cost an estimated $148 billion, while drug abuse and dependence cost an estimated $98 billion. The 1992 estimates for alcohol were 42 percent higher than the 1985 estimate (taking into account increases due to population growth and inflation).

Economic costs can be measured in several ways. When people die prematurely because of substance abuse problems, their wages are permanently lost. Not only do health-care costs increase as a result of substance abuse, but also society pays for the problem in terms of lost productivity and increased crime.

Premature Deaths. In 1992, there were an estimated 107,400 alcohol-related deaths in the United States. Many of the alcohol-related deaths were among people between the ages of 20 and 40. However, long-term, heavy drinking is also involved in numerous premature deaths among the older population. Total costs attributed to alcohol-related motor vehicle crashes were estimated to be $24.7 bil-

The economic costs of drug abuse and addiction are staggering. This study calculated "lost wages," or money that would otherwise have been earned if the person had not been addicted to drugs. It found that drug abuse represented lost wages of more than $77 million.

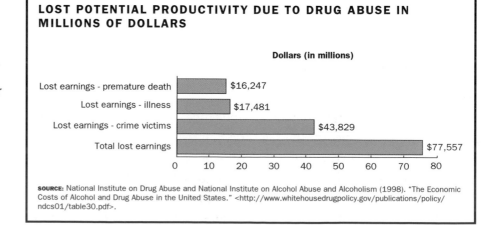

LOST POTENTIAL PRODUCTIVITY DUE TO DRUG ABUSE IN MILLIONS OF DOLLARS

Dollars (in millions)

Lost earnings - premature death	$16,247
Lost earnings - illness	$17,481
Lost earnings - crime victims	$43,829
Total lost earnings	$77,557

0 10 20 30 40 50 60 70 80

SOURCE: National Institute on Drug Abuse and National Institute on Alcohol Abuse and Alcoholism (1998). "The Economic Costs of Alcohol and Drug Abuse in the United States." <http://www.whitehousedrugpolicy.gov/publications/policy/ndcs01/table30.pdf>.

lion. This included $11.1 billion from premature death and $13.6 billion from automobile and other property destruction.

Health-Care Costs. In 1992, total estimated spending for health-care services was $18.8 billion for alcohol problems and the medical consequences of heavy drinking. Specialized services for the treatment of alcohol problems cost $5.6 billion. These services included **detoxification** and **rehabilitation** programs as well as prevention, training, and research expenditures. Costs of treatment for health problems caused by alcohol were estimated at $13.2 billion.

Lost Productivity. In 1992 an estimated $67.7 billion in lost potential productivity was caused by alcohol abuse. This lost productivity took the form of work not performed, including household tasks, and was measured in terms of lost earnings and household productivity. The alcohol abusers themselves and the people with whom they lived shouldered most of these costs. About $1 billion was for victims of **fetal alcohol syndrome** who had survived to adulthood and were mentally impaired. This study did not estimate the burden of drug and alcohol problems on work sites or employers.

Crime. The costs of crime attributed to alcohol abuse were estimated at $19.7 billion. These costs include reduced earnings due to imprisonment, crime careers, and victims of crimes whose ability to earn an income has been reduced. The costs also include criminal justice and seizure of drug shipments. Alcohol abuse is estimated to have contributed to 25 to 30 percent of violent crime.

Before 1996, people could collect welfare benefits if they were impaired as a result of drug or alcohol abuse or dependence. The study estimated that 3.3 percent of people who received welfare benefits in 1992 did so for this reason. These benefits totaled $10.4 billion. In 1996, new welfare reform laws changed the rules as to who is eligible for welfare. Alcohol or drug dependence can no longer be the main reason for a person to receive benefits.

Who Pays?

Much of the economic burden of substance abuse and dependence falls on the population that does not abuse drugs or alcohol. Economic costs to governments for alcohol problems were $57.2 billion in 1992, compared with $15.1 billion for private insurance, $9 billion for victims, and $66.8 billion for alcohol abusers and members of their households. Society bears these costs in a variety of ways, including

detoxification
process of removing a poisonous, intoxicating, or addictive substance from the body

rehabilitation
process of restoring a person to a condition of health or useful activity

fetal alcohol syndrome set of birth defects that affect a child's growth and behavior as a result of prenatal alcohol exposure

PERCENTAGE OF WORKING AGE POPULATION REPORTING SUBSTANCE USE IN 1999 BY EMPLOYMENT STATUS

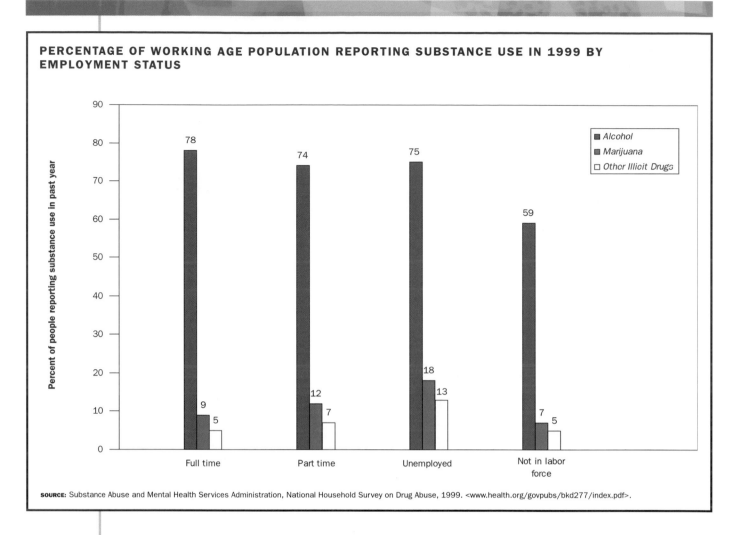

SOURCE: Substance Abuse and Mental Health Services Administration, National Household Survey on Drug Abuse, 1999. <www.health.org/govpubs/bkd277/index.pdf>.

Although many substance users are employed, users of marijuana and other illicit drugs are more likely to work part time or be unemployed.

alcohol-related crimes and trauma (for example, motor vehicle crashes); government services (such as criminal justice and highway safety); and various social insurance programs (such as private and public health insurance, life insurance, tax payments, pensions, and social welfare insurance).

In Conclusion

Substance abuse and dependence are costly to the nation in resources used for care and treatment of persons suffering from these disorders, lives lost prematurely, and reduced productivity. Data show clearly that the measurable economic costs of alcohol and drug abuse continue to be high. SEE ALSO ACCIDENTS AND INJURIES FROM ALCOHOL; ACCIDENTS AND INJURIES FROM DRUGS; ALCOHOL: COMPLICATIONS OF PROBLEM DRINKING; BABIES, ADDICTED AND DRUG-EXPOSED; COMPLICATIONS FROM INJECTING DRUGS; CRIME AND DRUGS; FETAL ALCOHOL SYNDROME (FAS); MEDICAL EMERGENCIES AND DEATH FROM DRUG ABUSE; SUBSTANCE ABUSE AND AIDS; SUICIDE AND SUBSTANCE ABUSE; WORKPLACE, DRUG USE IN.

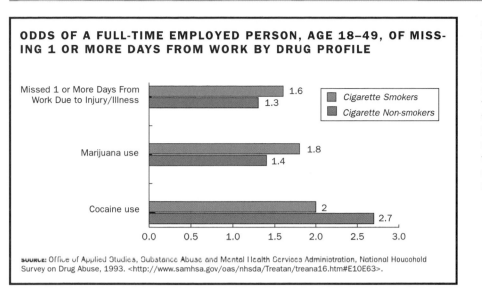

ODDS OF A FULL-TIME EMPLOYED PERSON, AGE 18–49, OF MISSING 1 OR MORE DAYS FROM WORK BY DRUG PROFILE

Missed 1 or More Days From Work Due to Injury/Illness — 1.6 / 1.3

Marijuana use — 1.8 / 1.4

Cocaine use — 2 / 2.7

■ Cigarette Smokers
■ Cigarette Non-smokers

SOURCE: Office of Applied Studies, Substance Abuse and Mental Health Services Administration, National Household Survey on Drug Abuse, 1993. <http://www.samhsa.gov/oas/nhsda/Treatan/treana16.htm#E10E63>.

According to one study by the Substance Abuse and Mental Health Administration, cigarette users are more likely to miss a day from work due to illness or injury than non-users are, but not as likely to miss a day when compared to cocaine users.

Crack

Crack (sometimes called crack cocaine) is the form of cocaine that is smoked. The white powder that people buy illegally as cocaine cannot be smoked, because it is destroyed at the temperatures required for smoking. Cocaine can be converted to crack by adding an **alkaline**, then heating the mixture, resulting in a pellet-sized, cakelike solid substance that can be smoked. Crack takes its name from the cracks formed in the solid as it dries. This form of cocaine is less expensive than powder cocaine and is available for purchase on the street.

alkaline similar in chemical composition to the alkali chemicals; possessing a pH greater than 7

Smoking cocaine began with the use of a preparation of cocaine called freebase. Soon after this form of cocaine became popular, single doses of crack cocaine already prepared for smoking became available through the illegal drug market. Although crack can be smoked in tobacco cigarettes or marijuana cigarettes, it is generally smoked in a special crack pipe.

Users adopted the smoking method of taking cocaine because smoking delivers the drug's effects quickly. Blood levels of cocaine peak rapidly when the drug is smoked, producing the cocaine "rush." The speed and duration of the effects are comparable to taking the drug by injection. Users of crack prefer smoking because it does not require the paraphernalia—syringes, needles, and so on—needed for injecting drugs.

Crack is an extremely dangerous substance because of its **toxicity**. Also, crack is dangerous because it is easy to use and available in single doses to almost anyone because of its relatively low price. The easier a drug is to obtain and the more rapidly it takes effect, the more

toxicity condition of being poisonous or dangerous to people

likely it is that the drug will be abused. SEE ALSO COCAINE; STREET VALUE.

Creativity and Drugs

Some young people have an image of artists, writers, actors, and others in the creative and performing arts as heavy users or abusers of drugs and alcohol. What follows from that image is the idea that drug use stimulates creativity or improves the artistic experience. However, there is little scientific evidence that alcohol and drug use actually increase creativity.

psychedelic substance that can cause hallucinations and/or make its user lose touch with reality

In particular, people have taken **psychedelic** drugs, such as lysergic acid diethylamide (LSD), mescaline, and methylene dioxyamphetamine (MDA) to increase their appreciation of art, to improve artistic techniques, and to enhance creativity. Marijuana, too, has been used to enhance creativity, to heighten one's sense of meaningfulness, and to expand one's range of perceptions. Countless people worldwide have used alcohol to loosen their inhibitions, to become more spontaneous, and to encourage originality.

psychoactive term applied to drugs that affect the mind or mental processes by altering consciousness, perception, or mood

One reason drugs are thought to inspire creativity is that **psychoactive** substances can produce altered states of consciousness. People on drugs think differently—they no longer distinguish between cause and effect, and they accept ideas that logically contradict each other. Often even their sense of time changes. They experience their emotions in a different way, and feel as though the boundary between themselves and the world dissolves. This sense of merging with the world is often described as a feeling of "oneness," and people may feel that they have been reborn. They may also have illusions and hallucinations, and at the same time feel that they see things more clearly.

After going through these altered states, it is not surprising that people may believe certain drug experiences lead to greater creativity. However, having creative thoughts while on a drug does not necessarily lead to the act of creating. In fact, drugs usually interfere with translating those thoughts into paintings or poems or musical compositions.

Do new perceptions experienced while on a drug spur more artistic creations? The creative process involves discovery and insight, as well as discipline to create something lasting. A lasting creative product has the qualities of novelty, surprise, uniqueness, originality, and

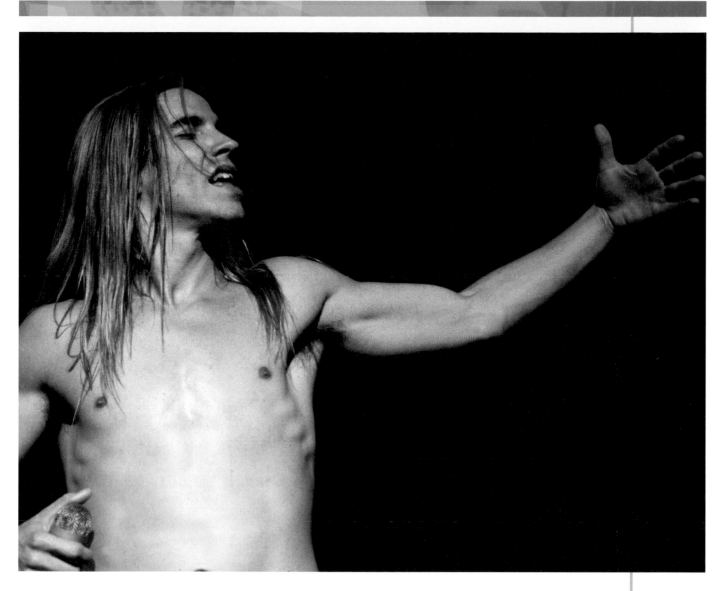

Anthony Kiedis, of the band Red Hot Chili Peppers, stopped using drugs after his bandmate and best friend, Hillel Slovak, died of a heroin overdose.

beauty. There is no evidence that alcohol and drugs actually contribute to the creative process, or that they result in more creative products. A person may feel that he or she has had original perceptions while on a drug; however, that sense of originality is related to the altered state of being on the drug. Once the drug's effects fade, the novelty wears off, and thus the perceptions experienced as part of a drug high contribute nothing toward a creative work of lasting benefit or value.

Only a few studies have explored the effect of drugs on creativity. The ones that exist show that drugs actually diminish rather than enhance creativity. This is especially true when drugs are taken in large amounts and over an extended period of time.

In a study conducted in 1946, a researcher asked seventeen artists who drank to describe how alcohol affected their work. All but one regarded the short-term effects of alcohol as harmful to their work, although they sometimes drank in order to overcome technical difficulties. In general, the artists said alcohol increased their sense of freedom when they approached their work but decreased their ability to get the work done in a skillful way. In a 1990 study involving thirty-four people in the arts, another researcher found that more than 75 percent of artists or performers who drank heavily felt that alcohol had negative effects on their creative activity, particularly when they drank while working.

Drugs and alcohol may actually interfere with an individual's ability to express creativity, because alcohol and drugs:

- May make users drowsy or sedated
- May hinder an individual's ability concentrate
- May interfere with coordination
- May blow out of proportion the importance of insignificant thoughts or details

Furthermore, the pursuit of more drugs and alcohol may take on more importance than the individual's artistic pursuit.

Given that no proof exists to show that drugs or alcohol enhance creativity, why are they used more widely within the artistic professions than among the general population? Probably the answer lies in the reasons why other people use drugs: to increase enjoyment of social occasions, to relax, to have pleasurable feelings.

Writers, artists, actors, or musicians may write about, portray, or act out certain aspects of their drug experiences. But this does not mean that these experiences are essential for the creative process. Creative people often use all aspects of their experiences, whether drug-induced or not, in a creative way. They try to translate personal visions and insights within their own fields of expression into art that other people can appreciate. Drug-induced experiences have little value or meaning for anyone other than, perhaps, substance users themselves. SEE ALSO LYSERGIC ACID DIETHYLAMIDE (LSD) AND PSYCHEDELICS.

Crime and Drugs

Drugs and crime: These two words are often linked, but does an increase in drug use automatically mean an increase in the number of crimes committed? The role of drugs in crime is of great public and political concern. Fear that an increase in drug use will contribute to an increase in crime rates has led individuals and communities to seek answers to urgent questions about the drugs-crime relationship. Recently, significant advances in research have furthered our understanding of this issue.

Research conducted before 1980 did not give an accurate picture of drug-related crime. These earlier studies relied on official arrest records as indicators of criminal activity. However, later studies showed that less than 1 percent of crimes committed by drug abusers result in arrest. More realistic estimates of drug-related crime must rely on confidential self-report data. By this method, researchers ask questions directly of people involved in crime or drug use. To ensure that the respondents answer truthfully, the researchers guarantee that answers will not lead to prosecution. These self-reports offer a clearer picture of the extent of criminal behavior among drug users.

In addition, the Bureau of Justice Statistics ☎ National Crime Victimization Survey asks victims of violent crime whether the offender appeared to be under the influence of drugs or alcohol. In the most recent survey, about 28 percent of victims of violent crimes perceived that their offender was under the influence of drugs or alcohol. Note that 42 percent of victims could not tell, and only 30 percent reported that the offender did not appear to be under the influence of drugs or alcohol.

The Criminal Behavior of Drug Abusers

In 1997, the National Institute of Justice established the Arrestee Drug Abuse Monitoring (ADAM) Program to measure drug use among people who have been arrested. To take this measurement, booking facilities in thirty-five U.S. cities collect voluntary and anonymous urine samples at the time of arrest. The researchers then calculate the percentage of arrestees who had urine tests that were positive for drug use. In addition, researchers conduct interviews with the arrestees about drug use and criminal activity. By combining drug testing with self-report data from interviews, the ADAM program gives researchers a powerful tool for collecting evidence of patterns of drug abuse. Data from the ADAM program reveal that there is no single national drug problem, but rather different local drug problems that vary from city to city.

One of the factors that experts in the field of drugs and crime have identified is that frequency of drug use increases criminal activity. This is especially true for crimes involving property (such as theft or vandalism), and for people who are addicted to heroin, who abuse cocaine, and who abuse more than one drug (multiple drug users).

ESTIMATED NUMBER OF DRUG OFFENDERS IN FEDERAL, STATE, AND LOCAL JAILS

	Drug offenders	Percent of total inmates
Federal	55,984	59% (95,323)
State	236,800	21% (1,141,700)
Jail	152,000	26% (592,462)

SOURCES: Bureau of Justice Statistics, 'Prisoners in 1999'; U.S. Department of Justice, August 2000; Federal Bureau of Prisons Quick Facts; Bureau of Justice Statistics 'Drug Use, Testing, and Treatment in Jails.' <http://www.whitehousedrugpolicy.gov/publications/pdf/94406.pdf>.

Nearly six in every ten prisoners in federal prisons are drug offenders. Most drug abusers, however, are not arrested.

☎ See *Organizations of Interest* at the back of Volume 1 for address, telephone, and URL.

Heroin and Other Narcotics

narcotic addictive substance that relieves pain and induces sleep or causes sedation; prescription narcotics includes morphine and codeine; general and imprecise term referring to a drug of abuse, such as heroin, cocaine, or marijuana

Studies show that the use of **narcotics** such as heroin leads to increases in property crime and robbery. The simplest explanation for this result is that addicts steal because they need cash to support their drug habits. In addition, many heroin addicts turn to crimes such as prostitution to support their habits. While this trend may not be reflected in increased prostitution rates, it is nevertheless an important link between heroin use, crime, and public health, since injecting drug use and HIV infection are involved.

Most of the crime associated with heroin appears to be related not to heroin addicts but to drug trafficking—getting the drug into the country and distributing it to dealers and users. This is especially true of violent crime associated with heroin. Heroin addicts are less likely to commit violent crime than to commit property crime. Only a small percentage of all addict crime is violent crime (approximately 1 percent to 3 percent). However, the actual number of violent crimes is still relatively large because addicts commit so many crimes. Researchers have also suggested that heavy heroin use and, more recently, heavy cocaine abuse have contributed to record numbers of homicides in large cities in the United States. Some of this increase may be attributed to heroin users, but most of it is likely the result of drug trafficking. Violent competition between drug dealers has resulted in many murders and the deaths of innocent bystanders.

Non-narcotics

Non-narcotic drugs include cocaine, marijuana, PCP, amphetamines, and barbiturates. The relationship between use of these drugs and criminal behavior is difficult to determine because people who use them often also use narcotics. It is not always possible to disentangle the drugs' separate relationships to criminal activity. Despite these difficulties, research has made significant advances in understanding how non-narcotic drugs relate to crime.

Cocaine. When researchers studied a sample of 1,725 adolescents nationwide, they found that cocaine use had a strong connection with crime. Only 1.3 percent of the adolescents reported using cocaine in the year preceding the interview. Yet the cocaine users were responsible for 60 percent of all minor thefts, 57 percent of felony thefts, 41 percent of all robberies, and 28 percent of felony assaults committed by the entire sample.

In studies of youths with multiple charges for delinquent behavior and female crack-cocaine abusers, the subjects who reported us-

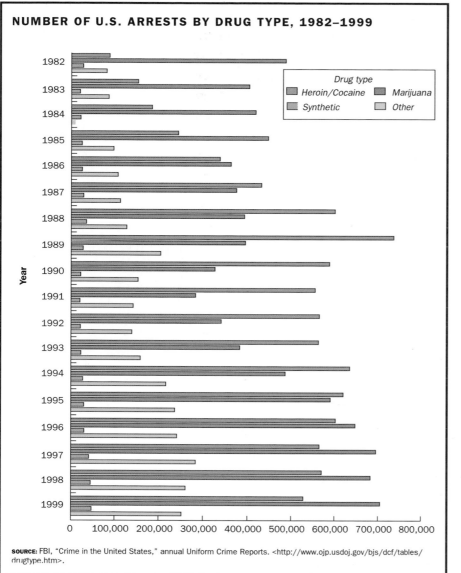

NUMBER OF U.S. ARRESTS BY DRUG TYPE, 1982–1999

Drug type
Heroin/Cocaine   Marijuana
Synthetic   Other

Year: 1982, 1983, 1984, 1985, 1986, 1987, 1988, 1989, 1990, 1991, 1992, 1993, 1994, 1995, 1996, 1997, 1998, 1999

0   100,000   200,000   300,000   400,000   500,000   600,000   700,000   800,000

SOURCE: FBI, "Crime in the United States," annual Uniform Crime Reports. <http://www.ojp.usdoj.gov/bjs/dcf/tables/drugtype.htm>.

Between 1982 and 1999, the number of heroin and cocaine arrests increased from less than 90,000 (in 1982) to more than half a million (in 1999).

ing cocaine most frequently committed more property and violent crimes than subjects who used crack less frequently. Out of a sample of 254 seriously delinquent youths, 184 crack dealers (86% of whom used crack every day) were responsible for 45,563 property crimes (an average of 231 per user) during the year preceding the interview. In contrast, the seventy subjects who were not crack dealers and who used crack less frequently (approximately three times per week) averaged 135 property crimes per year. In addition, the heavy cocaine users averaged ten robberies per year, compared with one per year for the other subjects.

According to the 2000 ADAM report, cocaine use among adult arrestees remained high, with variations among cities. Atlanta, New York City, Miami, Tucson, and Laredo, Texas, had the highest rates of cocaine use among male adult arrestees (40% or higher). In twelve other sites, however, cocaine use among male adult arrestees was less than 25 percent.

Other Non-narcotic Drugs. People who use only one non-narcotic drug, such as amphetamines, barbiturates, marijuana, or PCP, do not have high crime rates. In contrast, people who use these drugs in combination frequently have high crime rates. Use of a single drug may be related to such offenses as disorderly conduct or driving while impaired, but single use is not associated with other types of crime.

Marijuana. According to the 1999 ADAM report, marijuana remains a very popular drug among arrestees, particularly among young males between 15 and 20 years old. However, the use of marijuana is not connected with an increase in crime. The exceptions are sale of the drug and disorderly conduct or driving while impaired. Marijuana is often used in combination with other drugs. In such cases, it may be the other drugs' effects that play a role in criminal activity.

Amphetamines. Studies of drug abusers in different ethnic groups report that amphetamine use is related to violent crime in some individuals. In the general population, however, research shows little or no relationship between amphetamine use and crime. The 2000 ADAM report indicated that arrestees who use methamphetamine live mostly in the western part of the United States, although they are increasingly found in midwestern states as well. In other locations, tests showed virtually no methamphetamine use among arrestees.

Phencyclidine (PCP). The relationship between PCP and violence is still somewhat unclear. In the 1970s and early 1980s, studies claimed a strong link between PCP use and violent behavior. However, these studies were seriously flawed. The current view is that PCP use may cause violent behavior in a small proportion of users. PCP is not included in the ADAM report because it is rarely detected among arrestees.

Money Laundering

Laundering of money obtained through the sale of illegal drugs is an increasing component of crime in the United States. Money laundering is a process in which criminals convert the cash obtained through crime into a form they can use. **Drug traffickers** typically take hundreds of thousands of dollars in drug proceeds to a financial institution and exchange it for a cashier's check, which is much easier and much less suspicious to carry around (or out of the country)

drug traffickers people or groups who transport illegal drugs

than suitcases full of cash. In another scenario, the trafficker takes the cash to the bank, deposits it into an account, and then sends it by wire transfer to a bank in a foreign country, usually one in which banks promise a high degree of secrecy to their customers. Money laundering can also involve disguising where the money came from, avoiding paying taxes on it, and making it possible to transport.

Drug traffickers must be able to launder the money they collect in order to profit from their trade. This has led many governments that are unable to stop the actual drug trade to focus on breaking the drug networks by targeting money-laundering practices.

Theories on the Drugs–Crime Relationship

For many years experts in the field of drugs and crime believed in one of two opposing theories. The first theory states that drug addicts are criminals to begin with, and drug addiction is simply another form of a criminal lifestyle. The second theory states that addicts are not criminals but instead are forced into committing crime to support their drug habits.

More recent theories take the middle ground. Evidence shows that there is great variation in terms of which drug users commit crimes and when. Some addicts had been heavily involved in crime prior to addiction, whereas others were extensively involved in crime only when addicted. Drug users who are also criminals may have characteristics that **predispose** them to criminal activity.

predispose to be prone or vulnerable to something

Drug use and crime are often connected as a result of many different influences. Studies now examine that connection from many angles, rather than in a straight line between one cause and one effect. Thus research looks into many factors contributing to individuals' drug use and/or criminal activity, such as:

- The family: Did individuals lack parental supervision? Did they experience parental rejection, family conflict, and a lack of discipline? Did the parents use drugs and/or commit crimes?
- Association with peers who used drugs or committed crimes
- Dropping out of school
- Failure at tasks such as school or work
- Discipline problems
- Early antisocial behavior (acting out in ways that are not considered typical, expected, or acceptable)

Not all drug abusers are alike, and varying combinations of factors probably put certain individuals at risk of criminal behavior.

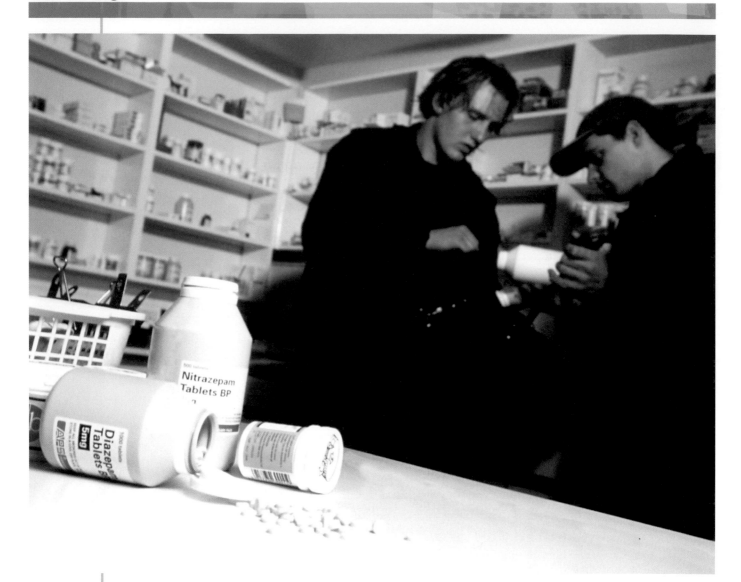

Because pharmaceutical drugs have street value, it is not uncommon for drugstores to encounter shoplifting or to be burglarized.

psychology scientific study of mental processes and behaviors

More research is needed to explain how certain types of drug abuse increase the frequency of criminal activity. Also, most theories focus on the period of adolescence, without examining factors that influence behavior during childhood and adulthood.

One of the major experts in the field of crime and drugs is Paul Goldstein. Goldstein formed a theory about drugs and violence based on studies of violent drug-related crimes in New York City. He studied descriptions of these crimes by both the perpetrators and the victims. According to this theory, drugs and violence can be related in three separate ways:

1. Violent crime results from the short- or long-term **psychological** and biological effects of a particular drug, most notably crack cocaine and heroin.

2. Violent crime is committed as a way to obtain money to buy drugs, mainly expensive addictive drugs such as heroin and cocaine.

3. Violent crime is the result of aggressive patterns of interaction found in the circles of illegal drug dealing and distribution. Examples include killing or assaulting someone for failure to pay debts; for selling "bad," or impure, drugs; or for operating on someone else's drug-dealing turf.

The U.S. Department of Justice's Bureau of Justice Statistics ☎ collects statistics about drug-related crimes from many agencies. According to the BJS, in 1999, 13 percent of all jail inmates and 24 percent of those convicted of property crime reported that they committed the crime to get money for drugs. The Uniform Crime Reporting Program of the Federal Bureau of Investigation reported that in 1999, 4.5 percent of the homicides in which circumstances were known were drug-related. Murders that occurred specifically during a drug felony, such as drug trafficking or manufacturing, are considered drug-related.

☎ See *Organizations of Interest* at the back of Volume 1 for address, telephone, and URL.

Who Commits the Most Serious Crimes?

In most cases, both drug use and crime begin in the early teens. The younger the individual is when first using a "soft" drug such as marijuana or committing a minor crime such as shoplifting, the more likely he or she will move on to "hard" drugs and more serious crimes. In general, criminal activity and drug use within the family, peer group, or community increases the risk that an individual will commit crimes at an early age.

Individuals who commit many different types of crime, including violent crime, at high rates, and who abuse many types of drugs, including heroin and cocaine, share certain characteristics. In general, the younger they are when first addicted to heroin and/or cocaine, the more frequent, persistent, and severe their criminal activity tends to be. This is true of both males and females, with one notable exception: Females who become addicted at an early age are more likely to commit nonviolent acts (such as prostitution, shoplifting, and other property crimes) at high rates, while males addicted early on are more likely to commit violent acts.

It is worth noting that, overall, both violent crime and property crime has been steadily declining in the United States for more than ten years. Violent crime rates have declined since 1994, and reached the lowest rate on record in 2000. Property crime rates have been declining for the past twenty years. During that same period, however, drug use among the arrestee population has remained consistently high, according to ADAM reports. Drugs and crime are likely to remain closely linked, whatever the crime rates. SEE ALSO COCAINE; FAMILIES AND DRUG USE; HEROIN; PHENCYCLIDINE (PCP); TERRORISM AND DRUGS.

Cutting and Self-Harm

Adolescents who cut themselves or engage in various other types of self-harming behavior often feel that their actions are very strange and unusual. Sometimes they are told that they are motivated by the desire to get attention. But in fact hurting themselves is their way of coping with difficult feelings. Self-harm occurs more often than one might think, and is usually done in private, with the hope that no one will ever find out about it. To explain self-harm, this entry defines the behavior and then discusses who engages in it and when, possible causes for this behavior, and how it can be treated.

What is Self-Harm?

Self-harm can take several forms, including cutting various parts of the body, most often the forearms or legs; head banging; skin picking; taking pills; and burning. (Self-harm is sometimes called self-injury or self-mutilation. However, because "mutilation" implies a frightening degree of severity, the term does not accurately represent the behavior.) It often occurs along with thoughts of wanting to be dead and/or killing oneself. Yet self-harm is very different from making a suicide attempt. While suicide attempts involve a wish to die, a young adult who acts on the urge to self-harm does not intend to cause death. Even so, self-harm behavior can at times be extremely dangerous, even if not intended. For example, a study led by Barbara Stanley in 2001 found that while suicide attempters with a history of self-injury perceived their suicide attempts as less serious than did suicide attempters without such a history, they were just as much at risk for dying and in fact suffered from greater **depression**. Therefore the behavior should always be taken very seriously.

Who Self-Harms?

Both adults and adolescents engage in self-harm. Adults who self-harm generally started doing so in adolescence. Recently, the number of acts of intentional self-harm not ending in death among adolescents has increased greatly. Armando R. Favazza and Karen Conterio in 1998 found that as many as 1,800 out of every 100,000

depression state in which an individual feels intensely sad and hopeless; may have trouble eating, sleeping, and concentrating, and is no longer able to feel pleasure from previously enjoyable activities; in extreme cases, may lead an individual to think about or attempt suicide

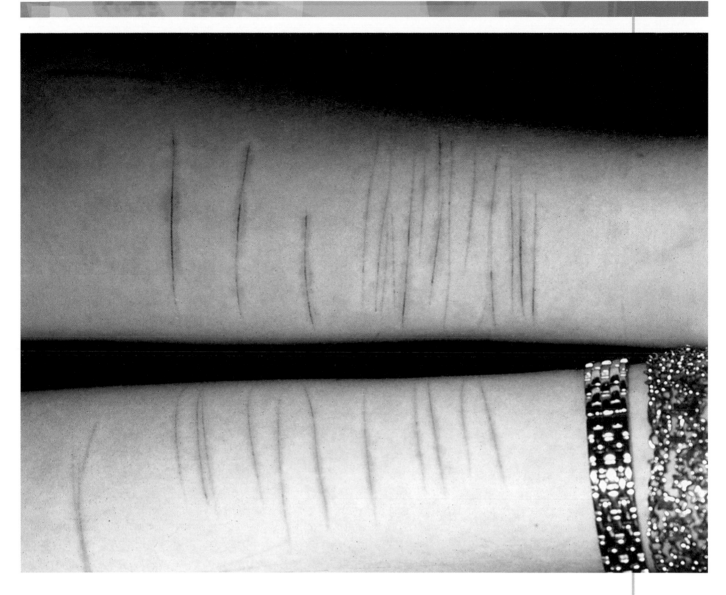

15- to-35-year-olds were deliberately hurting themselves. While some researchers say that there are no differences between males and females, others state that the behavior is more frequent in girls.

Adolescents who self-harm are in many ways similar to other kids. They sometimes have special strengths or skills, such as sensitivity and perceptiveness. However, they also often suffer from a variety of **psychological** or **psychiatric** difficulties, including depression and hopelessness, anxiety and anger, and personality disorders (having problems with difficult relationships and poor self-image). They may also have trouble in areas related to the body, such as with an eating disorder, having a clear sense of sexual identity, and/or substance abuse. Richard H. Schwartz and others in 1989 noted that many young self-harmers use alcohol, drugs, or both excessively. While certainly not true for everyone, self-harming adolescents can sometimes be aggressive toward others. Adolescents who suffer from major men-

Self-harm can take many forms—head banging, picking at the skin, taking pills, burning, and cutting one's skin. This behavior, often done secretly, is a very serious sign that the person needs help as soon as possible.

psychology scientific study of mental processes and behaviors

psychiatric deals with the study, treatment, and prevention of mental illness

schizophrenia psychotic disorder in which people lose the ability to function normally, experience severe personality changes, and suffer from a variety of symptoms, including confusion, disordered thinking, paranoia, hallucinations, emotional numbness, and speech problems

tal illnesses such as **schizophrenia** and who also self-harm tend to do so in a very different way than other self-harming adolescents. These young people often see their actions as a kind of religious act.

What Causes Self-Harm?

Many people believe that adolescents who harm themselves are trying to get attention or manipulate others, or that they are very disturbed. This may be true in some cases. But most often, the behavior is kept extremely private and secret. For most of the young people who self-harm, the behavior is a way to get relief from distressing feelings. Unfortunately, the relief obtained from self-injury is often only temporary. Usually a sense of shame and self-hatred quickly sets in after the act.

One researcher, Marsha M. Linehan, in 1993 wrote about self-harm as being an attempt to regulate emotions, meaning to feel more balanced and relaxed. Linehan suggested that self-harmers may have grown up in an environment that was not supportive, or that they may have a biological **predisposition** to the behavior.

predisposition condition in which one is vulnerable or prone to something

Scientists are studying some unusual differences in the brain chemistry of people who self-harm. Work by Maria Oquendo and J. John Mann in 2001 and Ronald Winchell and Michael Stanley in 1991 (among others) shows that adults, and perhaps adolescents as well, who engage in self-harm tend to have lower levels of a brain chemical called **serotonin**. Some studies have also shown that, in these people, other brain chemicals (norepinephrine, dopamine, prolactin, cortisal) function in an unusual way, or that their brains respond to these chemicals in an unusual way.

serotonin neurotransmitter associated with the regulation of mood, appetite, sleep, memory, and learning

Research into the causes of self-harm has considered the issue of whether self-harmers feel pain. Some people who practice self-harm say that they do not feel physical pain during the act. Ingrid Kemperman and others in 1997 found that this may be due to malfunctioning brain chemistry, such as the lower levels of serotonin. Self-harmers may have high levels of brain chemicals called **opioids**, which block the pain of their self-injury and instead cause a surging feeling of well-being.

opioid substance that acts similarly to opiate narcotic drugs, but is not actually produced from the opium poppy

Some people who self-harm have a higher threshold for pain in general, according to Martin Bohus in 2001, meaning they may experience less discomfort than the average person during any injury, even when they are not emotionally upset. On the other hand, at times self-harmers may experience and even welcome the feeling of pain as a way to help prove that their psychological pain (such as extremely distressing feelings of confusion, guilt, or self-doubt) is real.

They may also be trying to reverse a sense of deadness, to feel alive by feeling pain.

Certain factors in the life of an adolescent can contribute to a tendency to self-harm. These include life events that cause stress or **trauma**; problems with school, relationships, or family; the loss of parents; a history of physical or sexual abuse; serious illness and/or surgery; and violence and alcohol abuse in childhood. A crisis situation involving a relationship and the emotions of loss or anger can bring on self-harming behavior. Adolescents who self-harm while hospitalized for psychiatric reasons may do so out of a reaction to the imposition of an unwanted routine, or because they feel abandoned or ignored by their family and/or hospital personnel and employees. Adolescents who have had several different caretakers in their lives are also more likely to engage in self-harm. This suggests that self-harming adolescents may have trouble forming secure and trusting attachments to others, according to J. M. Vivona and others in 1995. Self-harm may also be triggered by too much or too little emotional involvement in a family, as well as the absence of someone the young person can confide in.

Some experts believe there are psychoanalytical explanations for self-harm. Psychoanalysis seeks to uncover a person's early experiences that may have affected their patterns of behavior without their being aware of it. For example, if in the person's childhood a caretaker, whether a parent or someone else, tended to criticize the child frequently, this criticism may contribute in later life to a desire to self-harm. Other psychoanalytic explanations of self-harm, such as that of S. Doctors in 1981, include having a poorly defined sense of self, anxiety about sex, a desire to separate from one's parents, or a conflicted relationship with one's body.

Self-harm among adolescents has sometimes been referred to as contagious. Adolescents who self-harm may occasionally let friends in on their secretive behavior as a way of communicating with their peers and forming close, if only temporary, bonds. Unfortunately, sharing the secret often leads to the confidant's beginning to self-harm. Teenagers who live together or spend a lot of time together can put pressure on each other to follow the example of self-harm, according to Barent W. Walsh and Paul M. Rosen in 1988.

Treating Those Who Self-Harm

There are a number of forms of treatment for self-harm, many of which are considered quite effective. Some treatments directly target self-harm behavior. Other treatments focus on improving factors in

---

RELATED READING

Cut (2000) by Patricia McCormick, tells the fictional story of Callie, a young woman who habitually cuts herself. Her pattern of abuse lands her in a treatment center where, slowly, she comes to understand the reasons for her urges to commit self-harm and the role her family's problems play in it.

trauma injury or damage, either to the body or to the mind

"Any mistake I made was blown up. I began to scrutinize everything I did. I began to almost hate myself for any tiny screw-up and spend my nights analyzing myself."

"Prom night: Special time, pinnacle (besides graduation) of senior year. Just before, my first cut is made on my right wrist: immense release follows. My prom sucks. I hate myself the entire night. The next morning, I cut again and thus begins my downfall."

—Anonymous Teenage Girl

a person's life that often occur along with self-harm, such as poor self-image, trouble sustaining close relationships, and overeating.

Psychiatrists sometimes prescribe medications to treat self-harm. **Antidepressants**, such as tricyclics, MAO inhibitors, and SSRIs, can address any accompanying feelings of sadness. **Neuroleptics** or mood stabilizers may be used to treat patients' occasional feelings of being out of touch with reality, anxiety, extreme sensitivity in relating to others, anger, and depression. **Benzodiazepines**, a type of anti-anxiety medication, are used occasionally. As mentioned earlier, research suggests that people who self-harm produce high levels of brain opioids that prevent them from feeling the pain of their self-injury. To counter this, some researchers (including A. Roth, R. Ostroff, and R. Hoffman in 1990) have studied the use of the drug naltrexone, which can block the rewards delivered by brain opioids and as a result increase the feeling of pain.

Another form of treatment for self-harm takes a psychological approach. A concern of this treatment is to keep patients who self-harm safe yet also to ensure that they do not become overly reliant on hospitalization. Patients need to set realistic and flexible goals, and therapists must be careful not to act out on their own feelings of frustration by blaming patients for not reaching these goals. Patients should not be made to feel that they have been rejected by their therapists.

Behavioral treatments have proven particularly effective with various forms of self-harm. An increasingly well-known form is dialectical behavior therapy (DBT), developed by Linehan specifically for self-harming patients with a diagnosis of **borderline personality disorder**. In this type of therapy, there is an emphasis on achieving a balance between acceptance and change, learning how to adapt to various life situations, and teamwork by therapists. Patients receive both individual and group treatment, generally on an **outpatient** basis.

Conclusion

The mental health community must pay more attention to the problem of self-harm. In addition, education by teachers and parents using sources in the media and the Internet can help to dispel myths about self-harm. All resources should be used to inspire hope and encourage recovery. If you or anyone you know suffers from this behavior, please make sure to get help as soon as possible. Organizations such as the American Psychological Association (http://www.apa.org) and the American Psychiatric Association (http://www.psych.org) can offer help. A web site, Mental-Health-Matters.com, and a telephone referral service, 1-800-lifenet, may also help. SEE ALSO BRAIN CHEM-

antidepressant medication used for the treatment and prevention of depression

neuroleptic one of a class of antipsychotic drugs, including major tranquilizers used in the treatment of psychoses such as schizophrenia

benzodiazepine drug developed in the 1960s as a safer alternative to barbiturates; most frequently used as a sleeping pill or an anti-anxiety medication

borderline personality disorder condition in which a person consistently has unstable personal relationships, negative self-image, unclear self-identity, recurring impulsivity, and problems with mood

outpatient person who receives treatment at a doctor's office or hospital but does not stay overnight

ISTRY; CONDUCT DISORDER; EATING DISORDERS; GENDER AND SUBSTANCE ABUSE; PERSONALITY DISORDER.

Date Rape Drug *See Robypnol*

Delirium Tremens *See Alcohol: Withdrawal*

Designer Drugs

Designer drugs are slightly altered imitations of known, dangerous drugs. They are synthesized, or formed, in laboratories and are designed to produce effects similar to the drugs they imitate. Examples include drugs like amphetamine and methamphetamine, such as MDA, MDMA (known as "ecstasy"), TMA, and MDE (also called "Eve"), or MBDB. Designer drugs are illegal and created solely for the purpose of recreational drug use. Although the goals are different, the process

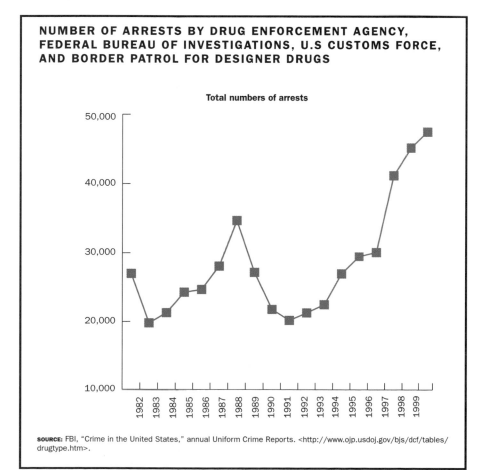

NUMBER OF ARRESTS BY DRUG ENFORCEMENT AGENCY, FEDERAL BUREAU OF INVESTIGATIONS, U.S CUSTOMS FORCE, AND BORDER PATROL FOR DESIGNER DRUGS

Total numbers of arrests

SOURCE: FBI, "Crime in the United States," annual Uniform Crime Reports. <http://www.ojp.usdoj.gov/bjs/dcf/tables/drugtype.htm>.

Designer drug use in the United States increased in the 1990s, but arrests for designer drug use also sharply increased during the same time period.

of creating designer drugs resembles the process of developing new and better drugs for medical purposes. This process applies the principles of basic chemistry to change the structure of a drug molecule. Many useful new drugs or changes in older drugs have resulted in improved health care.

The people who make illegal designer drugs range from cookbook amateurs to highly skilled chemists. Designer drugs may be made in the United States or smuggled in from other countries. When designer drugs are made in the United States, the ingredients necessary may be imported or may be illegally purchased or stolen. These illegal substances are produced in secret to avoid federal laws that regulate and control drugs. The street drugs that emerge from this illegal practice are unknown substances that may be toxic (poisonous) and may pose serious health consequences for the drug user. The drug user has no way of knowing what he or she is taking.

The best-known case of designer drug use leading to tragic consequences involves MPTP. A chemist attempted to synthesize a drug not covered by the Controlled Substances Act. He hoped to profit by selling the new drug without breaking any existing laws. The drug he created resembled heroin, but it contained a substance called MPTP. This substance was created by accident because of the chemist's careless mistakes. Drug users who bought the drug on the street developed a syndrome that resembled Parkinson's disease. In this disease, the muscles become rigid; people develop a tremor (shaking) and have trouble with motor skills such as walking and writing. MPTP was later found to be the cause of the syndrome. This discovery came too late for the drug users, because there is no known cure for the disease.

narcotic addictive substance that relieves pain and induces sleep or causes sedation; prescription narcotics includes morphine and codeine; general and imprecise term referring to a drug of abuse, such as heroin, cocaine, or marijuana

Other designer drugs that have resulted in serious health hazards on the street are drugs designed to imitate fentanyl (Sublimaze). This potent and extremely fast-acting **narcotic** painkiller is a known drug of abuse. Fentanyl-like designer drugs caused a number of deaths from drug overdoses.

hallucinogenic substance that can cause hallucinations, or seeing, hearing, or feeling things that are not there

Not every designer drug is thought up by chemists in illegal labs. Some are synthesized originally for medical uses but are never sold for that purpose. One example is the **hallucinogenic** drug LSD, which was formed as part of a project to create medicines but was later found not to have medical uses. Many hallucinogenic designer drugs such as MDA, MDMA or ecstasy, and MDEA or Eve, are toxic and have caused deaths. Users of these drugs may develop restlessness, agitation, sweating, high blood pressure, and heart problems. MDA causes **neurological** damage in rats, and may well cause similar damage in humans.

neurological relating to the nervous system

The widespread illegal production and use of designer drugs could result in an epidemic of neurological disorders. People who take drugs without knowing the drug's toxic effects are risking their long-term health for the sake of a brief high. SEE ALSO CLUB DRUGS; ECSTASY; LYSERGIC ACID DIETHYLAMIDE (LSD) AND PSYCHEDELICS.

Detoxification

The term "detoxification" describes the process that a drug- or alcohol-dependent person goes through when reducing the level of the substance in his or her body, or eliminating it entirely. Chronic (long-term) use of a drug can result in **physical dependence**. Stopping the use of that drug can cause a **withdrawal** syndrome. The goal of detoxification is to help the drug abuser make a safe and comfortable transition from withdrawal to being drug-free.

The detoxification process usually takes place in a supportive environment, often a hospital or clinic. It might also involve the use of medications to control or suppress symptoms and signs of withdrawal. The level of care and whether medications are used depends on which substance was abused and the severity of the withdrawal syndrome. It also depends on medical complications the person might have as a result of the drug or other conditions. The most severe complications of withdrawal occur from substances such as alcohol and **sedative-hypnotics** (such as the barbiturate Seconal and the benzodiazepine Valium). Detoxification is generally the first step in the process of recovering from alcohol or drug addiction. SEE ALSO ADDICTION: CONCEPTS AND DEFINITIONS; ALCOHOL: WITHDRAWAL; BENZODIAZEPINE WITHDRAWAL; COCAINE: WITHDRAWAL; NONABUSED DRUGS WITHDRAWAL; TREATMENT TYPES: AN OVERVIEW.

physical dependence condition that may occur after prolonged use of a particular drug or alcohol, in which the user's body cannot function normally without the presence of the substance; when the substance is not used or the dose is decreased, the user experiences uncomfortable physical symptoms

withdrawal group of physical and psychological symptoms that may occur when a person suddenly stops the use of a substance or reduces the dose of an addictive substance

sedative-hypnotic drug that has a calming and relaxing effect; "hypnotics" induce sleep

Diagnosis of Drug and Alcohol Abuse: An Overview

Diagnosis is the process of identifying and labeling specific disease conditions. Diagnostic criteria are standardized groups of signs and symptoms used to decide whether an individual has a particular disease or not. If a person has a certain number of symptoms from the list of possible criteria, then the diagnosis can be made. Once a diagnosis is made, the health-care provider and patient can begin to make decisions about appropriate treatment.

abuse related to drug use, describes taking drugs that are illegal, or using prescription drugs in a way for which they were not prescribed; related to alcohol use, describes drinking in a fashion that is damaging to the drinker or to others

dependence psychological compulsion to use a substance for emotional and/or physical reasons

intoxication loss of physical or mental control because of the effects of a substance

withdrawal group of physical and psychological symptoms that may occur when a person suddenly stops the use of a substance or reduces the dose of an addictive substance

illicit something illegal or something used in an illegal manner

Mental health professionals often treat patients who abuse drugs or alcohol. By consulting diagnostic manuals, medical professionals can make accurate diagnoses of substance use disorders, such as **abuse** or **dependence**. They can evaluate signs and symptoms (for example, acute **intoxication**, **withdrawal**, and delirium, or mental confusion), and laboratory data (such as blood alcohol content or liver function tests) and use these as a basis for planning treatment.

Two reference works, the *International Classification of Diseases* and the *Diagnostic and Statistical Manual of Mental Disorders*, are periodically revised to reflect important research findings that affect the accurate diagnosis of various conditions. Alcoholism and drug addiction have been defined at various times as medical diseases, mental disorders, social problems, and behavioral conditions.

Patient Histories

One of the first steps toward treating a person with substance use problems is to ask the individual for a history of drug and alcohol use. Unfortunately, patients with alcohol and drug problems often do not provide accurate information about their own past or present use. They are often embarrassed by or ashamed of their substance abuse, or are afraid of getting themselves into trouble with the law. Although they want help for the medical complications of substance abuse (such as injuries or depression), they may not be ready to give up alcohol or drug use entirely. Many people provide only a hazy picture of their behavior, hiding the full extent of their alcohol or drug use. Therefore, the medical professional obtaining a patient's history must be highly skilled, non-threatening, nonjudgmental, and very perceptive.

Taking a history of a person's illness usually follows a standard approach. This consists of:

- identifying the chief complaint
- evaluating the present illness
- reviewing past history
- reviewing physical functioning (such as blood pressure and cardiovascular health)
- asking about family history of similar disorders
- discussing the patient's psychological health and how well he or she is getting along with others in society.

A history of the present illness usually begins with questions about the use of alcohol, drugs, and tobacco. The questions should cover prescription drugs as well as **illicit** drugs, and the kinds of drugs used, the amount used, and the way the drug was taken (smoking, injec-

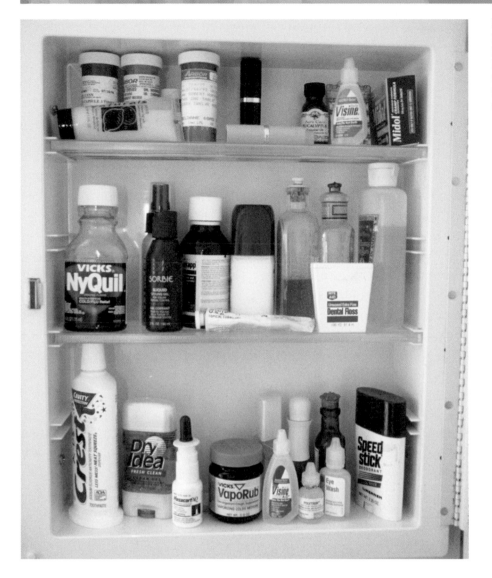

Drugs are used for many reasons, including medical reasons. Drug abuse occurs when it is being used for pleasure or from a compulsive need.

tion, and so on). Questions about alcohol use should refer specifically to the amount and frequency of use of major types (wine, spirits, beer). A thorough physical examination is important, because each substance has specific effects on certain organs and body systems. For example, alcohol can affect the liver, stomach, and cardiovascular systems. Drugs often produce abnormalities in vital signs such as temperature, pulse, and blood pressure. Evidence of substance use disorders can often be seen in the person's mental state. For example, poor personal hygiene, an inappropriate mood (sad, **euphoric**, irritable, anxious), illogical thought processes, and memory problems can all be symptoms of disorders.

The physical examination can be followed by laboratory tests, which sometimes aid in early diagnosis before severe or irreversible damage has taken place. Many drugs can be detected in the urine for twelve to forty-eight hours after their consumption. An estimate of

euphoric experience of intense, giddy happiness and well-being, sometimes occurring baselessly and out of sync with the circumstances

blood alcohol concentration can be made directly by blood test or indirectly by means of a breath or saliva test. Elevated levels of a liver enzyme, gamma glutamyl transpeptidase, can indicate liver damage from **chronic**, heavy alcohol intake.

Diagnosing Dependence

There are three essential features of dependence on substances: (1) the development of **tolerance**; (2) the presence of withdrawal symptoms when the drug dose is lowered or drug use is stopped; and (3) compulsive use of a substance.

Tolerance. Tolerance occurs when a person must take increasing amounts of a drug to obtain the effects originally produced by lower doses. Physical tolerance involves changes in a person's cellular functioning. Alcoholics can drink amounts of alcohol (such as a quart of vodka) that would be sufficient to incapacitate or kill nontolerant drinkers. Tolerance can also be psychological. An example of psychological tolerance is when the marijuana smoker or heroin user no longer experiences a "high" after the initial dose of the substance.

Withdrawal. Withdrawal is characterized by a group of symptoms that occur when a person stops taking a drug or lowers the dose. Some common minor withdrawal symptoms are restlessness, fatigue, and an inability to sleep. More serious withdrawal symptoms include **hallucinations** and **depression**. Some drugs, such as marijuana and hallucinogens, do not typically produce a withdrawal syndrome after use is stopped.

Withdrawal symptoms from alcohol occur within hours after a person has stopped drinking. These include shaking, rapid heartbeat, increased blood pressure, nausea, and vomiting. In some cases, patients may also have seizures or hallucinations. In addition to physical withdrawal symptoms, anxiety and depression are also common. Some chronic drinkers never have a long enough period of abstinence to permit withdrawal to occur.

Using a substance to relieve withdrawal symptoms is a clear sign of physical dependence. For example, taking a drink of alcohol in the morning to relieve nausea or the "shakes" is one of the most common signs of physical dependence in alcoholics.

Compulsive Use. Compulsive use of a substance refers to an individual's failure to abstain from using the substance, in spite of the negative consequences of that use. For example, an alcoholic may want to stop drinking, but—despite repeated attempts—he or she is

chronic continuing for a long period of time

tolerance the National Institute of Drug Abuse defines tolerance as a condition in which higher and higher doses of a drug or alcohol are needed to produce the effect or "high" experienced from the original dose

hallucination seeing, hearing, feeling, tasting, or smelling something that is not actually there, like a vision of devils, hearing voices, or feeling bugs crawl over the skin; may occur due to mental illness or as a side effect of some drugs

depression state in which an individual feels intensely sad and hopeless; may have trouble eating, sleeping, and concentrating, and is no longer able to feel pleasure from previously enjoyable activities; in extreme cases, may lead an individual to think about or attempt suicide

unable to do so. Not only can the individual not stop using the drug, he or she cannot even regulate the amount of alcohol or drug consumed on a given occasion. For instance, the cocaine addict vows to snort only a small amount, but then continues until the entire supply is used up. Or the alcoholic cannot stop drinking before becoming intoxicated.

Diagnosing Substance Abuse

Substance abuse is different from substance dependence. The criteria for substance abuse do not include tolerance, withdrawal, or a pattern of compulsive use. Instead, the major criterion for substance abuse is harmful use of a substance. The harm can be physical (such as fatty liver or hepatitis) or psychological (such as depression). A diagnosis of substance abuse can also be made in the case of hazardous use of a substance, such as driving while under the influence of alcohol or drugs.

The diagnosis of abuse is designed mainly for people who have recently begun to experience alcohol or drug problems, and for chronic users who do not show symptoms of dependence. For example, a diagnosis of substance abuse might be made in these cases:

- A pregnant woman who keeps drinking alcohol even though her physician has told her that it could damage the fetus.
- A college student whose weekend binges result in missed classes, poor grades, or alcohol-related traffic accidents.
- A middle-aged beer drinker who regularly drinks a six-pack each day and develops high blood pressure and fatty liver but no symptoms of dependence.
- An occasional marijuana smoker who has an accidental injury while intoxicated.

Diagnostic Tests

Physicians and researchers use various approaches to identify and assess people who may be abusing drugs or alcohol. One approach is to use brief screening instruments or tests—usually self-report questionnaires—to determine the possible presence of substance use disorders.

CAGE. One test that is commonly used to screen adults for alcohol abuse and/or dependence is called CAGE, which consists of four simple questions (asking about signs of compulsive use and withdrawal):

1. Have you ever felt the need to *cut* down on your drinking?
2. Do you get *annoyed* at criticism by others about your drinking?

THE HOLD OF DRUGS

One sign of addiction is that the drugs come to mean more than anything else in the user's life. "I wanted a new experience," said Sean, a 17-year-old who is recovering from his addiction to cocaine. He recalls how the drug took over his life: "The only thing on my mind was coke. I was forgetting all of my other responsibilities and losing friends quick. I was only hanging out with those five people [who I did coke with]. I wasn't going to school."

3. Have you ever felt *guilty* about your drinking or something you have done while drinking?

4. Have you ever felt the need for a drink early in the morning (or as an "*e*ye opener")?

Answering "yes" to two or more items on the CAGE questionnaire suggests the presence of problem drinking (and possibly dependence).

MAST. The Michigan Alcoholism Screening Test includes twenty-five items that help determine symptoms and consequences of a person's alcohol use. Items include information about guilt regarding drinking habits; experiences with blackouts following drinking; symptoms of delirium tremens (a delirium with tremors and shaking); loss of control; family, social, employment, and legal problems following bouts of drinking; and help-seeking behaviors (such as attending Alcoholics Anonymous ☎ meetings or going into a hospital due to drinking). There are also shorter questionnaires that are based on the MAST, including the 13-item Short-MAST and the 10-item Brief-MAST.

SMST. The Self-Administered Alcoholism Screening Test is a 35-item questionnaire that uses yes-or-no questions to try to define the probability that a person is an alcoholic.

ADS. The Alcohol Dependence Scale can help define how severely dependent an individual is on alcohol. This test covers questions that explore an individual's inability to control his or her drinking (compulsion), episodes of withdrawal, and loss of control due to drinking.

T-ACE. Heavy maternal drinking is a major pregnancy risk and a significant public health problem. Babies born with fetal alcohol syndrome may have facial deformities and an abnormal brain. To address the problem of drinking during pregnancy, a screening test, known as the T-ACE, was developed to determine which mothers are most at risk. The T-ACE is a brief, simple questionnaire given to women by health-care providers. It is similar to the CAGE test, in that it also asks about *a*nnoyance (by others), attempts to *c*ut down on alcohol use, and its use as an "*e*ye opener" in the morning. However, instead of *g*uilt, it asks about the number of drinks needed to feel the effects of alcohol, which can indicate the presence of *t*olerance.

The Drug Abuse Screening Test. The Drug Abuse Screening Test (DAST) is a questionnaire designed to indicate drug-related problems in certain groups of people, such as psychiatric patients, prison inmates, and employees in a workplace. The DAST takes approxi-

☎ See *Organizations of Interest* at the back of Volume 1 for address, telephone, and URL.

mately five minutes to administer and may be given as a written questionnaire or as an oral interview. The person taking the test is instructed that "drug abuse" refers to (1) the use of prescribed or over-the-counter drugs in excess of the directions and (2) any non-medical use of drugs. The drugs include marijuana, solvents or glue, tranquilizers, cocaine, LSD, and heroin. The questions do not include alcohol.

Diagnosing Adolescents

Adolescents are different from adults not only because their bodies are still developing, but also because they tend to live under quite different circumstances than adults do. For example, most of them are not yet married, they still attend school, and do not yet have full-time jobs. As a result, many of the questions contained in screening tests used to diagnose substance abuse in adults are not applicable to teenagers. Therefore, some of these tests have been modified—and some new ones have been developed—for use with this particular age group.

DAST-A. The DAST-A is a modified version of the DAST. It is a 27-item self-report screening instrument that directly asks adolescents about any negative consequences they may have had as a result of drug use. The DAST-A is very similar to the DAST; however, some questions have been changed to make them more relevant to an adolescent population. Instead of asking about spousal concerns, for instance, there are questions about concerns expressed by parents, boyfriends, or girlfriends. Similarly, items about work-related issues have been changed into questions referring to possible problems occurring at school.

RAFFT. The RAFFT test is a simple screening tool developed specifically to identify adolescents who may be abusing alcohol or drugs. It uses the following five questions:

1. Do you drink or take drugs to *r*elax, feel better about yourself, or fit in?

2. Do you ever drink or take drugs while you are *a*lone?

3. Do any of your closest *f*riends drink or take drugs?

4. Does a close *f*amily member have problems with alcohol or drugs?

5. Have you gotten into *t*rouble from drinking or taking drugs?

Other Tests for Adolescents. Many other tests have also been developed besides the above to screen adolescents for potential drug or alcohol abuse or dependence. One of these is the Personal Experience Screening Questionnaire, which is a relatively long (40-item) questionnaire that has been designed to measure the severity or degree of any alcohol or drug use problem by a teenager. Other commonly used tests include the Adolescent Alcohol Involvement Scale, the Adolescent Drinking Index, and the Rutgers Alcohol Problem Index.

Screening tests like these can help doctors and therapists determine if a person has been abusing drugs or alcohol. However, these instruments by themselves cannot be relied on to arrive at a diagnosis of substance abuse or dependence. Physicians must be well trained to recognize the signs and symptoms of drug abuse, and they should use their professional judgment to make an accurate diagnosis. Once they have done that, they can go on to the next step, which is to offer appropriate treatment to those in need. SEE ALSO ENTRIES ON SPECIFIC DRUGS; ADDICTION: CONCEPTS AND DEFINITIONS; DRUG TESTING METHODS AND ANALYSIS; FETAL ALCOHOL SYNDROME (FAS); RISK FACTORS FOR SUBSTANCE ABUSE.

Diagnostic and Statistical Manual (DSM)

The *Diagnostic and Statistical Manual of Mental Disorders* is a book used by medical professionals, insurance companies, and the court system to diagnose and define mental illnesses and disorders, including substance abuse and dependence. First published by the American Psychiatric Association in 1952 and revised periodically, the DSM is the most widely accepted reference work on the topic in the United States. The fourth edition of the DSM, known as the DSM-IV, was published in 1994, and a revision known as the DSM-IV-TR was published in 2000. The next full edition is expected to be published in 2006 or later. SEE ALSO DIAGNOSIS OF DRUG AND ALCOHOL ABUSE: AN OVERVIEW.

Distilled Spirits

Distillation is a process that separates alcohol (ethanol, also called ethyl alcohol or grain alcohol) from fermenting juices of grains, fruits, or vegetables. Distilled spirits (or, simply, spirits or liquors) are the alcoholic drinks formed by distillation. For example, the distillation of grapes results in wine, and the distillation of wine results in brandy, a spirit. Other distilled spirits include whiskey, rum, gin, and vodka. Distilled spirits are from 30 to 100 percent grain alcohol (60 to 200 proof), and the rest is mainly water. SEE ALSO ALCOHOL: HISTORY OF DRINKING; BEERS AND BREWS.

Dogs in Drug Detection

In 1970 the U. S. government faced a serious problem. The staff of inspectors in the U.S. Customs Service, responsible for ensuring that no dangerous or illegal materials entered the country, was on the decline. Sufficient funds were not available to increase this force. At the same time, a new flood of illegal **narcotics** was entering the United States, along with an increasing number of vehicles and passengers. A customs official suggested that "man's best friend," the dog, might provide the solution. Dogs can be trained to detect anything that produces an odor, including illegal narcotics. Dogs have been used ever since to detect not only narcotics but also currency, weapons, explosives, fruits, and meats.

narcotic addictive substance that relieves pain and induces sleep or causes sedation; general and imprecise term referring to a drug of abuse, such as heroin, cocaine, or marijuana.

Recently, many school districts have been using scent-trained dogs to detect drugs or other forbidden material (such as weapons) on school property, including inside students' lockers, in public areas, and in cars parked on school grounds. Schools that use detection dogs typically prepare students and staff for the program by explaining how searches will be conducted, what constitutes school property (such as lockers), and what will occur if drugs are detected.

The use of detection dogs in schools is controversial. Supporters argue that random, unannounced searches by dogs are an effective, safe way to help keep schools drug-free. They believe that these searches can prevent or deter students from bringing illicit drugs onto school grounds. Opponents claim that the use of drug-sniffing dogs violates students' Fourth Amendment rights (which protect citizens from unreasonable search and seizure). They believe that the searches create an unhealthy climate of mistrust.

Dog Selection and Training

When the dog training program first began, the U.S. Air Force supplied the Customs Service with technical expertise. Several key aspects of the training program are dog selection, development of a conditioned response, and odor integrity. Instructors in the original dog training program knew they had to start with a dog that displayed

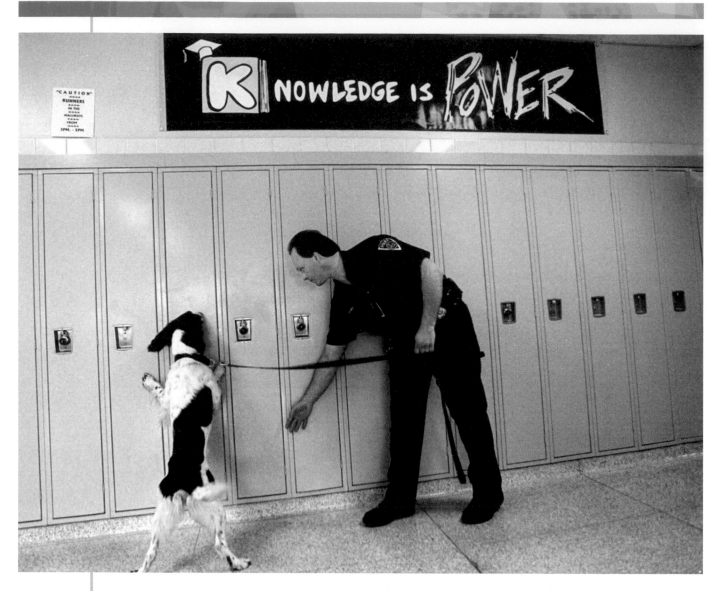

"CAUTION"
RUNNERS
IN THE
HALLWAYS
FROM
3PM. - 5PM.

KNOWLEDGE IS POWER

Roggie, a dog trained to detect narcotics, leads police officer Tom Kolbert to a locker during a search at John F. Kennedy High School in New York.

certain natural traits, retrieval motivation, and self-confidence. A dog displaying a natural desire to retrieve is the easiest to train to respond to the narcotic odor. Certain breeds are more suited to this type of training than others, especially sporting breeds such as golden retrievers, Labrador retrievers, German short-hair retrievers, and mixed breeds of these types. These dogs have had the retrieval drive bred into them over the centuries. In addition, these breeds are commonly found in animal shelters and humane societies used by the Customs Service as the primary source for dogs. Customs instructors select dogs scheduled to be put to sleep. Their selection benefits the shelters, while saving the lives of thousands of dogs that have gone on to perform a valuable service for the nation.

The training methods used by the Customs Service are similar to those of the Russian physiologist Ivan Pavlov (1849–1936). In his experiments with dogs, Pavlov observed that dogs salivate when food is placed in their mouths. He would give the dogs food while providing another **stimulus** such as a bell ringing. After a few repetitions, the dogs would salivate when they heard the bell ring, even without the food being present. The dogs had learned to associate the sound of the bell with food. This response was called a conditioned response.

The Customs Service instructors create a conditioned response to a drug odor. In a series of retrieval exercises, a dog retrieves an object with a specific drug's odor. After each retrieval, the dog plays a game of tug-of-war with its handler and receives physical praise. The dog soon associates the specific drug odor with the game and the physical praise. The dog is conditioned to respond to the drug odor because it wants to play and be praised.

During the training process, the integrity of the drug odor must be maintained to ensure the program's success. If anything other than the drug odor is present during the training program, the dog will pick up a combination of odors that it will then associate with a positive reward. As a result, the dog will not respond to the drug odor alone or will become confused when presented with it. All materials used in the training process must smell only like the specific drug in question. SEE ALSO LAW AND POLICY: CONTROLS ON DRUG TRAFFICKING.

Drinking Age

Before the twentieth century, few laws controlled the consumption of alcoholic beverages by youth. Laws prohibiting the sale of alcohol to minors were first put in place early in the twentieth century, as part of a broader trend of increasing legal controls on adolescent behavior. During the period known as Prohibition, from 1919 to 1933, the sale of alcohol to people of all ages was illegal. When Prohibition was repealed, all fifty states established legal minimum ages for the buying or drinking of alcohol, with most states setting the age at 21.

From the 1930s through the 1960s, the drinking age was not an issue of great public interest. However, in the 1970s a change in the voting age led to changes in the drinking age as well. In 1970 the 26th Amendment to the U.S. Constitution lowered the voting age in federal elections from 21 to 18. By 1974, all fifty states had lowered their voting ages for state elections to 18. As part of a trend to lower the "age of majority," twenty-nine states also lowered their minimum drinking ages, with most setting the age at 18 or 19.

Then, in the mid-1970s, studies emerged showing significant increases in the rate of young drivers' involvement in traffic accidents.

Although the number of teenagers who report having had their first alcoholic beverage before the age of 13 has fallen slightly, the number is still over 30 percent.

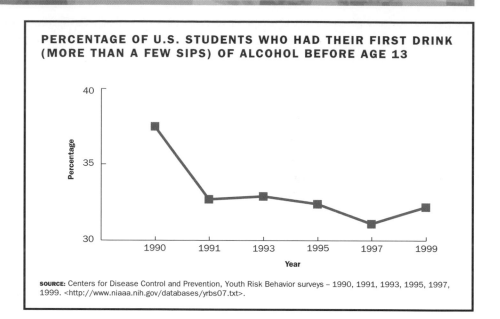

PERCENTAGE OF U.S. STUDENTS WHO HAD THEIR FIRST DRINK (MORE THAN A FEW SIPS) OF ALCOHOL BEFORE AGE 13

SOURCE: Centers for Disease Control and Prevention, Youth Risk Behavior surveys – 1990, 1991, 1993, 1995, 1997, 1999. <http://www.niaaa.nih.gov/databases/yrbs07.txt>.

☎ See *Organizations of Interest* at the back of Volume 1 for address, telephone, and URL.

This increase in accidents began almost immediately after the legal drinking age was reduced. Within a few years, states began to reverse the trend toward lower drinking ages. In October 1977, Maine became the first state to raise its legal drinking age, from 18 to 20. Several other states soon followed, and research studies completed by the early 1980s found significant declines in youth traffic-crash involvement when states raised their legal drinking age back to 20 or 21. Citizen-action groups such as Remove Intoxicated Drivers and Mothers Against Drunk Driving ☎ took action to reduce alcohol-related traffic accidents. They helped influence Congress to pass legislation in 1984 requiring that a portion of federal highway-construction funds be withheld from any state that did not have a legal drinking age of 21 by October 1986. By 1988, all the remaining states with a legal drinking age of below 21 had raised their drinking age to 21. Today, all states have a legal drinking age of 21, although rules regarding the purchase, possession, consumption, sales, and furnishing of alcohol to underage youth vary from state to state.

Car Crashes and Other Consequences

The legal drinking age became a major issue because of the serious consequences of drinking by young people. Many teenagers drink, and almost a third regularly get drunk. Youth drinking results in a great deal of damage. Car crashes are the leading cause of death for teenagers, and one-third to one-half of the crashes involve alcohol. Alcohol plays a role in 25 to 75 percent of the other leading causes of disability and death among youth, such as suicide, homicide, assault, drowning, and recreational injury.

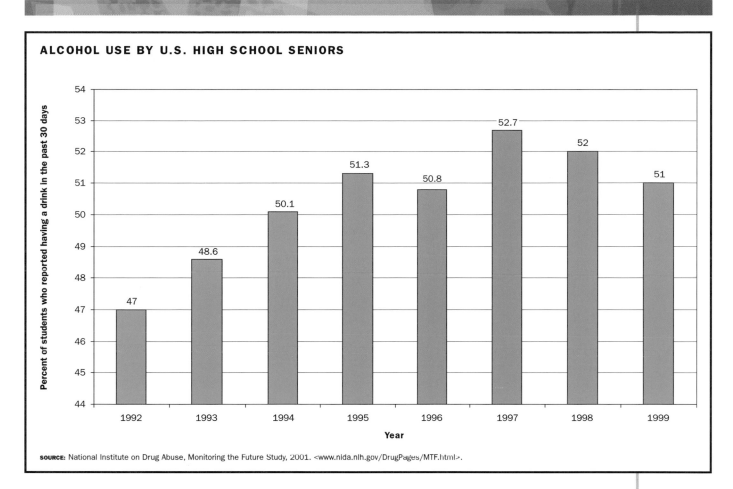

ALCOHOL USE BY U.S. HIGH SCHOOL SENIORS

SOURCE: National Institute on Drug Abuse, Monitoring the Future Study, 2001. <www.nida.nlh.gov/DrugPages/MTF.html>.

Injuries are only part of the problem. Early use of alcohol appears to affect many aspects of a person's development—physical, social, and mental. Alcohol use increases the odds of having unprotected sex (such as not using a condom). This in turn increases the chance of unwanted pregnancy and catching sexually transmitted diseases, including the human immunodeficiency virus (HIV), which causes AIDS. Many date rape situations involve individuals who have been drinking. The early use of alcohol increases the odds that a young person will move on to using other drugs, such as marijuana, cocaine, or heroin. Finally, the earlier a person starts a pattern of regular drinking, the higher the chance of later serious problems with alcohol, including **dependence**.

Of the many problems stemming from young people's drinking, the most obvious one, and the one that receives the most attention in debates on the legal drinking age, is the role of alcohol in traffic accidents. After the drinking age was lowered (in most cases from 21 to 18), traffic crashes involving young people increased significantly. In contrast, when the drinking age was raised again, traffic crashes among youths declined significantly. The National Highway Traffic Safety Administration estimates that, in the states that raised the

According to this study by the National Institute on Drug Abuse, alcohol use by high-school seniors, as recorded in the past thirty days, was on a slight decline in the late 1990s.

dependence psychological compulsion to use a substance for emotional and/or physical reasons

drinking age to 21 after 1982, the reduction in the number of car crashes alone saves 1,000 lives per year.

Raising the drinking age to 21 has also had an effect on problems other than traffic crashes. Vandalism dropped as much as 16 percent in four states that raised the drinking age. Studies also show significant reductions in the number of suicides, injuries to pedestrians, and other unintentional injuries. In a study of two Australian states that lowered the drinking age, increases in admissions to hospitals for alcohol-related injuries other than car crashes increased.

The drinking age appears to influence rates of drinking among young people. The most reliable studies show that raising the legal drinking age reduces young people's drinking. However, the age-21 policy does not eliminate youth drinking, particularly on college campuses. Surveys of college students tend to show that the drinking age has little effect on drinking patterns. In contrast, surveys of random samples of high school seniors and 18- to 20-year-olds across many states, including those entering college and those in the workforce, show that a higher legal drinking age does significantly reduce drinking.

Enforcement

Drinking among youth is now significantly down from its peak in 1980. Yet in surveys of high-school seniors, about half still report drinking in the past month, and about one-third report having had five or more drinks at a time at least once in the previous two weeks. Among the many reasons that youth continue to drink, one important reason is that alcohol remains easily available to them, despite the minimum drinking age law. Underage drinking very rarely results in arrests. More important, instances of drinking by underage youth very rarely result in any action being taken against a store, restaurant, or bar for selling or serving alcohol to a minor.

A number of research studies have stated that the problem of underage drinking can only be tackled by an approach that looks at the entire community in which underage drinkers live. Efforts to restrict underage drinking need to be directed at the adults, store-owners, and barkeepers that may potentially help supply underage drinkers with alcohol. Some communities have passed laws that make storekeepers and bartenders responsible for injuries or deaths inflicted by underage drinkers. In some states, an establishment's liquor license can be taken away. Private homeowners who allow alcohol to be served to underage drinkers can also be prosecuted for injuries that occur as the result of underage drinking. Law enforcement officials need to randomly spot-check establishments that sell and serve liquor to make sure that proof of age is checked before liquor is sold.

What are the Arguments against the Age-21 Policy?

Some have argued that it is illogical to set the legal age of drinking at 21 when other rights and privileges of adulthood, such as voting and signing legally binding contracts, begin at age 18. But we have many different legal ages, ranging from 12 to 21, for various activities—voting, driving, sale and use of tobacco, legal consent for sexual intercourse, marriage, access to contraception without parental consent, compulsory school attendance, and so forth. Minimum ages depend on the specific behavior involved. In the case of the drinking age, good policy must take into account the dangers of youth drinking.

Other critics of the age-21 policy have argued that a higher drinking age will increase drinking rates when young people finally get legal access to alcohol. The theory is that forbidding teenagers to drink will only strengthen their urge to drink when they reach the legal age. At 21, the theory goes, they will break loose and drink at significantly higher rates than they would have if they had been introduced to alcohol earlier. This theory is clearly not supported by research. One nationwide study found just the opposite results: people aged 21 to 24 drank at lower rates if they had to wait until 21 to have legal access to alcohol.

A related argument is that a minimum drinking age of 21 may reduce car crashes among teenagers, but this will only be a temporary effect if it simply delays those problems until the teenagers reach age 21. This argument is also false. The minimum age of 21 significantly reduces car crashes among people aged 18 to 20. There is no "rebound" effect at age 21. In fact, the higher legal age appears to produce benefits, in terms of reduced drinking, that continue into a person's early 20s.

Conclusion

The debate surrounding the legal age for drinking appears settled in the United States. Polls have shown that the majority of the public clearly supports a legal drinking age of 21. Even youth under the age of 21 support the age-21 policy. However, other countries (particularly in Europe, where drinking ages are typically set at 18) are now examining the research and experience of the United States with increasing interest. Professionals in the areas of public health and traffic safety, as well as citizens, are beginning to see the benefits of the age-21 drinking law in the United States, and they are beginning to debate in their own countries the most appropriate age for legal access to alcohol. SEE ALSO ACCIDENTS AND INJURIES FROM ALCOHOL; ADOLESCENTS, DRUG AND ALCOHOL USE; BINGE DRINKING; DRIVING, ALCOHOL, AND DRUGS; MOTHERS AGAINST DRUNK DRIVING (MADD); STUDENTS AGAINST DESTRUCTIVE DECISIONS (SADD).

Driving, Alcohol, and Drugs

Since the invention of the automobile, people have recognized that drinking alcohol could lead to traffic accidents. Injuries from motor vehicle accidents are now the leading cause of death for individuals ages 1 to 29, and alcohol is the single greatest cause of fatal vehicle crashes. In 2000 approximately 16,068 deaths in car accidents were linked to alcohol use and driving. In fact, more people are killed in automobile crashes involving alcohol than by firearms.

In 1968 the U.S. Department of Transportation made its first report to the U.S. Congress on traffic safety and alcohol. It revealed that more than 50 percent of fatal traffic collisions and 33 percent of serious injury traffic collisions were alcohol-related. By the late 1970s, citizen groups such as Mothers Against Drunk Driving, ☎ Students Against Driving Drunk (now calling itself Students Against Destructive Decisions), ☎ and Remove Intoxicated Drivers, had emerged to address the problem of drunk driving. These members—who included victims, their families, and concerned citizens—vigorously campaigned for new and tougher drunk-driving laws and punishments.

In the 1980s, Congress encouraged states to adopt stricter laws regulating drinking and driving. It did this by refusing to grant states federal funds to build or repair highways unless the states raised the legal age for drinking to 21. Ultimately, every state raised its drinking age accordingly. The states also passed a flood of legislation, providing for more and better law enforcement and a greater range of criminal penalties—from losing one's license to mandatory education in safe driving to jail terms. Public tolerance of driving under the influence of alcohol decreased sharply.

All these developments led to a significant decline in traffic fatalities related to use of alcohol, from a high of 57 percent of all fatal crashes in 1982 to 38.3 percent in 1999. Unfortunately, 2000 saw a reversal of that trend: 16,653 people were killed in crashes involving alcohol, representing 40 percent of the 41,821 people killed in all traffic crashes that year. Alcohol remains the single largest factor in traffic fatalities and serious injuries. The National Highway Traffic Safety

☎ See *Organizations of Interest* at the back of Volume 1 for address, telephone, and URL.

Administration estimates that three out of ten Americans will be involved in an alcohol-related crash sometime during their lives.

Driving Under the Influence

The terms "driving under the influence" (DUI), "driving while intoxicated" (DWI), and "driving while impaired" are legal terms. In some states, they are used interchangeably, and someone who is taken to court for any of these three offenses faces the same penalties and sentencing. In other states, they represent different blood alcohol levels, with DWI a more serious offense than DUI. People who are found to be DWI may get stiffer penalties and sentences than people who are found to be DUI. Furthermore, in some states young people under 21 who are arrested have stricter blood alcohol guidelines than do adults.

Some states also have a classification called "extreme DUI" for blood alcohol greater than 0.15 percent. In Arizona, for example, a jail sentence for extreme DUI tends to be ten times as long as a jail sentence for regular DUI or DWI. When a suspect is arrested for drunk driving, he or she must take a Breathalyzer test. The breath machine measures the amount of alcohol in the breath and converts it into a measure of the amount of alcohol in the blood. In most states, a blood alcohol concentration (BAC) of 0.10 percent or above is classified as driving under the influence. Some states have further reduced the legal limit to 0.08 percent, but the U.S. Congress rejected legislation in 1998 that would have required all states to lower the drunken driving arrest threshold to 0.08 percent. Most other industrial nations have already set their legal limit at 0.08 or lower. Not surprisingly, in most states where 0.08 BAC laws have been added to existing controls on impaired drivers, they have led to reductions in alcohol-related fatalities.

In October 2000, Congress passed the Transportation Appropriations Bill, which sets 0.08 BAC as the national standard for impaired driving. The legal limit for BAC is still set by the states, not the federal government. But states that do not adopt 0.08 BAC laws by 2004 would have 2 percent of certain highway construction funds withheld. The penalty increases to 8 percent by 2007. States adopting the standard by 2007 would be reimbursed for any lost funds.

There is a strong **correlation** between a BAC greater than 0.05 percent and risk of serious injury or death while operating a motor vehicle. The figure on page 223 helps you see this relationship. The x axis shows increasing amounts of blood alcohol content. The y-axis illustrates increasing risk of accident. As you follow the curved line

correlation the relation of two or more things that is not naturally expected

States are allowed to set their own legal limits on blood alcohol content (BAC) for drivers. Most states have set BAC limits at 0.10 for adult drivers, although new evidence about driving accidents have compelled some states to lower this limit to 0.08. For drivers under the legal drinking age of 21, most states have set BAC limits of 0.02 or less.

DRUNK DRIVING BLOOD ALCOHOL LEVELS BY STATE

State laws for drivers under age 21			State laws for adults	
Blood Alcohol Concentration (BAC) Limits of 0.00	BAC Limit of 0.01	BAC Limit of 0.02	Blood Alcohol Concentration (BAC) Limits of 0.08	BAC Limit of 0.10
Alabama	California	Alaska	Alabama	Alaska
Arkansas	New Jersey	Arizona	California	Arizona
Illinois		Colorado	Florida	Arkansas
Maine		Connecticut		Colorado
		District of Columbia	Hawaii	Connecticut
Minnesota		Florida	Idaho	Delaware
			Illinois	
		Georgia	Kansas	District of Columbia
		Hawaii		Georgia
North Carolina		Idaho	Maine	Indiana
Oklahoma		Indiana		
Oregon			New Hampshire	Iowa
		Iowa		
Texas			New Mexico	Kentucky
Utah		Kansas	North Carolina	Louisiana
			Oregon	
		Kentucky		Maryland
		Louisiana	Utah	
				Michigan
		Maryland	Vermont	Minnesota
			Virginia	
		Massachusetts		Mississippi
			Washington	Missouri
		Michigan		Montana
		Missouri		
		Montana		Nebraska
				Nevada
		Nebraska		
		Nevada		New Jersey
		New Hampshire		New York
		New Mexico		North Dakota
		New York		
		North Dakota		Ohio
				Oklahoma
		Ohio		Pennsylvania
				Rhode Island
				South Dakota
		Pennsylvania		
		Rhode Island		Tennessee
		Tennessee		Texas
		Vermont		West Virginia
		Virginia		Wisconsin
		Washington		Wyoming
		West Virginia		

SOURCE: Insurance Institute for Highway Safety. <http://www.hwysafety.org/safety_facts/state_laws/dui.htm>.

upward along the *x*-axis, you can see that at BACs greater than 80 milligrams/100 milliliters, relatively small increases in BAC will lead to an increasingly greater risks of accident.

Most alcohol-related traffic collisions occur because the driver's attention, visual abilities, and perception are all impaired. These are considered information-processing errors. The second most frequent cause of alcohol-related collisions are errors in judgment, such as believing the car is traveling more slowly than it really is. Driving also requires divided-attention tasks, which means that the driver must monitor and respond to more than one source of information at the same time. For instance, drivers need to pay attention to where the

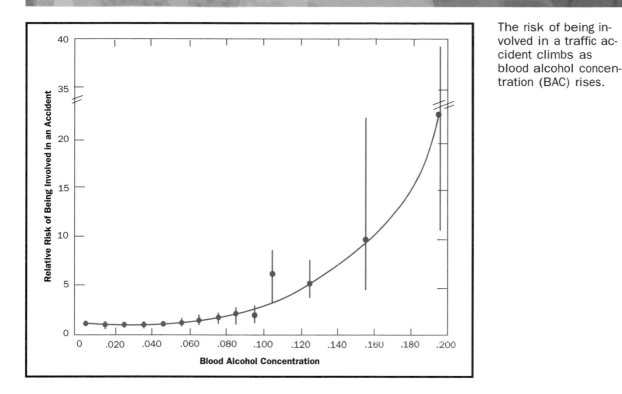

The risk of being involved in a traffic accident climbs as blood alcohol concentration (BAC) rises.

car is headed as well as what cars nearby are doing. Divided attention occurs in drivers with BAC levels as low as 0.02 percent. It is interesting to note that an adult male who drinks two twelve-ounce beers or two other standard drinks on an empty stomach will have a BAC of about 0.04 percent an hour later. Drivers under the influence of alcohol frequently fail to detect threats or dangers on the road around them.

Many studies have shown that any amount of alcohol in the system impairs a person's abilities. It is important to note that a person can have enough alcohol in the system to impair driving abilities even without showing any signs of being drunk, such as having slurred speech or appearing unsteady. He or she may not seem drunk but could still have a BAC high enough to increase the chances of having an accident. Recent studies have shown that impairment occurs at very low alcohol levels. Some researchers suggest that impairment begins as soon as alcohol is actually detectable in the bloodstream.

The Extent of the Problem

More than 1.4 million people are arrested each year for drunk driving. An unknown number of violators never get caught. Those most likely to be caught are usually the most dangerous of the drunk drivers: those who drive far above the speed limit, weave in and out of traffic, and cross into lanes of traffic going in the opposite direction. The toll in terms of personal and property damage caused by drunk drivers is staggering. Drunk drivers themselves, often in single-car collisions, account for a large number of motorists who are killed. Each year thousands of pedestrians and other motorists are also killed by drunk drivers, and tens of thousands are badly injured.

The Offender

Ninety percent of those arrested for drunk driving are white males. The highest percentage of this group are in their 20s. People who drive drunk are likely to be heavy drinkers and alcohol abusers, although light and moderate drinkers may also drive drunk on occasion, perhaps following a binge. The consensus of studies based on screening tests of drunk drivers is that about 50 percent arrested for this offense are alcohol abusers, about 35 percent are social drinkers, and the remainder fall in between.

The Crime of Drunk Driving

misdemeanor crime that is treated in the courts as a less serious crime than a felony

felony a very serious crime that usually warrants a more severe punishment than misdemeanor crimes

In most states, a first drunk-driving offense is a **misdemeanor**, and a second offense within a specified time period (up to ten years in some states) is a **felony**. In a few states, a first offense is treated as a traffic violation, a second offense a misdemeanor, and a third offense a felony. Punishments vary from state to state. The usual range of punishments includes loss of a driver's license for up to one year, fines of $500 to $1,000, and incarceration (or jail time) for up to thirty days. In the late 1980s, several states passed laws mandating at least forty-eight hours of incarceration for a first DWI offense and a longer time for a second or subsequent offense. Another penalty that is increasingly used is the automatic and immediate forfeiture of the driver's license at the police station when the suspect fails or refuses to take the breath test.

In many states, all drunk-driving offenders are routinely screened for alcoholism and alcohol abuse. Surveys such as the Michigan Alcoholism Screening Test (MAST) or the Mortimer-Filkins Questionnaire, the Driver Risk Inventory, the Substance Abuse Life Circumstance Evaluation, the Alcohol Use Inventory, or the Lovelace Comprehensive Screening Instrument are lists of questions about a person's drinking and/or drug habits. The person giving the test then uses these answers to create a score that helps identify which people have a chronic problem with drinking and driving, and who may be struggling with actual alcoholism. Drunk drivers found to be alcoholics or drug abusers may be assigned to treatment programs rather than be prosecuted. A judge can also direct the offender to participate in treatment as a condition of probation or in order to obtain a provisional or regular driver's license. In some states, the largest share of people entering drug treatment programs do so as the result of a court order.

Several million people have attended drinking-driver schools since the mid-1970s. Classes cover such subjects as the deterioration of driving skills at different BAC levels, the ineffectiveness of coffee or cold showers to "sober up," and criminal penalties for drunk driving. People taking these classes are also required to complete the MAST to determine whether they are alcohol abusers.

Deterring the Drinking Driver

Deterrence based on the threat of arrest, conviction, and punishment remains the chief strategy in the attack on drunk driving. State and local governments have established dozens of strike forces and passed hundreds of laws aiming to raise the costs to the offender of driving while intoxicated.

The number of traffic fatalities fell steadily from 1982 until 1992; since then the number has remained around 41,000 deaths per year. Fatalities related to drunk driving have clearly fallen steadily since 1982, when more than 25,000 deaths were due to alcohol-related accidents (57.3 percent), to 1999 (15,976 deaths, or 38.3 percent of all traffic fatalities). This trend appears to be slowing, however, since the percent of alcohol-related traffic fatalities actually rose slightly in 2000. There may be reasons for this other than deterrence, including general reductions in alcohol consumption and abuse, and more responsible public attitudes toward sober driving. However, the effect of deterrence, even if small, cannot be ruled out as a factor in the decline.

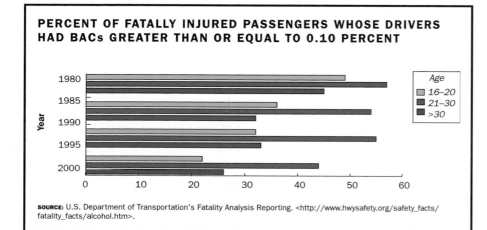

PERCENT OF FATALLY INJURED PASSENGERS WHOSE DRIVERS HAD BACs GREATER THAN OR EQUAL TO 0.10 PERCENT

SOURCE: U.S. Department of Transportation's Fatality Analysis Reporting. <http://www.hwysafety.org/safety_facts/fatality_facts/alcohol.htm>.

Since 1980, after states dropped legal blood alcohol concentration to 0.10 percent and lower and mandated stiffer penalties for drunk driving, the number of fatally injured passengers has fallen by half.

Other Strategies to Fight Drunk Driving

In addition to deterrence, states and localities have implemented many other anti-drunk-driving strategies. Since all these strategies are being used simultaneously, it is impossible to credit any reductions to one strategy over another.

"Vehicular homicide" is a term used to describe a situation in which one person kills another; the weapon in this instance is the vehicle driven by the killer. Even though the driver may not have intended to kill someone, if he or she drives while under the influence of drugs and/or alcohol, the driver can be charged with vehicular homicide. All but three states have vehicle-specific homicide statutes that allow impaired drivers to be tried on homicide charges. Two states (North Carolina and Kentucky) have even allowed cases of drivers charged with vehicular homicide to be tried as capital murder cases, meaning that the driver faced the death penalty.

Some courts have required a convicted drunk driver to pay punitive damages to victims in an accident. In this case, a jury determines an amount of money the convicted drunk driver must pay the accident victim to make up for his or her loss. Some states permit the drunk driver's automobile insurance to cover the costs of punitive damages. In this case the punishment has no deterrent effect, as the money does not come out of the driver's own pocket.

liable responsible

In some states, legislatures and courts have declared that businesses that sell alcohol can be held **liable** for causing drunk-driving injuries. Called Dramshop Laws, these regulations vary from state to state. In most cases they make sellers of alcohol to underage or intoxicated persons liable for any injuries they cause to themselves or others. A few state courts have even made social hosts, such as a person who gives a party where alcohol is served, liable for the alcohol-related traffic injuries caused by their guests.

An essential strategy for controlling drunk drivers is taking away their licenses to drive. Several studies have shown that drunk drivers who lose their driver's licenses are less likely to have a recurrence than drunk drivers who are fined, sent to jail, or assigned to mandatory treatment programs. Nevertheless, many people continue to drive even after their licenses are suspended (temporarily taken away) or revoked (taken away permanently). This should not be a surprise given how vital automobiles are to most people's economic and social lives. Several states also have laws that authorize taking away a person's vehicle, but these sanctions are rarely used, perhaps because automobiles are among our most valued, expensive pieces of private property.

"Opportunity blocking" refers to anticrime strategies that change the environment to reduce the opportunities of committing particular offenses. The best opportunity-blocking strategy for drunk driving involves fixing the defendant's vehicle so that it cannot be started until he or she blows alcohol-free breath into a tube affixed to the vehicle. Such equipment is now available, and several jurisdictions have begun experimental programs. Other opportunity-blocking strategies include setting the drinking age at 21 and new laws and regulations on bars, taverns, and stores that sell alcoholic beverages.

Many educational programs are designed to stop drunk driving. These include public-service announcements on radio and television and educational materials for primary and secondary schools. The effects of such programs are very difficult to evaluate. However, communities that are aware of the problem of alcoholism are more likely to offer effective rehabilitation strategies and other treatment services to drunk drivers.

Driving and Drugs

The role of alcohol in traffic and other injuries is well documented, but determining the effects of other drugs, both legal and illegal, on driving is more difficult. This is true for three reasons: (1) Few drivers who are not involved in crashes volunteer to provide blood samples so their drug levels can be compared with drug levels in blood samples obtained from collision victims; (2) It is very difficult to determine how drug levels in the blood are related to the drug's actions in the brain, and it is those actions in the brain that cause impaired behavior; and (3) It can be difficult to determine how the interactions of various combinations of drugs, with or without alcohol, may contribute to impairment.

One study was designed to get around the first problem. Researchers studied only drivers who had been in crashes. They divided the drivers into two groups—those who were responsible for the crash and those who were not—and studied blood samples from each. The drivers who caused crashes had higher levels of prescription drugs, such as antidepressants and tranquilizers, or over-the-counter drugs, such as antihistamines or cold medicines, in their blood than the other drivers.

Other researchers examined the presence of drugs in blood specimens from 1,882 fatally injured drivers. Drugs, both illicit and prescription, were found in 18 percent of the fatalities. Marijuana was found in 6.7 percent, cocaine in 5.3 percent, tranquilizers in 2.9 percent, and amphetamines in 1.9 percent of these fatally injured drivers. Crash-responsibility rates increased significantly as the number of drugs in the driver increased. Many drug users used several drugs simultaneously, and these drivers had the highest collision rates.

Marijuana. The most frequently used illegal drug in the United States since the mid-twentieth century is marijuana. It is also the drug most often used by drivers. More studies have been performed to understand its effects on drivers than on any other drug. Many of these studies, both those conducted on the road and with driving simulators, indicate that marijuana impairs coordination, tracking (the ability of the eyes to follow movement), perception, and vigilance. A 1999 study, however, concluded that there was no evidence that marijuana alone increased either fatal or serious injury crashes. The evidence was inconclusive as to whether marijuana in combination with alcohol caused more fatalities and serious injuries than did alcohol alone.

Prescription Drugs. Numerous experiments have been performed to evaluate the effects of prescription drugs on vision, attention, vigilance, and the performance of **psychomotor** skills such as tracking. When a prescription drug is shown to produce side effects, this finding has important implications for the use of drugs while driving.

A wide variety of studies have shown that many prescription tranquilizers, especially benzodiazepines such as Valium, impair attention and tracking. However, more recently introduced tranquilizers such as buspirone (tradename Buspar) showed little evidence of impairment.

Another class of **psychoactive** drugs, antidepressants, have long been known to impair performance on a variety of skills. This is especially true of amitriptyline (tradename Elavil). However, recently introduced types of antidepressants, such as Prozac and other selective serotonin reuptake inhibitors, such as Zoloft, Paxil, and Effexor, do not produce the same degree of impairment.

Scientists have shown that narcotic painkillers, such as codeine and Demerol, derived from opium (opiates) lead to decreased alertness in laboratory animals. However, some reports state that chronic use of narcotics produces **tolerance** to some of these side effects. This may explain why scientists have not found differences in crash rates between narcotic users and nonusers. Heroin addicts are often given methadone-maintenance treatment but this drug, a **synthesized** narcotic, does not usually lead to impairment.

Antihistamines. Some antihistamine drugs (such as Benadryl) show evidence of impairing skills performance in laboratory studies. Many people who have taken certain antihistamines report that their per-

psychomotor referring to processes of muscular movement directly influenced by mental processes

psychoactive term applied to drugs that affect the mind or mental processes by altering consciousness, perception, or mood

tolerance condition in which higher and higher doses of a drug or alcohol are needed to produce the effect or "high" experienced from the original dose

synthesize to produce artificially or chemically

formance becomes impaired and that they are drowsy. Recent **pharmacological** improvements have produced antihistamine drugs, such as loratadine (Claritin), that provide the benefits of antihistamine actions but, because they have difficulty crossing the blood-brain barrier, produce little impairment.

Stimulants. While there has been concern over increased use of stimulants, such as amphetamines and cocaine, by motor vehicle drivers, there is little experimental evidence that these drugs impair driving skills. In fact, most studies of these stimulants, as well as of caffeine, indicate that they improve skills performance. However, tolerance develops with chronic (long-term) use of stimulants, and the user must increase the dosage to get the desired effect. Thus, the dose levels examined in the laboratory may not be as high as those found among drivers. Also, an initial phase in which the user feels stimulated is followed by a phase in which depressant effects occur, including increased drowsiness and lack of alertness. Further study of stimulant drugs in relation to driving is needed, both for one-time use and chronic use. SEE ALSO ACCIDENTS AND INJURIES FROM ALCOHOL; ACCIDENTS AND INJURIES FROM DRUGS; ADDICTION: CONCEPTS AND DEFINITIONS; BREATHALYZER; COSTS OF SUBSTANCE ABUSE AND DEPENDENCE, ECONOMIC; DRINKING AGE; MOTHERS AGAINST DRUNK DRIVING (MADD); PREVENTION; STUDENTS AGAINST DESTRUCTIVE DECISIONS (SADD).

pharmacology
branch of science concerned with drugs and how they affect bodily and mental processes

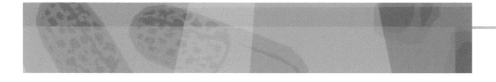

Photo and Illustration Credits

The illustrations and tables featured in *Drugs, Alcohol, and Tobacco: Learning About Addictive Behavior* were created by GGS Information Services. The images appearing in the text were reproduced by permission of the following sources:

Volume 1

AP/Wide World Photos, Inc.: **2, 26, 29, 70, 154, 214;** Custom Medical Stock Photo: **5, 80, 95, 101, 142;** The Advertising Archive Ltd.: **21;** © Prof. P. Motta/Dept. of Anatomy/University of "La Sapienza," Rome/Science Photo Library, National Audubon Society Collection/ Photo Researchers: **37;** © Roger Wood/ Corbis: **44;** © Francis G. Mayer/Corbis: **47;** © Pascal Goetgheluck / SPL / Photo Researchers, Inc.: **54;** Photograph by Robert J. Huffman. Field Mark Publications: **58;** © Photoedit: **60;** © Shepard Sherbell/Corbis: **63;** The Kobal Collection / Touchstone: **67;** © Photo Researchers, Inc.: **73, 163;** CNRI/SPL/ Photo Researchers, Inc.: **75;** © Sidney Moulds / SPL / Photo Researchers, Inc.: **105;** © Josh Sher/SPL/ Photo Researchers, Inc.: **109;** Image Works, Inc.: **116;** © Bettmann/Corbis: **121;** © Lowell Georgia/Corbis: **124;** Photograph by Secchi-Lecague/Roussel-UCLAF/CNRI/ Science Photo Library. © National Audubon Society Collection/Photo Researchers, Inc.: **133;** © Jim Varney / SPL / Photo Researchers, Inc.: **140, 196;**

NLM: **158;** © Bobbie Kingsley/SPL/ Photo Researchers, Inc.: **159;** The Library of Congress: **165;** © 1993 Peter Berndt M.D., P.A. Custom Medical Stock Photo, Inc.: **169;** © Photograph by Ken Settle: **189;** © Photo Researchers: **199;** Photograph by Robert J. Huffman. © Field Mark Publications: **207.**

Volume 2

AP/Wide World Photos, Inc.: **2, 18, 22, 45, 91, 121, 127, 134, 157, 208;** © AFP/Corbis: **26;** © Jacques M. Chenet/Corbis: **28;** © Earl and Nazima Kowall/Corbis: **31;** © Christophe Loviny/ Corbis: **33, 113;** Photo Researchers, Inc.: **43;** Custom Medical Stock Photo: **51;** © Bettmann/Corbis: **63;** Photograph by David H. Wells. © Corbis: **77;** © Sterling K. Clarren: **79;** © Phil Schermeister/ Corbis: **81;** The Kobal Collection / Columbia: **89;** UPI/Corbis Bettmann: **96;** Photograph by Will & Deni McIntyre. © Photo Researchers, Inc.: **101;** Custom Medical Stock Photo: **105, 185;** Photograph by Robert J. Huffman. © Field Mark Publications: **111;** © Reuters NewMedia Inc./Corbis.: **115, 165;** SAGA/Archive Photos, Inc.: **119;** © Scott Camazine & Sue Trainor/Photo Researchers, Inc.: **133;** Science Photo Library: **137;** © Daudicr, Jerrican / Photo Researchers, Inc.: **141;** © Galen Rowell/Corbis: **146;** © Corbis: **170;** © Richard Hutchings/Corbis: **179;** © CNRI/Phototake NYC: **181;** © Lester V.

Bergman/Corbis: **188;** © David Atlas: **197;** © Patrick Bennett/Corbis: **201;** © George Hall/Corbis: **212.**

Volume 3

© Annie Griffiths Belt/Corbis: **9;** © Michael S. Yamashita/Corbis: **20;** © Corbis: **26;** Custom Medical Stock Photo: **33, 85, 118;** American Cancer Society: **41;** AP/Wide World Photos, Inc.: **45, 58, 95, 103, 115, 127, 144, 149, 178;** © James Marshall/Corbis: **46;** Corbis-Bettmann: **52, 110, 124;** © Albert Matti: **54;** © Jennie Woodstock; Reflections Photolibrary/Corbis: **69;** © Joseph Sohm; ChromoSohm Inc./Corbis: **77;** Science Photo Library: **91;** © Dr. Tony Brain / SPL / Photo Researchers, Inc.: **98;** The Library of Congress: **112;** National Audubon Society Collection/Photo Researchers, Inc.: **137;** © Lester V. Bergman/Corbis: **139;** © Bettmann/Corbis: **142;** © LWA-Dann Tardif/Corbis: **158;** Photograph by Robert J. Huffman. © Field Mark Publications: **160;** Tony Freeman/ PhotoEdit: **186;** © Photoedit: **189;** © Scott Roper/Corbis: **205.**

Organizations of Interest

Adult Children of Alcoholics (ACOA)
ACA WSO
PO Box 3216
Torrance, CA 90510
310-534-1815 (message only)
<http://www.adultchildren.org>
meetinginfo@adultchildren.org

African American Parents for Drug Prevention (AAPDP)
4025 Red Bud Avenue
Cincinnati, OH 45229
513-961-4158
513-961-6719 (fax)

AIDS Hotline
American Social Health Association
PO Box 13827
Research Triangle Park, NC 27713
800-342-AIDS
<http://www.ashastd.org/nah>
hivnet@ashastd.org

AIDS National Information Clearinghouse
CDC NPIN
PO Box 6003
Rockville, MD 20849-6003
800-458-5231
<http://www.cdcnpin.org>
info@cdcnpin.org (reference services)
webmaster@cdcnpin.org (web site)

Alcohol Treatment Referral Hotline
107 Lincoln Street
Worcester, MA 01605
800-ALCOHOL
508-798-9446
<http://www.adcare.com>
info@adcare.com

Alcoholics Anonymous (AA)
General Service Office
PO Box 459
New York, NY 10163
212-870-3400
<http://www.alcoholics-anonymous.org>

American Council for Drug Education
164 West 74th Street
New York, NY 10023
800-488-3784
<http://www.acde.org>
acde@phoenixhouse.org

BACCHUS Peer Education Network and GAMMA
PO Box 100043
Denver, CO 80250
303-871-3068
<http://www.bacchusgamma.org>
bacgam@aol.com

Bureau of Alcohol, Tobacco, and Firearms
Office of Liaison and Public Information
650 Massachusetts Avenue, NW
Room 8290
Washington, DC 20226
202-927-8500
<http://www.atf.treas.gov/index.htm>
ATFMail@atfhq.atf.treas.gov

Clearinghouse of the National Criminal Justice Reference System
Bureau of Justice Assistance
PO Box 6000
Rockville, MD 20849
800-688-4252
<http://www.ncjrs.org>

Bureau of Justice Statistics
810 7th Street, NW
Washington, DC 20531
202-307-0765
800-732-3277
<http://www.ojp.usdoj.gov/bjs>
askbjs@ojp.usdoj.gov

Center for Mental Health Services Knowledge Exchange Network
PO Box 42490
Washington, DC 20015
800-789-2647
<http://www.mentalhealth.org>
ken@mentalhealth.org

Center for Substance Abuse Prevention
5600 Fishers Lane
Rockwall II Building, Suite 800
Rockville, MD 20857
301-443-8956
<http://www.samhsa.gov/centers/csap/csap.html>
info@samhsa.gov

Center for Substance Abuse Treatment
National Treatment Hotline
1-800-662-HELP
<http://www.samhsa.gov/centers/csat2002/csat_frame.html>

Centers for Disease Control and Prevention
Office on Smoking and Health
4770 Buford Highway, NE, MS-K50
Atlanta, GA 30341-3724
800-CDC-1311
<http://www.cdc.gov/tobacco>
tobaccoinfo@cdc.gov

Child Help USA
Childhelp USA National Headquarters
15757 N. 78th Street
Scottsdale, Arizona 85260
800-4-A-CHILD
<http://www.childhelpusa.org>

CoAnon Family Groups
PO Box 12722
Tucson, AZ 85732
800-898-9985 (Leave your name, number, and a brief message and someone will call you back.)
<http://www.co-anon.org>

Cocaine Anonymous (CA)
3740 Overland Ave., Suite C
Los Angeles, CA 90034
310-559-5833
<http://www.ca.org>
cawso@ca.org

DARE America
PO Box 512090
Los Angeles, CA 90051-0090
800-223-3273
<http://www.dare.com>

Drug Enforcement Administration (DEA)
Information Services Section
2401 Jefferson Davis Highway
Alexandria, VA 22301
202-307-1000
<http://www.dea.gov>

Employee Assistance Professional Administration
2101 Wilson Blvd., Suite 500
Arlington, VA 22201
703-387-1000
<http://www.eap-association.com>
info@eap-association.org

Families Anonymous
PO Box 3475
Culver City, CA 90231-3475
800-736-9805
<http://www.familiesanonymous.org>
famanon@FamiliesAnonymous.org

Food and Drug Administration (FDA)
5600 Fishers Lane
Rockville, Maryland 20857
888-463-6332
<http://www.fda.gov>

Gamblers Anonymous
International Service Office
PO Box 17173
Los Angeles, CA 90017
213-386-8789
<http://www.gamblersanonymous.org>
isomain@gamblersanonymous.org

Girls and Boys Town National Hotline
13943 Gutowski Road
Boystown, NE 68010
800-448-3000 (English and *Español*)

<http://www.girlsandboystown.org>
hotline@boystown.org

Higher Education Center for Alcohol and Other Drug Prevention
55 Chapel Street
Newton, MA 02458-1060
800-676-1730
617-928-1537
<http://www.edc.org/hec>

Indian Health Service
The Reyes Building
801 Thompson Avenue, Suite 400
Rockville, MD 20852-1627
301-443-2038
<http://www.ihs.gov>
feedback@ihs.gov

Institute for Social Research
University of Michigan
426 Thompson Street
PO Box 1248
Ann Arbor, MI 48106
734-764-8354
<http://www.isr.umich.edu>
MTFinfo@isr.umich.edu

Juvenile Justice Clearinghouse
PO Box 6000
Rockville, MD 20849
800-638-8736
<http://virlib.ncjrs.org/JuvenileJustice.asp>
askncjrs@ncjrs.org

March of Dimes
1275 Mamaroneck Avenue
White Plains, NY 10605
914-428-7100
<http://www.modimes.org>

Marijuana Anonymous
PO Box 2912
Van Nuys, CA 91404
800-766-6779
<http://www.marijuana-anonymous.org>
office@marijuana-anonymous.org

Mediascope
12711 Ventura Boulevard, Suite 440
Studio City, CA 91604
818-508-2080
<http://www.mediascope.org>
facts@mediascope.org

Mothers Against Drunk Driving (MADD)
National Headquarters
PO Box 541688
Dallas, TX 75354
800-438-6233
<http://www.madd.org>

Nar-anon Family
World Service Office
PO Box 2562
Palos Verdes, CA 90274
310-547-5800

Narcotics Anonymous (NA)
PO Box 9999
Van Nuys, CA 91409
818-773-9999
<http://www.na.org>

National Alliance for Hispanic Health
1501 Sixteenth Street, NW
Washington, DC 20036
800-725-8312
<http://www.hispanichealth.org>

National Alliance for the Mentally Ill
Colonial Place Three
2107 Wilson Boulevard, Suite 300
Arlington, VA 22201
703-524-7600
<http://www.nami.org>

National Association for Children of Alcoholics
11426 Rockville Pike
Suite 100
Rockville, MD 20852
888-554-2627
<http://www.nacoa.org>
nacoa@erols.com

National Association for Native American Children of Alcoholics (NANACOA)
1402 Third Avenue
Suite 1110
Seattle, WA 98101
800-322-5601
nanacoa@nanacoa.org

National Association of Alcoholism and Drug Abuse Counselors
1911 North Fort Myer Drive
Suite 900

Arlington, VA 22201
800-548-0497
<http://www.naadac.org>
naadc@naadc.org

**National Association of Anorexia
Nervosa and Associated Disorders**
PO Box 7
Highland Park, IL 60035
847-831-3438
<http://www.anad.org>
anad20@aol.com

**National Association of State Alcohol
and Drug Abuse Directors**
808 17th Street NW
Suite 410
Washington, DC 20006
202-293-0090
<http://www.nasadad.org>
dcoffice@nasadad.org

**National Center for Victims
of Crime**
2111 Wilson Boulevard
Suite 300
Arlington, VA 22201
800-211-7996
<http://www.ncvc.org>

**National Clearinghouse on Child Abuse
and Neglect Information**
330 C Street, SW
Washington, DC 20447
800-394-3366
<http://www.calib.com/nccanch>
nccanch@calib.com

**National Council on Alcoholism and
Drug Dependence, Inc.**
20 Exchange Place
Suite 2902
New York, NY 10005
800-NCA-CALL
<http://www.ncadd.org>
national@ncadd.org

**The National Council on Problem
Gambling, Inc.**
208 G Street, NE
Washington, DC 20002
800-522-4700 (hotline)
<http://www.ncpgambling.org>
ncpg@ncpgambling.org

**National Crime Prevention Council
Online Resource Center**
1000 Connecticut Avenue, NW
13th floor
Washington, DC 20036
202-466-6272
<http://www.ncpc.org>

National Domestic Violence Hotline
PO Box 161810
Austin, TX 78716
800-787-3224
<http://www.ndvh.org>
ndvh@ndvh.org

National Eating Disorders Association
603 Stewart St., Suite 803
Seattle, WA 98101
206-382-3587
<http://www.NationalEatingDisorders.org>
info@NationalEatingDisorders.org

National Health Information Center
PO Box 1133
Washington, DC 20013
800-336-4797
<http://www.health.gov/nhic>
nhicinfo@health.org

**National Inhalant Prevention
Coalition**
2904 Kerbey Lane
Austin, TX 78703
800-269-4237
<http://www.inhalants.org>
nipc@io.com

**National Institute of Mental Health
(NIMH)**
NIMH Public Inquiries
6001 Executive Boulevard, Rm. 8184,
MSC 9663
Bethesda, MD 20892-9663
301-443-4513
<http://www.nimh.nih.gov>
nimhinfo@nih.gov

**National Institute on Alcohol Abuse and
Alcoholism**
6000 Executive Boulevard
Willco Building
Bethesda, MD 20892
301-443-3860
<http://www.niaaa.nih.gov>

National Institute on Drug Abuse (NIDA)
6001 Executive Boulevard
Room 5213
Bethesda, MD 20892
301-443-1124
<http://www.drugabuse.gov>
information@lists.nida.nih.gov

National Institutes of Health (NIH)
9000 Rockville Pike
Bethesda, MD 20892
301-496-4143
<http://www.nih.gov>

National Maternal and Child Health Clearinghouse
Health Resources and Services
Administration
U.S. Department of Health and Human
Services
Parklawn Building
5600 Fishers Lane
Rockville, MD 20857
<http://www.ask.hrsa.gov>
ask@hrsa.gov

National Organization on Fetal Alcohol Syndrome
216 G Street, NE
Washington, DC 20002
800-666-6327
<http://www.nofas.org>
information@nofas.org

National Resource Center on Homelessness and Mental Illness
Policy Research Associates, Inc.
345 Delaware Avenue
Delmar, NY 12054
800-444-7415
<http://www.nrchmi.com/>
nrc@prainc.com

National Safety Council
1121 Spring Lake Drive
Itasca, IL 60143
800-621-7615
<http://www.nsc.org>

National Women's Health Information Center
8550 Arlington Boulevard
Suite 300
Fairfax, VA 22031

800-994-9662
<http://www.4woman.org>

Office for Victims of Crime Resource Center
Department of Justice
810 7th Street, NW
Washington, DC 20531
800-627-6872
<http:/www.ojp.usdoj.gov/ovc>

Office of Minority Health Resource Center
PO Box 37337
Washington, DC 20013
800-444-6472
<http://www.omhrc.gov>

Office of National Drug Control Policy (ONDCP)
Executive Office of the President
750 17th Street, NW
Washington DC 20503
202-395-6700
<http://www.whitehousedrugpolicy.gov>
ondcp@ncjrs.org

Office on Smoking and Health (see Centers for Disease Control and Prevention)

ONDCP's Drug Policy Information Clearinghouse
PO Box 6000
Rockville, MD 20849
800-666-3332
<http://www.whitehousedrugpolicy.gov/
publications/index.html>

Overeaters Anonymous
PO Box 44020
Rio Rancho, NM 87124-4020
505-891-2664
<http://www.overeatersanonymous.org>
info@overeatersanonymous.org

Partnership for a Drug-Free America
405 Lexington Avenue
Suite 1601
New York, NY 10174
212-922-1560
<http://www.drugfreeamerica.org>

PRIDE
4684 S. Evergreen
Newaygo, MI 49337

800-668-9277
<http://www.prideyouthprograms.org>
prideyouth@ncats.net

Psychomedics, Inc
5832 Uplander Way
Culver City, CA 90230
800-522-7424

Rational Recovery
PO Box 800
Lotus, CA 95651
800-303-2873
<http://www.rational.org>
home@rational.org

Safe and Drug-Free Schools
Department of Education
Federal Building No. 6
400 Maryland Avenue, SW
Washington, DC 20202
202-260-3954 for information on grant
applications
800-624-0100 for drug prevention materials
202-260-3954
<http://www.ed.gov>
customerservice@inet.ed.gov

Secular Organizations for Sobriety
SOS Clearinghouse
5521 Grosvenor Boulevard
Los Angeles, CA 90066
310-821-8430
<http://www.secularsobriety.org>

**Self-Help and Information Exchange
Network (SHINE)**
c/o Voluntary Action Center
Suite 420

538 Spruce Street
Scranton, PA 18509
570-961-1234
570-347-5616
<http://www.vacnepa.org>

Skyshapers University
157 Chambers Street
10th floor
New York, NY 10007
800-759-9675
800-SKYSHAPERS
<http://www.skyshapers.com>
webmaster@skyshapers.com

**Students Against Destructive Decisions
(SADD)**
Box 800
Marlboro, MA 01752
800-787-5777
<http://www.saddonline.com>

**Substance Abuse and Mental Health
Services Administration (SAMHSA)**
5600 Fishers Lane
Rockville, MD 20857
301-443-6315
<http://www.samhsa.gov>

**Working Partners for an Alcohol- and
Drug-Free Workplace**
Department of Labor
Office of Public Affairs
200 Constitution Ave., NW, Room
S-1032
Washington, DC 20210
202-693-4650
<http://www.dol.gov/dol/workingpartners
.htm>

Selected Bibliography

General Texts About Alcohol and Drug Abuse

Alcohol and drug abuse take a terrible toll on teenagers. Unfortunately, studies show that more and more teenagers are using drugs and alcohol and suffering the consequences of that use. Substance abuse puts teenagers at a much greater risk for a wide variety of problems, including:

- school problems
- criminal behavior
- traffic accidents
- sexual activity at a young age
- depression and other psychiatric conditions
- victimization
- death by suicide, murder, drowning, fire

Articles and Nonfiction Books

"Alcohol: How It Affects You." *Current Health* 1, vol. 21, no. 5 (Jan. 1998).

Drug Dangers Series (Berkeley Heights, NJ: Enslow Publishers, 2001), including:

Alcohol Drug Dangers

Amphetamine Drug Dangers

Crack and Cocaine Drug Dangers

Diet Pill Drug Dangers

Ecstasy and Other Designer Drugs Drug Dangers

Herbal Drugs Drug Dangers

Heroin Drug Dangers

Inhalant Drug Dangers

LSD, PCP, Hallucinogen Drug Dangers

Marijuana Drug Dangers

Speed and Methamphetamine Drug Dangers

Steroid Drug Dangers

Tobacco and Nicotine Drug Dangers

Tranquilizer, Barbiturate, and Downer Drug Dangers

Gofen, E. "Alcohol in the Life of a Teen." Current Health 2, vol. 17, no. 2 (Oct. 1990).

"Illicit Drug Use by Teens Rising." *Alcoholism Report* 22, no. 2 (Feb./Mar. 1994).

Kuhn, Cynthia, et al. *Buzzed: The Straight Facts About the Most Used and Abused Drugs from Alcohol to Ecstasy.* New York: Norton, 1998.

Roza, Greg, ed. *Encyclopedia of Drugs and Alcohol.* New York: Franklin Watts, 2001.

Schuckit, Marc Alan. *Educating Yourself About Alcohol and Drugs: A People's Primer.* New York: Plenum Press, 1998.

"Survey Illustrates Wide Reach of Drugs in Teens' Lives." *Alcoholism and Drug Abuse Weekly* 10, no. 26 (June 29, 1998).

"Teens' Steroid Use Linked to Their Use of Other Drugs." *Addiction Letter* 11, no. 11 (Nov. 1995).

"Teens Who Do Not Try Drugs Are Better-Adjusted, Study Says." *Alcoholism and Drug Abuse Weekly* 8, no. 21 (May 20, 1996).

"Withdrawal Symptoms May be Worse for Teens." *Addiction Letter* 12, no. 1 (Jan. 1996).

"Young Teens and Drugs Use." *Current Health* 1, vol. 17, no. 2 (Oct. 1993).

Fiction of Interest

Anonymous. *Go Ask Alice.* Minneapolis: Econo-Clad Books, 1998.

Childress, Alice. *A Hero Ain't Nothin' but a Sandwich.* New York: Avon, 1995.

Draper, Sharon M. *Tears of a Tiger*. New York: Simon and Schuster, 1996.

Glovach, Linda. *Beauty Queen*. New York: Harper-Collins, 1998.

Greene, Shep. *The Boy Who Drank Too Much*. New York: Bantam Doubleday Dell, 1981.

Keizer, Garrett. *God of Beer*. New York: HarperCollins, 2002.

Web Sites

"For Tweens and Teens." National Center on Addiction and Substance Abuse at Columbia University.

<http://www.casacolumbia.org/info-url1940/info-url_list.htm?section=For%20Tweens%20%26%20Teens>.

"Mind Over Matter: The Brain's Response to Marijuana, Opiates, Inhalants, Hallucinogens, Methamphetamine, Nicotine, Stimulants, Steroids." National Institute on Drug Abuse, National Institutes of Health. Last updated September 14, 2001. <http://www.nida.nih.gov/MOM/MOMIndex.html>.

Overcoming Substance Abuse

Many substance users think they will never get addicted. But once substance abuse becomes a stranglehold, it can be exceedingly difficult for the user to struggle free. Although a wide variety of treatments are available, researchers are constantly searching for ways to help users break their addiction and to help former addicts avoid slipping back into substance abuse.

Articles and Nonfiction Books

"Alcohol and Drug Interventions for Teens Should Consider Peer Use, Peer Pressure." *DATA: The Brown University Digest of Addiction Theory and Application* 14, no. 5 (May 1995).

"Alcohol Interventions for Teens Should Address Social Factors." *DATA: The Brown University Digest of Addiction Theory and Application* 14, no. 7 (July 1995).

Chiu, Christina. *Teen Guide to Staying Sober*. New York: Rosen Publishing Group, 1995.

"Gender-Specific Substance Abuse Treatment Promising." *DATA: The Brown University Digest of Addiction Theory and Application* 20, no. 7 (July 2001).

Landau, Elaine. *Hooked: Talking About Addiction*. Brookfield, CT: Millbrook Press, 1995.

Moe, Barbara A. *Drug Abuse Relapse: Helping Teens to Get Clean Again*. Drug Abuse Prevention Library. New York: Rosen Publishing Group, 2000.

Roos, Stephen. *A Young Person's Guide to the Twelve Steps*. Center City, MN: Hazelden Information and Educational Services, 1993.

"Youth Treatment Study Shows Good Results, Parallels Findings for Adult Outcomes." *Alcoholism and Drug Abuse Weekly* 13, no. 27 (July 16, 2001).

Web Site

"Principles of Drug Abuse Treatment: A Research-Based Guide." National Institute on Drug Abuse, National Institutes of Health.

<http://www.nida.nih.gov/PODAT/PODAT1.html>.

When Parents Abuse Alcohol or Drugs

Most studies show that having a substance-abusing parent can affect children from birth on into adulthood. Babies of substance abusers can be born addicted to drugs or suffering from fetal alcohol syndrome. Children living in a home with substance-abusing parents are more likely to suffer from anxiety, depression, and behavior problems. Rates of child abuse and neglect are higher in homes with substance-abusing parents. Teenage children of substance abusers have a higher risk of themselves turning to drugs or alcohol. Adults from alcoholic homes or homes where drugs were used have more problems with anxiety and depression, greater difficulties with relationships, and a high risk of becoming addicted to alcohol or drugs.

Articles and Nonfiction Books

"Depression in Children Linked to Parents' Alcoholism." *Alcoholism and Drug Abuse Weekly* 8, no. 27 (July 1, 1996).

Emshoff, James G., and Ann W. Price. "Prevention and Intervention Strategies With Children of Alcoholics" (part 2 of 2). *Pediatrics* 103, no. 5 (May 1999).

Foltz-Gray, Dorothy. "An Alcoholic in the Family." *Health* 11, no. 5 (July/Aug. 1997).

Hornik-Beer, Edith Lynn. *For Teenagers Living with a Parent Who Abuses Alcohol/Drugs.* iUniverse.com, 2001.

Johnson, Jeannette L., and Michelle Left. "Children of Substance Abusers: Overview of Research Findings" (part 2 of 2). *Pediatrics* 103, no. 5 (May 1999).

Leite, Evelyn, and Pamela Espeland. *Different Like Me: A Book for Teenagers Who Worry about Their Parents' Use of Alcohol/Drugs.* Center City, MN: Hazelden Information and Educational Services, 1989.

Price, Ann W., and James G. Emshoff. "Breaking the Cycle of Addiction: Prevention and Intervention With Children of Alcoholics." *Alcohol Health and Research World* 21, no. 3 (1997).

Shuker, Nancy. *Everything You Need to Know About an Alcoholic Parent.* New York: Rosen Publishing Group, 1998.

"Substance Abuse Programs for Parents." *Brown University Child and Adolescent Behavior Letter* 11, no. 2 (Feb. 1995).

Tomori, Martina. "Personality Characteristics of Adolescents with Alcoholic Parents." *Adolescence* 29, no. 116 (winter 1994).

Ullman, Albert D., and Alan Orenstein. "Why Some Children of Alcoholics Become Alcoholics: Emulation of the Drinker." *Adolescence* 29, no. 113 (spring 1994).

Fiction of Interest

Bauer, Joan. *Rules of the Road.* New York: Putnam, 1998.

Gantos, Jack. *Joey Pigza Loses Control.* New York: HarperTrophy, 2002.

Web Sites

"Alateen: Hope and Help for Young People Who Are the Relatives and Friends of a Problem Drinker."

<http://www.al-anon.org/alateen.html>.

National Association for Children of Alcoholics.

<http://www.nacoa.org/kidspage.htm>.

Alcohol and Drug Policy, Drug Trafficking, and Crime

The United States and other concerned countries work to rewrite policy and law in an effort to regulate alcohol and tobacco use, to decrease drug production and drug trafficking, and to cut down on drug-related crime. The dangerous consequences of drug use range from its effects on individuals (increased risk of murder, suicide, and motor vehicle accidents) to its effects on entire nations. In recent years, many events have brought the link between drug trafficking, money laundering, and terrorism to the world's attention.

Articles and Nonfiction Books

"Alcohol Most Common 'Date-Rape' Drug: Study." *Alcoholism Report* 26, no. 3 (March 1998).

Grosslander, Janet. *Drugs and Driving.* New York: Rosen Publishing Group, 2001.

Hyde, Margaret O. *Drug Wars.* New York: Walker and Company, 2000.

"Let's Redefine U.S. Drug Policy to One of Harm Reduction." *DATA: The Brown University Digest of Addiction Theory and Application* 16, no. 2 (Feb. 1997 supplement).

Levine, Herbert M. *The Drug Problem: American Issues Debated.* New York: Raintree/Steck Vaughn, 1997.

Leviton, Susan, and Marc A. Schindler. "Drug Trafficking and the Justice System" (part 2 of 2). *Pediatrics* 93, no. 6 (June 1994).

"SAMHSA Study Links Treatment to Drops in Drug Use, Crime." *Alcoholism and Drug Abuse Weekly* 8, no. 36 (Sept. 16, 1996).

Stewart, Gail B. *Drug Trafficking.* Detroit: Gale Group, 1990.

"Study of Probationers Reveals High Drug Use." *Alcoholism and Drug Abuse Weekly* 10, no. 15 (April 13, 1998).

Fiction of Interest

Kehret, Peg. *Cages.* New York: Pocket Books, 1993.

Smith, Roland. *Zach's Lie.* New York: Hyperion Books, 2001.

Web Sites

Drug Enforcement Administration.

<http://www.dea.gov>.

Office of National Drug Control Policy.

<http://www.whitehousedrugpolicy.gov>.

Smoking

It has been known for years that smoking is deadly. Studies show that if the current rate of tobacco use holds steady, five million U.S. children who were aged 18 or under in 2000 will die prematurely as adults due to complications of the smoking habit they started during their teen years.

Articles and Nonfiction Books

"African-American Teens at High Risk from Smoking." *Alcoholism and Drug Abuse Weekly* 13, no. 10 (Mar. 5, 2001).

Hyde, Margaret O. *Know About Smoking.* New York: Walker and Company, 1995.

Kowalski, Kathiann M. "Tobacco's Toll on Teens." *Current Health* 2, vol. 23, no. 6 (Feb. 1997).

McMillan, Daniel. *Teen Smoking: Understanding the Risk.* Berkeley Heights, NJ: Enslow Publishers, 1996.

"Restricting the Movies Teens Watch May Impact Tobacco Use." *Brown University Child and Adolescent Behavior Letter* 18, no. 5 (May 2002).

"Study: Parents and Peers Influence Smoking, Drinking." *Alcoholism and Drug Abuse Weekly* 13, no. 6 (Feb. 5, 2001).

"Teens: Smoking Isn't Good. Quitting Isn't Easy." *Current Health* 2, vol. 20, no. 8 (Apr. 1994).

"Teen Smoking May Hint at Other Risky Behavior." *Health Letter on the CDC*, December 22–December 29, 1997.

"Teens Who Exhibit Problems More Likely to Smoke." *Alcoholism and Drug Abuse Weekly* 14, no. 10 (Mar. 11, 2002).

Williams, Mary E. *Teens and Smoking.* Detroit: Gale Group, 2000.

Fiction of Interest

Cossi, Olga. *The Magic Box.* New York: Pelican, 1989.

Web Sites

Campaign for Tobacco Free Kids.

<http://www.tobaccofreekids.org>.

"The Surgeon General's Report for Kids About Smoking." National Center for Chronic Disease Prevention and Health Promotion, Centers for Disease Control and Prevention.

<http://www.cdc.gov/tobacco/sgr/sgr4kids/sgrmenu.htm>.

Gambling

Gambling is spreading among younger teens and even children, mainly because of the ever-increasing number of online gambling web sites. For those people who are susceptible to becoming addicted to gambling, the ease of gambling online is a particular danger. The social costs of gambling problems among adults include increased rates of crime, financial downfall leading to bankruptcy, higher divorce rates, and a greatly increased chance of becoming addicted to alcohol or drugs.

Articles and Nonfiction Books

Cozick, Charles P., and Paul A. Winters. *Gambling.* Detroit: Greenhaven Press, 1995.

Dolan, Edward F. *Teenagers and Compulsive Gambling.* New York: Franklin Watts, 1994.

"Gambling Common Among Marijuana-Smoking Teens." *Brown University Child and Adolescent Behavior Letter* 17, no. 12 (Dec. 2001).

Haddock, Patricia. *Teens and Gambling: Who Wins?* Berkeley Heights, NJ: Enslow Publishers, 1996.

Rafenstein, Mark. "Why Teens Are Becoming Compulsive about Gambling." *Current Health* 2, vol. 26, no. 8 (Apr./May 2000).

"Teens and Gambling." *Current Health* 2, vol. 26, no. 8 (Apr./May 2000 teacher's edition).

Fiction of Interest

Hautman, Pete. *Stone Cold.* New York: Simon and Schuster, 1998.

Web Sites

"Questions and Answers About the Problem of Compulsive Gambling and the Gamblers Anonymous Recovery Program." Gamblers Anonymous.

<http://www.gamblersanonymous.org/qna.html>.

"Youth Problem Gambling." International Centre for Youth Gambling Problems and High-Risk Behaviors, McGill University, Montreal, Canada.

<http://www.education.mcgill.ca/gambling/en/problemg.htm>.

Other Conditions That May Influence Substance Abuse

A number of other psychiatric conditions may occur along with substance abuse, including depression, bipolar disorder, obsessive-compulsive disorder, eating disorders, cutting (self-harm or self-mutilation), anxiety, and conduct disorders. Why are these conditions associated with each other? Is there something similar genetically about people with substance abuse and other psychiatric problems? Is there something about the brain structure or the brain chemistry of some individuals that makes them more susceptible to these disorders, as well as to substance abuse? Do people begin using alcohol or taking drugs in order to treat the symptoms of other psychiatric illnesses?

Articles and Nonfiction Books

Cobain, Bev, et al. *When Nothing Matters Anymore: A Survival Guide for Depressed Teens.* Minneapolis: Free Spirit Publishing, 1998.

Costin, Carolyn. *The Eating Disorder Sourcebook: A Comprehensive Guide to the Causes, Treatments, and Prevention of Eating Disorders.* New York: McGraw Hill, 1999.

Farley, Dixie. "On the Teen Scene: Overcoming the Deficit of Attention." *FDA Consumer* 31, no. 5 (July/Aug. 1997).

Hallowell, Edward M., and John J. Ratey. *Driven to Distraction: Recognizing and Coping With Attention Deficit Disorder from Childhood Through Adolescence.* New York: Simon and Schuster, 1995.

Levonkron, Steven. *Cutting: Understanding and Overcoming Self-Mutilation.* New York: Norton, 1999.

McLellan, Tom, and Alicia Bragg. *Escape from Anxiety and Stress.* Broomall, PA: Chelsea House Publishing, 1988.

Normandi, Carol Emery, and Lauralee Roark. *Over It: A Teen's Guide to Getting Beyond Obsession With Food and Weight.* Novato, CA: New World Publishing, 2001.

Rapoport, Judith L. *The Boy Who Couldn't Stop Washing: The Experience and Treatment of Obsessive Compulsive Disorder.* New York: New American Library, 1997.

"Study Finds Co-morbid Eating Disorders among Women Who Abuse Substances." *DATA: The Brown University Digest of Addiction Theory and Application* 20, no. 1 (Jan. 2001).

"Study: Use of Ritalin for ADHD Reduces Substance Abuse Risk." *Children's Services Report* 3, no. 16 (Aug. 23, 1999).

"Teens with Depression Gravitate to Smoking." *Mental Health Weekly* 7, no. 1 (Jan. 6, 1997).

Fiction of Interest

Gantos, Jack. *Joey Pigza Swallowed the Key.* New York: Farrar Straus Giroux, 1998. (Concerns ADHD.)

Hesser, Terry Spencer. *Kissing Doorknobs.* New York: Bantam Books, 1999. (Concerns obsessive-compulsive disorder.)

Jenkins, A. M. *Damage.* New York: HarperCollins, 2001. (Concerns depression.)

Levonkron, Steven. *The Best Little Girl in the World.* New York: Warner Books, 1979. (Concerns eating disorders.)

Levonkron, Steven. *The Luckiest Girl in the World.* New York: Penguin, 1998. (Concerns cutting.)

McCormick, Patricia. *Cut.* New York: Scholastic, 2002. (Concerns cutting.)

Newman, Leslie. *Fat Chance.* New York: Putnam, 1996. (Concerns eating disorders.)

Willey, Margaret. *Saving Lenny.* New York: Bantam Books, 1991. (Concerns depression, codependence.)

Web Sites

"Attention Deficit Hyperactivity Disorder." National Institute of Mental Health, National Institutes of Health.

<http://www.nimh.nih.gov/publicat/adhd.cfm>.

"Eating Disorders: Facts about Eating Disorders and the Search for Solutions." National Institute of Mental Health, National Institutes of Health.

<http://www.nimh.nih.gov/publicat/eatingdisorder.cfm>.

"Let's Talk about Depression," National Institute of Mental Health, National Institutes of Health.

<http://www.nimh.nih.gov/publicat/letstalk.cfm>.

Prevention of Alcohol or Drug Abuse

The issue of preventing substance abuse is as complicated as it is important. Effective prevention seems to involve helping young people learn how to manage peer pressure and develop a strong and confident sense of self.

Articles and Nonfiction Books

Alexander, Ruth Bell. *Changing Bodies, Changing Lives: A Book for Teens on Sex and Relationships.* New York: Times Books, 1998.

Benson, Peter L., et al. *What Teens Need to Succeed: Proven, Practical Ways to Shape Your Own Future.* Minneapolis: Free Spirit Publishing, 1998.

Covey, Sean. *Seven Habits of Highly Effective Teens: The Ultimate Teenage Success Guide.* New York: Simon and Schuster, 1998.

"Improving Substance Abuse Prevention, Assessment, and Treatment Financing for Children and Adolescents." *Pediatrics* 108, no. 4 (Oct. 2001).

Palmer, Pat, and Melissa Alberti Froehner. *Teen Esteem: A Self-Direction Manual for Young Adults.* Atascadero, CA: Impact Publishers, 2000.

Scott, Sharon. *How to Say No and Keep Your Friends: Peer Pressure Reversal for Teens and Preteens.* Amherst, MA: Human Resource Development Press, 1997.

Web Sites

"CASA's Tips for Staying Drug-Free." National Center on Addiction and Substance Abuse at Columbia University.

<http://www.casacolumbia.org/info-url1940/info-url_show.htm?doc_id=20812>.

"A Guide for Teens: Does Your Friend Have an Alcohol or Drug Problem?" National Clearinghouse for Alcohol and Drug Information, Substance Abuse and Mental Health Services Administration, Department of Health and Human Services.

<http://www.health.org/govpubs/phd688>.

For Parents and Teachers

Parents have a lot of influence over their children. While parents cannot fully control their children's behavior, studies have shown that close-knit families provide some protection against alcohol and drug abuse in children. It is also clear that the use or abuse of substances by a child's parent or parents can increase that child's risk of beginning to use or abuse substances. Still, some children who come from warm, supportive homes and whose parents do not themselves abuse substances may stumble into alcohol or drug use. How can parents (and teachers) identify such problems and get their child the help he or she so desperately needs?

Articles and Nonfiction Books

Babbit, Nikki. *Adolescent Drug and Alcohol Abuse: How to Spot It, Stop It, and Get Help for Your Family.* Sebastopol, CA: Patient-Centered Guides, 2000.

Biederman, Joseph, et al. "Patterns of Alcohol and Drug Use in Adolescents Can Be Predicted by Parental Substance Use Disorders." *Pediatrics* 106, no. 4 (Oct. 2000).

Cappello, Dominic, and Xenia G. Becher. *Ten Talks Parents Must Have with Their Children about Drugs and Choices.* New York: Hyperion, 2001.

"Does Your Child Have a Gambling Problem?" *Brown University Child and Adolescent Behavior Letter* 12, no. 3 (Mar. 1996).

"'Hands-On' Parenting Reduces Teens' Substance Abuse Risk." *Nation's Health* 31, no. 4 (May 2001).

Kuhn, Cynthia. *Just Say Know: Talking with Kids about Drugs and Alcohol.* New York: Norton, 2002.

Nolen, Billy James. *Parents, Teens, and Drugs.* Baltimore: American Literary Press, 2000.

"Parents Can Influence When, How Teens Use Alcohol and Marijuana." *DATA: The Brown University Digest of Addiction Theory and Application* 19, no. 6 (June 2000).

"Program Helps Parents Cope with Substance-Abusing Teens." *DATA: The Brown University Digest of Addiction Theory and Application* 20, no. 7 (July 2001).

Wood, Barbara. *Raising Healthy Children in an Alcoholic Home.* New York: Crossroad/Herder and Herder, 1992.

Web Sites

Mothers Against Drunk Driving (MADD).

<http://www.madd.org/under21/0,1056,1108,00.html>.

Safe and Drug-Free Schools Program, U.S. Department of Education.

<http://www.ed.gov/offices/OESE/SDFS>.

Glossary

abstinence complete avoidance of something, such as the use of drugs or alcoholic beverages

abstinent to completely avoid something, such as drug or alcohol use

abuse related to drug use, describes taking drugs that are illegal, or using prescription drugs in a way for which they were not prescribed; related to alcohol use, describes drinking in a fashion that is damaging to the drinker or to others

abuse potential chance, or likelihood, that a drug will be abused

acute having a sudden onset and lasting a short time

addiction state in which the body requires the presence of a particular substance to function normally; without the substance, the individual will begin to experience predictable withdrawal symptoms

advocate to support or defend a cause or a proposal

aesthete one who has a deep appreciation for beauty, especially in the arts or nature

aggression hostile and destructive behavior, especially caused by frustration; may include violence or physical threat or injury directed toward another

aggressive hostile and destructive behavior

agonist chemical that can bind to a particular cell and cause a specific reaction

AIDS stands for acquired immunodeficiency syndrome, the disease caused by the human immunodeficiency virus (HIV); in severe cases, it is characterized by the profound weakening of the body's immune system

alcoholism disease of the body and mind in which an individual compulsively drinks alcohol, despite its harmful effects on the person's career, relationships, and/or health; leads to dependence on alcohol, and the presence of withdrawal symptoms when alcohol use is stopped; can be progressive and fatal; research indicates the disease runs in families, and may be genetically inherited

alkaline similar in chemical composition to the alkali chemicals; possessing a pH greater than 7

amino acids organic molecules that make up proteins

amphetamine central nervous system stimulant, used in medicine to treat attention-deficit/hyperactivity disorder (ADHD), narcolepsy (a sleep disorder), and as an appetite suppressant

analgesic broad drug classification that includes acetaminophen, aspirin, ibuprofen, and addictive agents such as opiates

analog a different form of a chemical or drug structurally related to a parent chemical or drug

androgenic effects effects on the growth of the male reproductive tract and the development of male secondary sexual characteristics

anesthetic an agent or event that causes anesthesia, or the loss of sensation and/or consciousness

anorectic a substance that decreases a person's appetite

anorexia nervosa eating disorder characterized by an intense and irrational fear of gaining weight, resulting in abnormal and unhealthy eating patterns, malnutrition, and severe weight loss

antagonist an agent that counteracts or blocks the effects of another drug

anticonvulsant drug that relieves or prevents seizures

antidepressant medication used for the treatment and prevention of depression

antipsychotic drugs drugs that reduce psychotic behavior, but often have negative long-term side effects

antisocial personality disorder a condition in which people disregard the rights of others and violate these rights by acting in immoral, unethical, aggressive, or even criminal ways

antitrust relating to laws that prevent unfair business practicies, such as monopolies

anxiety disorder condition in which a person feels uncontrollable angst and worry, often without any specific cause

archaeological relating to the scientific study of material remains from past human life and activities

attention-deficit/hyperactivity disorder ADHD is a long-term condition characterized by excessive, ongoing hyperactivity (overactivity, restlessness, fidgeting), distractibility, and impulsivity; distractibility refers to heightened sensitivity to irrelevant sights and sounds, making some simple tasks difficult to complete

autopsy examination of a body after a person has died, to determine the cause of death or to explore the results of a disease

ayahuasca an intoxicating beverage made from *Banisteriopsis caapi* plants, which contain dimethyltriptamine or DMT

barbiturate highly habit-forming sedative drugs that decrease the activity of the central nervous system

behavioral therapy form of therapy whose main focus is to change certain behaviors instead of uncovering unconscious conflicts or problems

benign harmless; also, noncancerous

benzodiazepine drug developed in the 1960s as a safer alternative to barbiturates. Most frequently used as a sleeping pill or as an anti-anxiety medication

binge relatively brief period of excessive behavior, such as eating an usually large amount of food

binge drinker a man who consumes 5 or more drinks on a single occasion; or a woman who consumes 4 or more drinks on a single occasion

biopsy procedure in which a body tissue, cells, or fluids are removed for examination in a laboratory

black market sale and purchase of goods that are illegal, such as drugs like heroin

blood alcohol concentration (BAC) amount of alcohol in the bloodstream, expressed as the grams of alcohol per deciliter of blood; as BAC goes up, the drinker experiences more psychological and physical effects

borderline personality disorder condition in which a person consistently has unstable personal relationships, negative self-image, unclear self-identity, recurring impulsivity, and problems with mood

bulimia nervosa literally means "ox hunger"; eating disorder characterized by compulsive overeating and then efforts to purge the body of the excess food, through self-induced vomiting, laxative abuse, or the use of diuretic medicines (pills to rid the body of water)

buprenorphine new medication that has proven to reduce cravings associated with heroin withdrawal, and may also be helpful in treating cocaine addiction

cannabis plants and/or drug forms of the Indian hemp plant, *Cannabis sativa*, also known as marijuana

carcinogen substance or agent that causes cancer

cartel group that controls production and/or price of a good such as diamonds, oil, or illegal drugs

catatonia psychomotor disturbance characterized by muscular rigidity, excitement, or stupor

central nervous system comprised of brain and spinal cord in humans

cerebellum a large part of the brain, which helps with muscle coordination and balance

cerebral cortex surface layer of gray matter in the front part of the brain that helps in coordinating the senses and motor functions

chronic continuing for a long period of time

cirrhosis chronic, scarring liver disease that can be caused by alcohol abuse, toxins, nutritional deficiency, or infection

civil libertarian person who believes in the right to unrestricted freedom of thought and action

cleft palate congenital (present at birth) cleft or separation in the roof of the mouth

clinical trial scientific experiment that uses humans, as opposed to animals, to test the efficacy of a new drug, medical or surgical technique, or method of diagnosis or prevention

clitoris small erectile organ in females at front part of the vulva

club drug group of drugs commonly reported to be used by young people at clubs or "raves" to increase stamina and energy and/or extend the euphoric effects of alcohol

codependence situation in which someone (often a family member) has an unhealthy dependence on an individual with an addiction; the dependent relationship allows the addicted individual to be manipulative, and is often characterized as "enabling" the addict to continue his or her addiction

codependent person who has an unhealthy dependence on another person with an addiction

coma state of very deep and sometimes prolonged unconsciousness

comorbid two or more disorders that occur at the same time in a person

compensation an amount of money or something else given to pay for loss, damage or work done

completed suicide suicide attempt that actually ends in death

compound pure substance that is made up of two or more elements, but possesses new chemical properties different from the original elements

compulsion irresistible drive to perform a particular action; some compulsions are performed in order to reduce stress and anxiety brought on by obsessive thoughts

condom covering worn over the penis, used as a barrier method of birth control and disease prevention

conduct disorder condition in which a child or adolescent exhibits behavioral and emotional problems, often finding it difficult to follow rules and behaving in a manner that violates the rights of others and society

convulsion intense, repetitive muscle contraction

correlate to link in a way that can be measured and predicted

correlation relation of two or more things in a way that can be measured and predicted

corroborate to independently find proof or support

corticosteroid medication that is prescribed to reduce inflammation and sometimes to suppress the body's immune responses

crack cocaine a freebase cocaine, or a cocaine that is specially processed to remove impurities; crack cocaine is smoked and is highly addictive

craving a powerful, often uncontrollable desire

debilitating something that interferes with or lessens normal strength and functioning

deficiency having too little of a necessary vitamin or mineral

deflect to cause somebody to change from what he or she usually does or plans to do

dehydration a state in which there is an abnormally low amount of fluid in the body

delirium mental disturbance marked by confusion, disordered speech, and sometimes hallucinations

delusion unshakable false belief that a person holds onto even when facts should convince the individual otherwise

dementia type of disease characterized by progressive loss of memory and the ability to learn and think

denial psychological state in which a person ignores obvious facts and continues to deny the existence of a particular problem or situation

dental dam piece of latex used to protect the mouth; can be used in dentistry, or can be used to prevent the oral transmission of sexually transmitted diseases

dependence psychological compulsion to use a substance for emotional and/or physical reasons

dependent someone who has a psychological compulsion to use a substance for emotional and/or physical reasons

depletion state of being used up or emptied

depressant chemical that slows down or decreases functioning; often used to describe agents that slow down the functioning of the central nervous system; such agents are sometimes used to relieve insomnia, anxiety, irritability, and tension

depressed someone who feels intensely sad and hopeless

depression state in which an individual feels intensely sad and hopeless, may have trouble eating, sleeping, and concentrating, and is no longer able to feel pleasure from previously enjoyable activities; in extreme cases, it may lead an individual to think about or attempt suicide

deprivation situation of lacking the basic necessities of life, such as food or emotional security

detoxification process of removing a poisonous, intoxicating, or addictive substance from the body

dietary supplement product used to supplement an individual's normal diet, by adding a specific vitamin, mineral, herb, or amino acid, or by increasing the general caloric intake; often available without a prescription; usually not subjected to rigorous clinical testing

dilution process of making something thinner, weaker, or less concentrated, typically by adding a diluting material (often a liquid such as water); can also refer to the result of diluting, a weakened solution

disordered state characterized by chaotic, disorganized, or confused functioning; may refer to problems with a person's individual thought processes or problems within a system, such as a family

distillation process that separates alcohol from fermenting juices

diuretic drug that increases urine output; sometimes called "water pill"

divine relating to or proceeding from God or a god

Down syndrome form of mental retardation due to an extra chromosome present at birth often accompanied by physical characteristics, such as sloped eyes

downers slang term for drugs that act as depressants on the central nervous system, such as barbiturates

drug traffickers people or groups who transport illegal drugs

drug trafficking act of transporting illegal drugs

dysphoria depressed and unhappy mood state

ecstasy designer drug and amphetamine derivative that is a commonly abused street drug

efficacy ability to produce desired results

endocrine system cells, tissues, and organs of the body that are active in regulating bodily functions, such as growth and metabolism

enthusiast supporter

enzyme protein produced by cells that causes or speeds up biological reactions, such as those that break down food into smaller parts

epidemic rapid spreading of a disease to many people in a given area or community at the same time

euphoria state of intense, giddy happiness and well-being, sometimes occurring baselessly and at odds with an individual's life situation

euphoric someone who experiences a state of intense, giddy happiness and well-being, sometimes occurring baselessly and out of sync

excise tax tax that a government puts on the manufacture, sale, or use of a domestic product

expertise expert advice or opinions expressed by a person with recognized skill or knowledge in a particular area

exploitation condition in which one uses another person for one's own selfish advantage

export to send merchandise to another country as part of commercial business

expulsion act of forcing somebody out of a group or institution, such as a school or club

felony very serious crime that usually warrants a more severe punishment than those crimes considered misdemeanors

gastrointestinal tract entire length of the digestive system, running from the stomach, through the small intestine, large intestine, and out the rectum

half-life amount of time it takes for one-half of a substance to undergo a process, such as to be broken down or eliminated

hallucination seeing, hearing, feeling, tasting, or smelling something that is not actually there, like a vision of devils, hearing voices, or feeling bugs crawl over the skin; may occur due to mental illness or as a side effect of some drugs

hallucinogen a drug, such as LSD, that causes hallucinations, or seeing, hearing, or feeling things that are not there

hallucinogenic describing a substance that can cause hallucinations, or seeing, hearing, or feeling things that arcn't there

heritable trait that is passed on from parents to offspring

homicide murder

hormone chemical substance, produced by a gland, that travels through the blood or other body fluids to another part of the body where it causes a physiological activity to occur

hyperactivity overly active behavior

hypersensitivity state of extreme sensitivity to something

hypnotic drug that induces sleep by depressing the central nervous system

illicit something illegal or something used in an illegal manner

immune system human body's system of protecting itself against foreign substances, germs, and other infectious agents; protects the body against illness

impair to make worse or to damage, especially by lessening or reducing in some way

impotence inability to get or maintain an erection

impotency condition in which one is unable to get or maintain an erection

impulsive acting before thinking through the consequences of the action

impulsivity state in which someone acts before thinking through the consequences of their actions

incentive something, such as a reward, that encourages a specific action or behavior

induce to bring about or stimulate a particular reaction

induction process of formally admitting somebody into a position or organization

infertility inability to have children

ingenuity inventive skill or imagination

inhalant legal product that evaporates easily, producing chemical vapors; abusers inhale concentrated amounts of these vapors to alter their consciousness

inpatient person who stays overnight in a facility to get treatment

interpret to explain the meaning of or make a judgment about technical information or data

interpretation judgment or explanation about technical information

intervention act of intervening or positioning oneself between two things; when referring to substance abuse, the term means an attempt to help an addict admit to his or her addiction, recognize the ill effects the addiction has had on the addict and on his or her relationships, and get help to conquer the addiction

intoxicant food or drink capable of diminishing physical or mental control

intoxicated someone whose physical or mental control has been diminished

intoxicating a food or drink capable of diminishing physical or mental control

intoxication loss of physical or mental control because of the effects of a substance

invasive in the context of medical actions, describing a procedure in which a part of the body is entered; relating to an infection or a cancer, describing a disease that has spread from its original site in the body

LAAM (Levo-Alpha-Acetylmethadol) a synthetic opiate used to treat heroin addiction by blunting the symptoms of withdrawal for up to 72 hours

laxative product that promotes bowel movements

legitimate meeting or conforming to legal or recognized standards

lethargy state of being slowed down, sluggish, very drowsy, lacking all energy or drive

liable responsible

licit legal; permitted by law

lobbying activities aimed at influencing public officials, especially members of the legislature

logo an identifying symbol (as for advertising) that a company uses as a way of gaining recognition

LSD lysergic acid diethylamide, known for its hallucinogenic properties

lucrative something with the potential to make a lot of money

malaria disease caused by a parasite in the red blood cells, passed to humans through the bite of mosquitoes

malnutrition unhealthy condition of the body caused by not getting enough food or enough of the right foods or by an inability of the body to appropriately break down the food or utilize the nutrients

marijuana dried leaves and flowers of female *Cannabis sativa* plants, smoked or eaten for its intoxicating effect

market share percentage of the total sales of a product that is controlled by a company

media means of mass communication, such as newspapers, magazines, radio or television

mescaline hallucinogenic drug that is the main active agent found in mescal buttons of the peyote plant

metabolic describing or related to the chemical processes through which the cells of the body breakdown substances to produce energy

metabolism chemical processes through which the cells of the body break down various substances to produce energy and allow the body to function

methadone potent synthetic narcotic, used in heroin recovery programs as a non-intoxicating opiate that blunts symptoms of withdrawal

misdemeanor crime that is treated in the courts as a less serious crime than a felony

money laundering activity in which a person or group hides the source of money that has been illegally obtained

monopoly situation that exists when only one person or company sells a good or service in a given area

morphine primary alkaloid chemical in opium, used as a drug to treat severe, acute, and chronic pain

narcotic addictive substance that relieves pain and induces sleep or causes sedation; prescription narcotics includes morphine and codeine; can refer to a drug of abuse, such as heroin, cocaine, or marijuana

neuroleptic one of a class of antipsychotic drugs, including major tranquilizers, used in the treatment of psychoses like schizophrenia

neurological relating to the nervous system

neuron nerve cell that releases neurotransmitters

neuropathic relating to a disease of the nerves

neurotransmitter chemical messenger used by nerve cells to communicate with other nerve cells

nicotine alkaloid derived from the tobacco plant that is responsible for smoking's addictive effects

noninvasive not involving penetration of the skin

norm behavior, custom, or attitude that is considered normal, or expected, within a certain social group

obscene morally offensive; describes something meant to degrade or corrupt

obsessed someone who experiences repeated thoughts, impulses, or mental images that are irrational and that the person cannot control

obsession repeating thoughts, impulses, or mental images that are irrational and that an individual cannot control

obsessive-compulsive disorder anxiety disorder in which a person cannot prevent dwelling on unwanted thoughts, accting on urges, or repeating rituals

opiate drug derived directly from opium and used in its natural state, without chemical modification; examples of opiates are morphine, codeine, thebaine, noscapine, and papaverine

opioid substance that acts in a way similar to opiate narcotic drugs, but is not actually produced from the opium poppy

oppositional defiant disorder psychiatric condition in which a person repeatedly shows a pattern of negative, hostile, disobedient, and/or defiant behavior, without serious violation of the rights of others

optimism a positive outlook

outpatient person who receives treatment at a doctor's office or hospital but does not stay overnight

overdose excessively high dose of a drug, which can be toxic or even life-threatening

paranoia excessive or irrational suspicion, illogical mistrust

paranoid someone who is excessively or irrationally suspicious

paranoid psychosis symptom of mental illness characterized by changes in personality, a distorted sense of reality, and feelings of excessive and irrational suspicion; may include hallucinations (seeing, hearing, feeling, smelling, or tasting something that is not truly there)

paraphernalia equipment that enables drug users to take the drugs, such as syringes and needles

periodic occuring at regular intervals or periods

peyote a cactus that can be used to make a stimulant drug

pharmaceuticals legal drugs that are usually used for medical reasons

pharmacology branch of science concerned with drugs and how they affect bodily and mental processes

philanthrophy acts performed with the desire to improve humanity, especially through charitable activities

physical dependence condition that may occur after prolonged use of a particular drug or alcohol, in which the user's body cannot function normally without the presence of the substance; when the substance is not used, or when the dose is decreased, the user experiences uncomfortable physical symptoms

physically dependent someone who takes drugs for relief of uncomfortable physical symptoms, rather than for emotional or psychological relief

physiological relating to the functions and activities of life on a biological level

physiology branch of science that focuses on the functions of the body

placebo effect improvement in an individual's symptoms that is not due to the specific treatment offered; for example, a patient may report that his or her pain has improved after taking a sugar pill, which contains no active medicinal ingredients

placenta in most mammals, the organ that is attached to the mother's uterus and to the fetus's umbilical cord; it is responsible for passing nutrients and oxygen from the mother to the developing fetus

predispose to be prone or vulnerable to something

predisposition condition in which one is vulnerable or prone to something

prenatal existing or occurring before birth; refers also to the care a woman receives while pregnant

problem drinking when a person's drinking disrupts life and relationships, causing difficulties for the drinker

productivity quality of yielding results or benefits

prohibit to forbid

promiscuity having many sexual partners

proportional properly related in size; corresponding

prostate gland located near the bladder and urethra in men, it secretes the fluid that contains sperm

psychedelic substance that can cause hallucinations and/or make its user lose touch with reality

psychiatric relating to the branch of medicine that deals with the study, treatment, and prevention of mental illness

psychiatry branch of medicine that deals with the study, treatment, and prevention of mental illness

psychoactive drugs that affect the mind or mental processes by altering consciousness, perception, or mood

psychology scientific study of mental processes and behaviors

psychometric relating to the technique of measuring mental abilities

psychomotor referring to processess of muscular movement directly influenced by mental processes

psychosis mental disorder in which an individual loses contact with reality and may have delusions (unshakable false beliefs) or hallucinations (the experience of seeing, hearing, feeling, smelling, or tasting things that are not actually present)

psychosocial relates to both life experiences as well as mental processes

psychostimulant medication that is prescribed to control hyperative and impulsive behaviors

psychotherapeutic drugs drugs used to relieve the symptoms of mental illness such as depression, anxiety and psychosis

psychotherapy treatment of a mental or emotional condition during which a person talks to a qualified therapist in order to understand his or her problems and change problem behaviors

psychotropic substance that affects mental function

quinine substance used to treat malaria

rave organized gathering of young people that includes loud, pulsing "house" music and flashing lights

receptor specialized part of a cell that can bind a specific substance; for example, a neuron has special receptors that receive and bind neurotransmitters

recidivism tendency to relapse into previous criminal behavior

recreational drug use casual and infrequent use of a substance, often in social situations, for its pleasurable effects

regulate to bring under the control of law or authorized agency

rehabilitate to restore or improve someone to a condition of health or useful activity

rehabilitation process of restoring a person to a condition of health or useful activity

reinforced to make something stronger by repeating an activity or by adding extra support

relapse term used in substance abuse treatment and recovery that refers to an addict's return to substance use and abuse following a period of abstinence or sobriety

repeal to revoke or cancel

repression the effort of the mind to block unpleasant or painful thoughts or desires; or, an act in which one person or group keeps another group in a lower, less advantageous position

resent to feel anger, bitterness or ill will towards someone or something

residue the quantity of some substance or material left over at the end of a process; a remainder of something

resuscitation revival from unconsciousness; restoring energy, vitality

risk an increased probability of something negative happening

Rohypnol medication that causes sleep, banned in the United States but used illegally as a club drug; also known as a "date rape" drug

sanction punishment imposed as a result of breaking a law or rule

schizophrenia psychotic disorder in which people lose the ability to function normally, suffer from severe personality changes, and suffer from a variety of symptoms, including confusion, disordered thinking, paranoia, hallucinations, emotional numbness, and speech problems

sedated describing someone who took a medication that reduced excitement

sedation process of calming someone by administering a medication that reduces excitement, often called a tranquilizer

sedative a medication that reduces excitement, often called a tranquilizer

sedative-hypnotic drug that has a calming and relaxing effect; "hypnotics" induce sleep

self-harm repeated dangerous behaviors, such as cutting the skin, headbanging, or taking pills

self-medicate when a person treats an ailment, mental or physical, with alcohol or drugs rather than see a physician or mental health professiona

serotonin neurotransmitter associated with the regulation of mood, appetite, sleep, memory, and learning

shamanism religion whose leaders perform rituals of magic, divination, and healing and act as intermediaries between reality and the spirit world

skeletal system the bones and related parts that serve as a framework for the body

sober in relation to drugs and alcohol, refers to abstaining from alcoholic beverages or intoxicants; describes a state in which someone is not under the influence of drugs or alcohol

sociologist someone who studies society, social relationships, and social institutions

sophisticated knowledgeable about the ways of the world, self-confident

specimen a sample, as of tissue, blood, or urine, used for analysis and diagnosis

spina bifida one of the more common birth defects in which the backbone never closes or its coverings stick out through the opening

sterility condition in which one is unable to conceive a child

steroid specific chemical compound; certain types of steroids are produced naturally by the body (such as sex and stress hormones); other types of steroids are laboratory-produced drugs used to treat a variety of illnesses and to reduce swelling

stigma the shame or disgrace attached to something regarded as socially unacceptable

stimulant drug that increases activity temporarily; often used to describe drugs that excite the brain and central nervous system

stimuli things that excite the body or part of the body to produce specific responses

stimulus anything that excites the body or part of the body to produce a specific response

stupor state of greatly dulled interest in the surrounding environment; may include relative unconsciousness

synapse the gap between communicating nerve cells through which impulses pass from one nerve cell to another

synthesize to produce artificially or chemically

testimonial statement that backs up a claim or support a fact

testosterone hormone produced in higher amounts in males that is responsible for male characteristics such as muscle-building and maintaining sexual organs, and during puberty causes hair growth and a deepening voice

tetanus rare but often fatal disease that affects the brain and spinal column

therapeutic healing or curing

tic repetitive, involuntary spasm that increases in severity when it is purposefully surpressed; may be motor (such as muscle contractions or eye blinking) or vocal (such as an unintended yelp or use of an expletive)

tolerance condition in which higher and higher doses of a drug or alcohol are needed to produce the effect or "high" experienced from the original dose

Tourette's syndrome chronic tic disorder involving multiple motor and/or vocal tics that cause distress or significant impairment in social, occupational, or other important areas of functioning

toxic something that is poisonous or dangerous to people

toxicity condition of being poisonous or dangerous to people

toxicology study of the nature, effects, and detection of poisons and the treatment of poisoning

trance state of partial consciousness

tranquilizer drug that decreases anxiety and tension

trauma injury or damage, either to the body or to the mind

trivialize to treat something as less important or valuable than it really is

Twelve Steps program for remaining sober developed by Alcoholics Anonymous; adopted by many other groups, such as Narotics Anonymous

ulcer irritated pit in the surface of a tissue, often on the stomach lining

unethical something that is morally questionable

uppers slang term for amphetamines, drugs that act as stimulants of the central nervous system

variable something that can change or fluctuate

vascular relating to the transport of fluids (such as blood or lymph fluid) through tubes in the body; frequently used to refer to the system of blood vessels

vulnerable at greater risk

withdrawal group of physical and psychological symptoms that may occur when a person suddenly stops the use of a substance or reduces the dose of an addictive substance

Volume 1 Index